Nutrition and the Eye

—

For Elsevier Butterworth-Heinemann:

Commissioning editor: Robert Edwards
Development editor: Kim Benson
Project manager: Jane Dingwall
Design: Stewart Larking
Illustrations: Peter Cox

Nutrition and the Eye

A Practical Approach

Edited by

Frank Eperjesi BSc(Hons) PhD MCOptom DipOrth FAAO MHEA PGCertHE

University Lecturer, Director of Optometry Programme, Research Optometrist, Division of Optometry, School of Life and Health Sciences, Aston University, Birmingham, UK

Stephen Beatty MB(Hons) MMSc FRCOphth MD

Consultant Ophthalmic Surgeon, Waterford Regional Hospital and Associate Lecturer, Waterford Institute of Technology, Waterford, Republic of Ireland

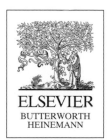

ELSEVIER
BUTTERWORTH
HEINEMANN

EDINBURGH LONDON NEW YORK OXFORD PHILADELPHIA ST LOUIS SYDNEY TORONTO 2006

BUTTERWORTH
HEINEMANN

© 2006, Elsevier Limited. All rights reserved.
First published 2006

ISBN-13: 978 0 7506 8816 1
ISBN-10: 0 7506 8816 5

British Library Cataloguing in Publication Data
A catalogue record for this book is available from the British Library.

Library of Congress Cataloging in Publication Data
A catalog record for this book is available from the Library of Congress.

Note
Knowledge and best practice in this field are constantly changing. As new
research and experience broaden our knowledge, changes in practice,
treatment and drug therapy may become necessary or appropriate.
Readers are advised to check the most current information provided (i) on
procedures featured or (ii) by the manufacturer of each product to be
administered, to verify the recommended dose or formula, the method and
duration of administration, and contraindications. It is the responsibility of
the practitioner, relying on their own experience and knowledge of the
patient, to make diagnoses, to determine dosages and the best treatment for
each individual patient, and to take all appropriate safety precautions. To
the fullest extent of the law, neither the Publisher nor the Editors assume
any liability for any injury and/or damage to persons or property arising
out of or related to any use of the material contained in this book.

The Publisher

Working together to grow
libraries in developing countries

www.elsevier.com | www.bookaid.org | www.sabre.org

ELSEVIER   BOOK AID
            International   Sabre Foundation

ELSEVIER   your source for books,
            journals and multimedia
            in the health sciences
www.elsevierhealth.com

The
Publisher's
policy is to use
paper manufactured
from sustainable forests

Printed in China

Contents

Preface

A mass of evidence generated over the last 30 years or so has led to the widely held belief that there is a direct relationship between nutrition and many types of ocular disease. Furthermore, recent research has shown that the course of the most common blinding eye disease in the developed world, age-related macular degeneration, can be modified through the use of specific nutritional supplements. Current texts in this area are very much focused on research and there is little available in the form of advice for the front-line eye care clinician. We have attempted to remedy this by writing a text in which we have distilled those research findings with a practical emphasis into a digestible format.

Our aim, therefore, is to present in a readily accessible way a comprehensive guide and up-to-date reference source so as to enable the front-line eye care professional to give patients sound, evidence-based nutritional advice. In order to achieve this we have drawn on the academic knowledge and clinical expertise of diet specialists, ophthalmologists and optometrists.

An introduction to the field of nutrition sets the scene; we then go on to discuss nutrients and micronutrients with respect to the eye and with respect to vision. This is followed by a section on the ophthalmic manifestations of nutritional deficiencies and then a section on the physiological and pathological effects of ocular senescence, with particular emphasis on the role that nutrition plays in this ageing process; here we discuss in some detail the relationship between nutrition and common ocular diseases such as dry-eye syndrome, glaucoma, cataract and age-related macular disease. This is then followed by evidence in support of dietary modification and/or supplementation in the prevention and/or management of ocular disease. The penultimate section reviews contraindications and offers guidance on avoiding potential adverse reactions associated with dietary modification, and we then offer some broad conclusions in the final section.

We hope that this book will be of use in routine eye care practice so that the patient can be better informed about all possible options with respect to nutrition and vision.

Frank Eperjesi
Stephen Beatty

Acknowledgement

We thank Kim Benson at Elsevier for her patience and support.

Contributors

Rasha Al Taie MBChB FRCSI MSc
Waterford Regional Hospital
Waterford
Ireland

Hannah Bartlett BSc(Hons) PhD MCOptom
Division of Optometry
School of Life and Health Sciences
Aston University
Birmingham
UK

Stephen Beatty MB(Hons) MMSc FRCOphth MD
Waterford Institute of Technology
Macular Pigment Laboratory
Waterford
Ireland

Usha Chakravarthy PhD
Institute of Clinical Science
Department of Ophthalmology and Vision Science
Belfast
UK

Geraldine J Cuskelly PhD
Wellcome Research Laboratories
Department of Medicine
Queen's University Belfast
Belfast
UK

Frank Eperjesi BSc(Hons) PhD MCOptom DipOrth FAAO
MHEA PGCertHE
Division of Optometry
School of Life and Health Sciences
Aston University
Birmingham
UK

Ruth Hogg BSc(Hons) PhD MCOptom
Ophthalmic Research Centre
Royal Victoria Hospital
Belfast
UK

Kumari Neelam MBBS DNB FRCS(Glasgow)
Waterford Regional Hospital
Waterford
Ireland

John Nolan BSc(Hons)
Waterford Institute of Technology
Macular Pigment Laboratory
Waterford
Ireland

Orla O'Donovan BSc(Hons) PhD
Waterford Institute of Technology
Waterford
Ireland

Jayne V Woodside
Department of Medicine
Royal Victoria Hospital
Belfast
UK

Ian S Young BSc(Hons) PhD
Wellcome Research Laboratories
Department of Medicine
Royal Victoria Hospital
Belfast
UK

Abbreviations

α-TTP	α-tocopherol transfer protein	EMS	Eger Macular Stressometer
AD	Alzheimer's disease	ERG	electroretinogram
AFC	alternative forced choice	FABPs	fatty acid-binding proteins
AI	adequate intake	FACITs	fibril-associated collagens
AMD	age-related macular degeneration	FAD	flavin adenine dinucleotide
AREDS	Age-Related Eye Disease Study	FAO	Food and Agricultural
ARI	average requirement intake		Organization of the United
ARM	age-related maculopathy		States
ATP	adenosine triphosphate	Fe	iron
AVED	ataxia with vitamin E	FNB	Food and Nutrition Board
BDES	Beaver Dam Eye Study	G6PD	glucose-6-phosphate
BMES	Blue Mountains Eye Study		dehydrogenase
BMI	body mass index	GA	geographic atrophy
BMR	basal metabolic rate	GABA	γ-aminobutyric acid
CAREDS	Carotenoids in Age-Related Eye	GAGs	glycosaminoglycans
	Disease Study	GBE	ginkgo biloba extract
CARMA	Celtic Age-Related Maculopathy	GI	gastrointestinal
	Arrestation	GPCRs	G-protein-coupled receptors
CFF	critical flicker fusion	GSH	reduced glutathione/glutathione
CI	confidence interval		peroxidase
CNV	choroidal neovascularisation	GSSG	oxidized glutathione/glutathione
CNVM	choroidal neovascular membrane		disulphide
COMA	Committee on Medical Aspects of	H_2O_2	hydrogen peroxide
	Food Policy	HCl	hydrochloric acid
CRF	case report form	HDL	high-density lipoproteins
CS	contrast sensitivity	HMP	hexose monophosphate pathway
Cu	copper	HRQL	health-related quality of life
DHA	docosahexaenoic acid	HRT	hormone replacement therapy
DRI	dietary reference intake	ICAM-1	intercellular adhesion molecule-1
DRV	dietary reference value	ICG	indocyanine green
EAR	estimated average requirement	IOP	intraocular pressure
EFAs	essential fatty acids	IPL	inner plexiform layer

IRBP	interphotoreceptor retinol-binding protein	PEM	protein–energy malnutrition
IU	international units	PERG	pattern-evoked electroretinograms
L	lutein	PPRPE	preserved para-arteriolar retinal pigment epithelium
LAST	Lutein Antioxidant Supplementation Trial	PRI	population reference intake
LCPUFAs	long-chain polyunsaturated fatty acids	PSC	posterior subcapsular
		PSRT	photostress recovery time
LDL	low-density lipoproteins	PUFA	polyunsaturated fatty acids
LGN	lateral geniculate nucleus	PVD	posterior vitreous detachment
LMWA	low-molecular-weight antioxidants	RBP	retinol-binding protein
		RCT	randomised controlled trial
LRNI	lower reference nutrient intake	RDA	recommended daily allowance
LTI	lowest threshold intake	RDI	recommended dietary intake
MFA	monounsaturated fatty acids	RE	retinol equivalents
MII	metarhodopsin II	REACT	Roche European American Cataract Trial
MM	Macular Mapping		
Mn	manganese	RNI	reference nutrient intake
MP	macular pigment	ROI	reactive oxygen intermediates
MPOD	macular pigment optical density	ROP	retinopathy of prematurity
MT	metallothionein	ROS	rod outer segments
MTHFR	methylenetetrahydrofolate reductase	RP	retinitis pigmentosa
		RPE	retinal pigment epithelium
NADH	nicotinamide adenine dinucleotide	RR	relative risk
		SD	standard deviation
NADP	nicotinamide adenine dinucleotide phosphate	Se	selenium
		SENECA	Survey in Europe on Nutrition and the Elderly: A Concerted Action
NADPH	reduced nicotinamide adenine dinucleotide phosphate		
		SFA	saturated fatty acids
NEI-VFQ	National Eye Institute Visual Function Questionnaire	-SH	sulfhydryl
		SKILL	Smith-Kettlewell Institute low-luminance
NHANES	National Health and Nutrition Examination Survey		
		SOD	superoxide dismutase
NO	nitric oxide	TAP	Treatment of Age-Related Macular Degeneration with Photodynamic Therapy
NRC	National Research Council		
NSP	non-starch polysaccharides		
NTG	normal-tension glaucoma	TCA	tricarboxylic acid
O_2^-	superoxide	TM	trabecular meshwork
OCT	optical coherence tomography	TP	α-tocopherol
OD	oculus dexter (right eye)	TTT	transpupillary thermotherapy
OH*	hydroxyl radical	UL	upper intake level
ONOO⁻	peroxynitrite	UNU	United Nations University
OPL	outer plexiform layer	UV	ultraviolet
OR	odds ratio	VA	visual acuity
OS	oculus sinister (left eye)	VAD	vitamin A deficiency
P	placebo	VEGF	vascular endothelial growth factor
PDE	phosphodiesterase	VEP	visual evoked potential
PDT	photodynamic therapy	VLDL	very-low-density lipoproteins
PEDF	pigment epithelium-derived factor	WHI	Women's Health Initiative

WHI-OS	Women's Health Initiative Observational Study	XO	xanthine oxidase
		Z	zeaxanthin
WHO	World Health Organization	Zn	zinc
WHR	waist-to-hip ratio	Ω-3 LCPUFA	omega-3 long chain polyunsaturated fatty acids
XDH	xanthine dehydrogenase		

SECTION 1

Introduction to nutrition for eye care practitioners

Chapter **1.1**

Introduction to nutrition for eye care practitioners

Geraldine J Cuskelly and Ian S Young

INTRODUCTION AND DEFINITIONS

Eating is far more complicated than simply warding off hunger or having a pleasurable experience. It involves aspects of our psychological make-up, social group, mood and many external factors relating to the availability of food. Eating also does more than just keep us alive. When insufficient food or specific nutrients are supplied, some physiological adaptation may occur to minimise the consequences. Eventually, however, a deficiency state will arise.

At the beginning of the twentieth century the science of nutrition was directed at discovering the essential nutrients, studying the effects of insufficient intakes and determining the quantities needed to prevent deficiency states. Since then it has been gradually recognised that good nutrition is not simply a matter of providing enough of all the nutrients. We now realise that diets in the affluent developed countries, although apparently containing all the necessary nutrients, are probably contributing to many of the diseases afflicting these populations. Much research is focused on finding which nutrients are linked to which diseases, in an effort to promote a change in the dietary intake and hence an improvement in health. Since the 1970s a great deal of advice has been aimed at encouraging people to eat in a healthier way, thereby reducing disease. However, nutritionists have realised that altering people's food intake is complicated because diets are influenced by many factors other than the need to eat and the desire for well-being.

Arriving at a definition of nutrition is far from straightforward. Two rather different definitions have been suggested, describing nutrition as: 'the study of foods and nutrients vital to health and how the body uses these to promote and support growth, maintenance and reproduction of cells' and 'the study of the relationship between people and their food'.

The first definition deals only with the nutrients, what happens to them within the human body and what the results are if insufficient amounts are provided. However, people do not eat nutrients, they eat food. This first definition therefore ignores all the external factors that play a role in our approach to food, and that are crucial in any study of what people are eating. These factors are different for each individual, depending on cultural background and the circumstances of a person's life.

The second definition takes a much broader perspective, from the supply of food and all the influences thereon, to the individual's food selection and finally to the physiological and biochemical effects of the nutrients in the human body and the consequences for health and survival. It also recognises that nutritionists do not just work in the laboratory studying the effects of nutrients on biochemical and physiological functioning. They have an additional responsibility to translate their knowledge for those who produce, process and market the foods. Furthermore, nutritionists must be involved in the formulation of policy, which determines the customers' access to food. Finally, consumers need the help of nutritionists to enable them to make the best of the food available. Only by broadening our definition of the subject across the full range of human relationships with food can nutrition have its justified place in human well-being.

WHY IS NUTRITION IMPORTANT?

To answer this question, it is perhaps useful to consider the various levels at which nutrition can be studied. Table 1.1.1 illustrates some examples of the application of nutritional science in other fields of study. In each case, nutrition plays a specific role, and the emphasis required may differ from its application and meanings to different specialists. Nevertheless, all of these specialists working in their own particular field of expertise need to have knowledge of nutrition in order to apply the findings of their work to the nutritional context.

WHY IS NUTRITION INTERESTING?

There has been an upsurge of general interest in nutrition in the last 20 years; this has not just been among the scientific community, but also among

Table 1.1.1   Levels at which nutrition can be studied

Level of study	Areas of research	Examples of application
Macro/population studies	Government statistics	For formulation of policy, e.g. about agriculture or health
	Epidemiology	Study relationships between diet and disease
	Food producers	Respond to changes in consumer demand and lead demand
Individual/whole-person studies	Sociology	Study patterns of behaviour related to food
	Food science/technology	Identify changes in individual preferences for food and sensory qualities
	Medicine	Study influences of diet on the health of the individual and recovery from illness
Micro/laboratory studies	Physiology	Understand the role of nutrients in functioning of body systems
	Biochemistry	Investigate the biochemical role of nutrients in normal and abnormal functioning
	Molecular biology	Study gene–nutrient interactions

Data from Baresi ME (1997). Human nutrition: a health perspective. London: Arnold.[1]

the general public. First, it is notable that dietary intakes have been and are changing rapidly.[1] In the western world we have an ever-increasing selection of foods available to us. People can now eat every day the foods our ancestors had only on special occasions. New foods are appearing which have been developed by food technologists; sometimes these contain unusual ingredients that provide nutrients in unexpected amounts and this can be a problem for the nutritionist when giving advice. New processing techniques such as irradiation may affect the nutrients in food.[2]

In modern society meal patterns have become less rigid and many people no longer always eat meals at regular mealtimes. Family members may each have an independent meal at different times of the day.

Concerns about food safety and environmental issues have resulted in changes in dietary habits, the most notable amongst these being the rise in vegetarianism in the UK.[3] Health issues have been given a great deal of prominence in the media. Statistics show that populations in developed countries have excessive mortality and morbidity from many diseases related to diet, such as cardiovascular disorders,[4] bowel diseases and cancers,[5] as well as a high prevalence of obesity.[6] At the same time we are often shocked by images of starvation in other parts of the world where conflict, drought and other disasters have resulted in millions of people suffering acute malnutrition and starvation.

As more nutritionists are trained and the discipline becomes more widely studied, more knowledge is accumulated. However, as with all scientific research, more questions follow every finding. Consensus is being reached on some of the dietary involvements in disease, and advice can now be based on much firmer evidence. However, new research may cause current advice to be modified. New approaches to nutrition research, particularly from the field of molecular biology, are explaining observations made earlier at the whole-body level. Improved methods allow more sensitive and appropriate measurements to be made. For example, in the study of energy balance, the use of stable isotope-labelled water has provided a means of measuring energy expenditure in subjects during their normal lives.[7] This has provided a wealth of information about this important area of nutrition.

The media are very sensitive to public interest, so that news about nutritional findings receives a great deal of publicity. Unfortunately, the style of reporting may distort the scientific detail, so that what is eventually presented by the media may not accurately represent the findings. Moreover, excessive prominence may be given to very minor and insignificant findings, especially if they appear to contradict earlier results. Consequently, rather than being better informed, the public may become confused. It is essential, therefore, that those trained in nutrition have a clear understanding of nutritional issues, and are able to disentangle some of the inaccuracies presented by the media.

This section will introduce some important pivotal principles of nutrition, including: (1) how we decide how much of given nutrient(s) (and/or food) to consume; (2) how to achieve these nutrient requirements in diets of the general population in different countries; (3) how to assess the factors (absorption and nutrient bioavailability) that affect how we assimilate food and nutrients; and finally (4) how to assess optimal nutritional status clinically and biochemically.

Chapter 1.2

Optimal nutrition

Geraldine J Cuskelly and Ian S Young

Estimates of requirements are essentially based upon current intakes in an apparently healthy population.[8] The level of nutrient intake required to achieve optimal nutritional status will, therefore, vary depending upon the definition, and the defining marker, of health. When requirements were first formulated, health was defined as an absence of clinical deficiency symptoms.[1] However, in recent times, we have come to realise the benefits of optimising a nutrient's status, not only to prevent a related deficiency disease, but also to minimise the risk of disease(s) not traditionally associated with deficiency of the nutrient. Which physiological or biochemical marker chosen is therefore crucial. The principle is illustrated in Figure 1.2.1.

For example, in the case of vitamin C, traditionally, prevention of scurvy was the marker used to define requirements (level B). Serum vitamin C may be used to assess requirements, in which case requirements will be defined as higher (levels C and D). Saturation of body pools (white blood cell levels) of vitamin C defines level E. Antioxidant properties of vitamin C have been highlighted in terms of their potential to prevent cardiovascular disease (level F).[9] If we define vitamin C requirements as the amount to prevent the common cold, we are defining a pharmacological dose (level G).[10] At higher levels, particularly in the case of fat-soluble vitamins and minerals, higher intakes may have detrimental or toxic effects (level H).

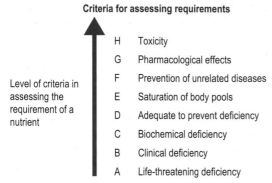

Criteria for assessing requirements

Level of criteria in assessing the requirement of a nutrient

H	Toxicity
G	Pharmacological effects
F	Prevention of unrelated diseases
E	Saturation of body pools
D	Adequate to prevent deficiency
C	Biochemical deficiency
B	Clinical deficiency
A	Life-threatening deficiency

Figure 1.2.1 Criteria for assessing requirements.

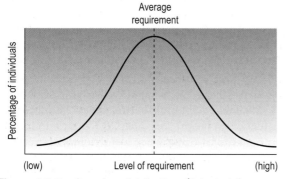

Figure 1.2.2 Gaussian distribution. (Adapted from Department of Health. Report on health and social subjects 41. Dietary reference values for food energy and nutrients for the United Kingdom. Committee on Medical Aspects of Food Policy. London: HMSO; 1991.[8])

DISTRIBUTION OF NUTRITIONAL REQUIREMENTS IN A POPULATION

When measurements of requirements are obtained from a sufficiently large population, the results are assumed to follow a typical normal (Gaussian) distribution curve, as shown in Figure 1.2.2.[8] This indicates that, for the majority, the requirement is around the mean for the group, but some have higher requirements and some have lower values. If the group is sufficiently large, then half will fall above the sample mean and half below it; this is simply a property of the distribution and not something peculiar to nutrition or requirements.

NUTRITIONAL REQUIREMENTS ASSESSED BY THE UK DIETARY REFERENCE VALUES PANEL

The definition of the recommended daily allowance (RDA) for a nutrient which was used in the previous Report of the UK Committee on Medical Aspects of Food Policy is 'the average amount of the nutrient which should be provided per head in a group of people if the needs of practically all members of the group are to be met'. This was framed in an attempt to make it clear that the amounts referred to are averages for a group of people and not amounts which individuals must consume.[8]

The UK dietary recommendations were revised in 1991 and the RDA was replaced with the dietary reference value (DRV). The most recent panel (1991) found no single criterion to define requirements for all nutrients. There are inherent errors in some of the data, for instance in individuals' reports of their food intake, and the day-to-day variation in nutrient intakes also complicates interpretation. Even given complete accuracy of a dietary record, its relation to habitual intake remains uncertain, however long the recording period. The food composition tables normally used to determine nutrient intake from dietary records contain a number of assumptions and imperfections.[11] Furthermore, there is uncertainty about the relevance of many biological markers, such as serum concentrations of a nutrient, as evidence of an individual's status for that nutrient.[12] Some nutrients may have a variety of physiological effects at different levels of intake. Which of these effects should form the parameter of adequacy is therefore to some extent arbitrary. For each nutrient the particular parameter or parameters that were used to define adequacy are given in the text of the report.[8]

Having established the range of nutritional requirements for a particular nutrient, it is necessary to define more precisely what would be an adequate level of intake to meet these requirements. Several options might be available (Figure 1.2.3). Setting the level at point A, which is above the range of individual requirements, would ensure that everyone's needs were met but might impose a risk in terms of excessive intakes if the

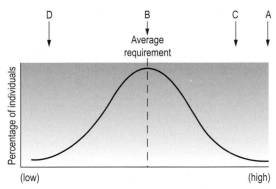

Figure 1.2.3 Dietary reference values. (Adapted from Department of Health. Report on health and social subjects 41. Dietary reference values for food energy and nutrients for the United Kingdom. Committee on Medical Aspects of Food Policy. London: HMSO; 1991.[8])

nutrient was harmful in large amounts. There would also be cost implications – should people be encouraged to buy sufficient food to meet this high level? An alternative might be to set the level at point B, which is the mean. By definition, this would imply that this level of intake would be insufficient for half of the population, but would be adequate for the other half. This would not be satisfactory for most nutrients. However, point B, which is defined as the estimated average requirement (EAR), is used as the reference value for energy intakes.[8] This is because it would clearly be undesirable to advise people to consume a level of energy which was above the needs of most of the population. In addition, the reference values are actually for use by groups. Within a group, there will be some whose energy needs are above, and some below the EAR. If the food provided, or consumed, contains an amount of energy which reaches the EAR, and the individuals eat to appetite, then one can assume that their energy needs are being met. If the mean energy provided or consumed lies below the EAR, this suggests that some of the group may not be reaching their EAR, and conversely a mean intake above the EAR implies an excessive intake of energy amongst some members of the group. However, judgements about individuals cannot be made by comparison with the EAR figure, as this is a group mean.

In practice, for the majority of nutrients the DRV Panel followed the pattern of previous committees and used a point which is towards the upper end of the distribution curve of nutritional requirements, at the mean + 2 standard deviations (SD). Because of the particular properties of this type of distribution curve, this point (C) covers the requirement figures for 97.5% of the population. It could be argued that this leaves 2.5% of the population outside the limits, and therefore at risk of an inadequate intake. However, in practice, it was felt that an individual would not have extremely high requirements for all nutrients, and it was thus unlikely that anyone would consistently fail to meet requirements across the range. Eating to satisfy appetite would be likely to ensure adequate intake.

Therefore, to summarise, point C was identified as the reference nutrient intake (RNI). In addition, the Panel identified point D, at the lower end of the requirement range. This represents the mean minus 2 SD, and covers the requirements of only 2.5% of the population, who fall below this level. Again it is possible that there are some people who have nutritional requirements consistently below this point. Individuals who are consuming an intake as low as this, are probably not meeting their nutritional requirement. This point has been called the lower reference nutrient intake (LRNI). It effectively represents the lowest level that might be compatible with an adequate intake.

Safe intakes

For some nutrients, which are known to have important functions in humans, the DRV Panel found insufficient reliable data on human requirements and were unable to set a DRV for these. However, they decided on grounds of prudence to set a safe intake, particularly for infants and children. The safe intake was judged to be a level or range of intake at which there is no risk of deficiency, and below a level where there is a risk of undesirable effects. The DRV tables[8] therefore provide three distinct figures for the majority of nutrients – the LRNI, EAR and RNI – which can be used as a yardstick to give a guide on the adequacy of diets. The Panel chose a new name for these figures, moving away from the RDA which was used previously.[13] It was felt that this had been too prescriptive, suggesting that the amounts given referred to what individuals must consume. The corollary of this was that intakes that fell below the RDA were deemed to be deficient. In setting the DRV with a range of figures, the Panel intended the range to be used, and therefore to provide more flexibility in assessing dietary adequacy.

Weights and standard age ranges

As requirements for most nutrients vary with both age and gender, the Panel has attempted to set DRVs for all such groups of the population. The Panel has sought new weight data for use in calculating DRVs for people of all ages in the UK. These weights are given in the report for each of the standard age groups.[8]

Specific examples of DRVs

DRVs for energy

RNIs for all nutrients, but not energy, can be set at the upper end of the range of requirements because an intake moderately in excess of requirements has no adverse effects, but reduces the risk of deficiency. For energy, however, this is not the case. Recommendations for energy have therefore always been set as the average of energy requirements for any population group. The Panel has therefore calculated EARs but not LRNIs or RNIs for energy.

DRVs for protein

The approach, derived from estimates of basic nitrogen requirements with additions for specific situations such as growth and pregnancy, and adopted by joint Food and Agricultural Organization of the USA (FAO)/World Health Organization (WHO)/United Nations University (UNU) Expert Consultation in 1985,[14] has formed the basis of the Panel's deliberations and enabled calculations of DRVs, including EARs.

Uses of DRVs

These DRVs apply to groups of healthy people and are not necessarily appropriate for those with different needs arising from disease, such as infections, disorders of the gastrointestinal tract or metabolic abnormalities. The DRVs for any one nutrient presuppose that requirements for energy and all other nutrients are met.

Assessing diets of individuals

The imprecision of most estimates of individuals' nutrient intakes and of nutritional status, and thus of the estimation of the DRVs themselves, means that caution should be used in applying the figures to the interpretation or assessment of individual diets. Even with a perfect measure of an individual's habitual intake of a nutrient (a difficult goal), the DRVs can give no more than a guide to the adequacy of diet for that individual.

If the habitual intake is below the LRNI, it is likely that the individual will not be consuming sufficient of the nutrient to maintain the function selected by the Panel as an appropriate parameter of nutritional status for that nutrient, and further investigation, including biological measures, may be appropriate. If the habitual intake is above the RNI, then it is extremely unlikely that the individual will not be consuming sufficient. If the intake lies between the two, then the chances of the diet being inadequate (in respect of the chosen function parameter for any nutrient) fall as the intake approaches the RNI. It is impossible to say with any certainty whether an individual's nutrient intake, if it lies between the LRNI and the RNI, is or is not adequate, without some biological measure.

Assessing diets of groups of individuals

When measures of individual diets are aggregated, one of the sources of imprecision is attenuated, that is, intra-individual day-to-day variability. Assuming that the inter-individual variability is random, then in a sufficiently large group, this source of imprecision is also diminished. Thus the group mean intake will more pre-

Table 1.2.1   Dietary reference intake reports published to date

Panel of nutrients	Reference
Calcium, phosphorus, magnesium, vitamin D and fluoride	FNB (1997)[17]
Thiamin, riboflavin, niacin, vitamin B_6, folate, vitamin B_{12}, pantothenic acid, biotin and choline	FNB (1998)[18]
Vitamin C, vitamin E, selenium and carotenoids	FNB (2000)[19]
Vitamin A, vitamin K, arsenic, boron, chromium, copper, iodine, iron, manganese, molybdenum, nickel, silicon, vanadium and zinc	FNB (2001)[20]
Energy, carbohydrate, fibre, fat, fatty acids, cholesterol, protein and amino acids	FNB (2002)[21]
Electrolytes and water	FNB (2004)[22]

FNB, Food and Nutrition Board.

cisely represent the habitual group mean intake than any of the individual measures will represent individual intakes.

OTHER INTERNATIONAL CRITERIA/STANDARDS

USA[15,16]

RDAs were revised in 1989 and are jointly produced by the Food and Nutrition Board, the National Academy of Sciences and the National Research Council. They are designed for the maintenance of good nutrition of practically all healthy people in the USA.

RDA is the average daily intake over time; it provides for individual variations among most normal persons living in the USA under the usual environmental stresses. Estimated safe intakes and adequate daily dietary intakes are given for some vitamins and minerals where there is less information on which to base allowances, and figures are provided in the form of ranges of recommended intakes. Since the toxic levels for many trace elements may not be much greater than the safe intakes, e.g. for copper, these safe levels should not be habitually exceeded.

The Institute of Medicine and Food and Nutrition Board are currently establishing a set of reference values to replace the previous RDAs for the USA and Canada. The new DRIs will encompass EAR, RDA, adequate intakes (AI) and tolerable upper intake levels (ULs). RDAs and AIs are nutrient levels that should decrease the risk of developing a nutrient-related condition with a negative functional outcome. AIs are used where insufficient evidence is available to calculate EARs and may be used as a goal for intake of individuals but should not be applied rigorously. Six reports have been published to date (Table 1.2.1[17–22]).

DRIs replace the Food and Nutrition Board's previous RDAs for healthy individuals.[23] Four levels of intake values are documented (Figure 1.2.4).

The EAR is the nutrient intake value that is estimated to meet the requirement defined by a specified indicator of adequacy (e.g. balance studies) in 50% of individuals in a life-stage and gender group. Hence, it is a median rather than an average. At this level of intake, the remaining 50% of the specified group would not have its nutrient needs met. For some groups, data had to be extrapolated to estimate the value. In deriving the EARs, contemporary concepts of reduction of disease risk were among the factors considered, rather than basing reference values solely upon prevention of nutrient deficiencies, unlike the UK DRVs. Because the EAR is a dietary intake value, it includes an adjustment for an assumed bioavailability of the nutrient. The EAR is used in setting the RDA.

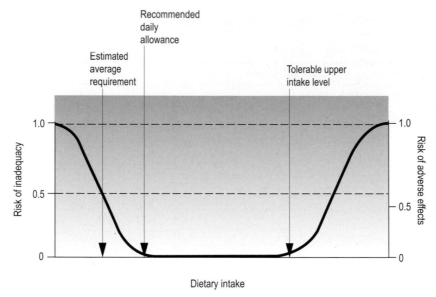

Figure 1.2.4   Principle of dietary reference intakes. EAR, estimated average requirement; RDA, recommended daily allowance; AI, adequate intake; UL, upper intake level. (Adapted from Bloch AS, Shils ME. Appendix A-22. In: Modern Nutrition in Health and Disease, 9th edn. Baltimore, MD: Williams & Wilkins; 1999, with permission.)

Table 1.2.2   Recommended daily allowances (RDAs) and dietary reference intakes (DRIs)

	Age (years)	Ascorbic acid[a] (mg)	Folacin/folate (µg)	Niacin (mg)	Riboflavin (mg)	Thiamin (mg)	Vitamin B_6 (mg)	Vitamin B_{12} (µg)
Children	4–6	40/45	200/75	12	1.1	0.9	0.9/1.1	1.5/1.0
	7–10	40/45	300/100	16/13	1.2	1.2/1.0	1.2	2.0/1.4
Males	15–18	45/60	400/200	20	1.8	1.5	2.0	3.0/2.0
	19–24	45/60	400/200	20/19	1.8/1.7	1.5	2.0	3.0/2.0
	25–50	45/60	400/200	18/19	1.6/1.7	1.4/1.5	2.0	3.0/2.0
	50+	45/60	400/200	16/15	1.5/1.4	1.2	2.0	3.0/2.0
Females	15–18	45/60	400/180	14/15	1.4/1.3	1.1	2.0/1.5	3.0/2.0
	19–24	45/60	400/180	14/15	1.4/1.3	1.1	2.0/1.6	3.0/2.0
	25–50	45/60	400/180	13/15	1.2/1.3	1.0/1.1	2.0/1.6	3.0/2.0
	50+	45/60	400/180	12/13	1.1/1.2	1.0	2.0/1.6	3.0/2.0

[a]First figure refers to the old RDA (1989) while the second figure refers to the new DRI.
Data from National Research Council, Food and Nutrition Board, Commission on Life Sciences. Recommended dietary allowances, 10th edn. Washington, DC: National Academy Press; 1989;[15] and Food and Nutrition Board – Institute of Medicine. Dietary reference intakes for thiamin, riboflavin, niacin, vitamin B_6, folate, vitamin B_{12}, pantothenic acid, biotin, and choline. Washington, DC: National Academy Press; 1998.[18]

The RDA is the daily dietary intake level that is sufficient to meet the nutrient requirements of nearly all (97–98%) of individuals in the life-stage and gender group. The RDA applies to individuals, not to groups. The EAR serves as the foundation for setting the RDA. If the SD of the EAR is known, the RDA is set at 2 SD above the EAR. If the data are insufficient to calculate an SD, a coefficient of variation of 10% is assumed, and the RDA = 1.2 × EAR. The RDA for a nutrient is a value to be used as a goal for dietary intake by individuals and is not intended for use in assessing the diets of either individuals or groups or for planning for groups. The 1989 RDAs are listed for comparison with the new DRIs in Table 1.2.2 for a selection of nutrients.

The AI is the value used when there is insufficient evidence to calculate an EAR. It is based on observed or experimentally determined approximations of the average intake of a defined population that appears to sustain a defined nutritional state such as normal circulating nutrient values or growth. AIs rather than EARs and RDAs are being proposed for all nutrients for infants to age 1 year[17,18], for calcium, vitamin D and fluoride[17] and for pantothenic acid, biotin and choline[18] for all life stages.

The tolerable UL is the maximal level of nutrient intake that is unlikely to pose risks of adverse health effects to almost all individuals in the target group. The term was chosen to avoid implying a possible beneficial effect and is not intended to be a recommended intake level. For most nutrients, the UL refers to total intakes from food, fortified food and nutrient supplements. In some instances, it may refer only to intakes from pharmacologic agents. The UL applies to chronic daily use. The relationship between these four dietary reference intakes is depicted in Figure 1.2.4.

Europe

European values were revised in 1993.[24] Carbohydrate, fat and non-starch polysaccharide population goals were not included, so those used here are from reference 25.

LTI	Lowest threshold intake
ARI	Average requirement intake
PRI	Population reference intake: mean requirement +2 SD. This is the value chosen for most of the tables
Acceptable range	Range of safe values given where insufficient information is available to be more specific.

World Health Organization, WHO (1974, 1990, 1996) WHO/FAO (1987), FAO/WHO (1988), FAO/WHO/UNU (1985)[14,26–30]

WHO requirements have been revised for groups of nutrients at different times. The trace elements are the most recent revision (1996); carbohydrate, fat and non-starch polysaccharides are 1990 values; vitamin A, iron, folate and vitamin B_{12} are FAO/WHO 1988 values; the values for vitamin E as α-tocopherol are from WHO/FAO in 1987; energy and protein are from FAO/WHO/UNU in 1985, and the values for other nutrients were set in 1974.

Population requirement safe ranges (1996)

Basal	Lower limit of safe ranges of population mean intakes
Normative	Population mean intake sufficient to meet normative requirements. This value is used most often in their tables
Maximum	Upper limit of safe ranges of population mean intakes.

Recommended intakes (1974)

Average requirement augmented by a factor that takes into account interindividual variability. The amounts are considered sufficient for the maintenance of health in nearly all people.

Chapter **1.3**

Food groups and types

Geraldine J Cuskelly and Ian S Young

A HEALTHY DIET – WHICH FOODS TO CHOOSE?

If we are interested in and committed to taking care of ourselves and others, the healthiness of our selection of food is paramount. However, healthiness is not the only feature we look for in our food. Most of us would be very reluctant to eat an unfamiliar food just because we were told it was healthy; the property of healthiness would be included in the general consideration of the food in deciding whether or not to include it in the diet.

However, food which constitutes a healthy diet is in the main not very different from that which makes up a less healthy diet – it is the balance of the parts making up the total meal or diet that is important. According to nutritionists, there are no bad foods; it is their place in the general picture of the diet that is important. Some foods provide only a very narrow range of nutrients, perhaps even just one. If such foods comprise a substantial part of the daily intake, the consumer will run the risk of not meeting nutritional requirements for a range of nutrients. Broccoli, for example, is regarded as a very nutritious food; however, a diet composed solely or predominantly of broccoli would be significantly deficient in many vital nutrients.

The greater the range of foods in the diet, the less likely there are to be gaps in the nutrient intake, and the more likely it is that consumers will meet their nutritional needs.[31] We are attracted by variety in foods, and would find a diet containing just one or two foods very monoto-

Table 1.3.1 Core, secondary and peripheral foods

Food category	Description
Core	The most important foods in the diet – the staple food of the region (normally a cereal or a root). Usually one or two foods only (in the UK, bread/cereals and potatoes tend to appear in most meals). Nutritionally a source of carbohydrate, some protein and a range of minerals and vitamins
Secondary	Enhance the meal, but not essential. May have specific perceived properties (e.g. protein-rich, healthy, promoting balance, suitable for particular ages/conditions in life). May include meat/fish, vegetables, pulses, fruit
Peripheral	Non-essential but pleasant to eat. Special-occasion foods, e.g. eaten at festivals, celebrations. May include biscuits, cakes, confectionery, alcoholic drinks, exotic fruit, sauces, drinks, e.g. tea/coffee

Data from Baresi ME. Human nutrition: a health perspective. London: Arnold; 1997.[1]

nous. This might result in a smaller intake of the foods. The converse is also true; when presented with a variety of foods, we move from one to another and are likely to eat more. The appearance of a tempting dessert after a filling meal can readily override feelings of satiety.[1]

Selecting several foods is therefore beneficial for our nutrient intake. Traditional meal patterns can help us to decide on combinations of foods to make up meals, as well as what foods to have at specific points of our day. The pattern of core, secondary and peripheral foods serves as a general guide (Table 1.3.1). It must be recognised that there is increasing variation in this pattern. It is possible that in the future meals may be quite different, although there are also signs of a traditionalist revival, which may take us back to old-established food patterns.

Chapter **1.4**

A healthy diet – how much to eat?

Geraldine J Cuskelly and Ian S Young

In addition to deciding on what foods to eat, each person makes a decision about the quantity to consume. From experience, we have learned what an adequate serving size is; of course this varies between individuals. Our ability to assess how much of a food we would like to eat relies on learned responses established during our childhood and added to whenever a new food has been introduced. The sensations arising from the stomach when a particular serving size has been eaten will be remembered and will help to determine our behaviour in the future. Other reflex pathways, linked to the metabolic consequences of the meal, may also be part of the regulatory process. It is believed that this type of learning is an important component of the control of food intake.[32]

The variability of normal serving sizes between individuals is a dilemma for those studying food intakes in populations. There is no such thing as an average serving size which would apply to everyone. However, for the sake of expediency, such a measure is quoted and used in many contexts. In relation to this average, it is recognised that different people will also have large and small servings. Interpretations of these are also subjective, and therefore variable.

Dieticians try to resolve this issue by using replica foods (food models), which generally represent the average serving.[33] Individuals may then indicate whether the amount they would consume is similar to this or different. Nutrition researchers use food photographs to assist subjects in defining amounts eaten.[34]

WHY DO WE NEED GUIDELINES?

All the research results and interpretations published in books, peer-review journals and in the wider literature of nutritional science cannot help the great majority of people in our countries until this mass of data is translated into information that most people can understand and accept. Food consumption patterns can become healthier in two ways: (1) from change in the foods that are available and affordable; and (2) from change in the foods people choose to eat and in the way they prepare them. What is needed ideally as the foundation of nutritional education and national food policy is a set of nutritional recommendations or dietary guidelines that are evidence-based, authoritative and comprehensible.

Evidence-based

Nutritional recommendations for a nation should be based on objective, unbiased and thorough reviews of all the evidence relating the nutrients, food components and foods to health or disease risk. Evidence-based medicine is now encouraged,[35] and meta-analysis is a recent powerful method in epidemiology,[36] but systematic reviews of nutrition and health have been appearing since the 1960s,[37] at first focused on diet and heart disease.

Authoritative

For most people to take notice of and accept national dietary recommendations, the recommendations have to be credible and be prepared by a committee of experts convened by a government department, national academy of science or professional association. Membership of the committee should have broad coverage (of scientific area and constituency), adequate independence and minimal commercial bias. One excellent model is the committee that prepared the Diet and Health report for the US National Research Council (NRC) in 1989.[15] It had 33 experts on the main committee and another 76 specialists recorded as providing input.

Comprehensible

Nutrition, like other scientific disciplines, has its own technical vocabulary, which is easily understood by professional groups but opaque to the general public. Dietary guidelines have to be comprehensible to the general public,[38] who are confused about terms like cholesterol, fat, fibre, polyunsaturated and energy. Guidelines must also be available in language meaningful to health professionals who can explain the above and other technical terms and the meanings of 'moderate in', 'low in' and 'plenty of' for individuals.

In public health nutrition, two major sets of messages are sent from a consensus of nutritional scientists to the rest of the population – politicians, government departments, food industry, farmers, health professionals, economists, journalists, school teachers, supermarkets, caterers, shoppers and consumers. Recommended dietary intakes (RDI) (in the case of the USA) are the first and older set. They advise the quantities of the essential nutrients that people ought to consume. These technical numbers have to be converted for ordinary people to more easily understand concepts such as food groups, meal plans or exchange lists. In underdeveloped countries and communities, food and nutritional policy must concentrate on striving to reach the RDIs for as many people and as many nutrients as possible. In affluent countries, intakes near the RDIs can be taken for granted for most people.

Other sets of authoritative statements, dietary guidelines, have emerged since the late 1960s and advise how to select from the many combinations of foods in adequate diets to give the best chances of long-term health. The variety of food products is bewildering, and the whole food system needs signposts – guidelines to healthier diets that can be used in nutritional education, planning by food companies and national nutrition policy.

FEATURES OF DIETARY GUIDELINES OR GOALS

Dietary guidelines aim to reduce the chances of developing chronic degenerative diseases rather than to provide enough of the essential nutrients (in the USA, that is the purpose of RDIs). While there is never more than one RDI (or RDA) committee and report in a country, there can be several sets of dietary guidelines at a time.[37]

Dietary goals or guidelines do not start from zero intake (as RDIs do) but from the present estimated national average diet. They deal with the optimal proportions of the energy-yielding macronutrients: how much carbohydrate? fat? protein? alcohol? and which types? They are not usually expressed as nutrients, but as food components, food groups or even eating behaviour. So, they are often a hybrid collection of recommendations.

Dietary goals or guidelines are not usually expressed as weight of nutrient per day, but as semiquantitative advice on consumption of a food component or on people's eating behaviour. If expressed quantitatively, this is mostly as a percentage of total energy, that is, nutrient density (e.g. total fat intake should be 30–35% of total energy). Dietary guidelines are targets for the population to aim for some time in the future. In some sets, the year is given or goals are progressive (e.g. total fat: intermediate goal, 35% energy; ultimate goal, 20–30%).[39] By contrast, RDIs are needed now and every day (although there are reserves in the body – large for some nutrients, small for others).

A few sets of dietary guidelines draw a distinction between general advice for the whole population and (usually more radical) advice for groups at risk. For example, the US Surgeon General's report[40] has five recommendations for most people and another four for some people. The recommendations of the WHO in Europe[41] give intermediate goals separately for the general population and for the cardiovascular high-risk group. Although most RDIs are relatively well established scientifically, guidelines are more provisional, being based on indirect evidence about the complex role of food components in causing multifactorial diseases with very long incubation periods. Dietary goals and guidelines, which primarily examine macronutrients, rely more on epidemiologic data than RDIs do. In addition, they depend on using food consumption patterns. The NRC Committee on Diet and Health[15] observed that the term 'insufficient data' could perhaps be applied to most issues concerning nutrition and

health. In particular, it characterises many of the relationships between diet and certain chronic diseases. The lack of certainty about causal associations and mechanisms of action is common and stems in part from attempts to relate a complex mixture such as diet to complex, multifactorial chronic diseases for which the pathophysiological, environmental and genetic predisposing factors are imprecisely understood. Despite such limitations, a large body of evidence has emerged in the past four decades concerning chronic diseases and their relationship to general dietary patterns or specific dietary components.[15]

Unlike RDIs, which give separate numbers for males and females and for different age groups and physiologic states, dietary guidelines have usually appeared to be the same for every man, woman and child. Of course, adjustments have to be made at the implementation stage. An international WHO symposium in Japan[41] concluded that, while countries could usually share their RDIs, dietary guidelines are most effective if the target group is defined. New Zealand has different dietary guidelines reports for infants,[42] children,[43] adolescents,[44] most adults,[45] healthy pregnant women[46] and healthy older people.[47] Most of these reports (except reference 45) do not appear to be the work of a large, representative committee. In Australia, there is a general dietary guidelines report[48] and a separate report for infants, children and adolescents.[49] Canada has a separate report on fat recommendations for children.[50] Although they are more recent than RDIs, dietary guidelines are better known by the general public. Their summary recommendations, written in deliberately simple language about major food components or food habits, appeal to journalists, consumer organisations and cookbook writers.

GOALS OR GUIDELINES?

The classic *Dietary Goals for the United States*[51] was addressed to the nation, and the recommendations were expressed in such technical terms as 'increase the consumption of complex carbohydrates and naturally occurring sugars from about 28% of energy intake to about 48% of energy intake'[51] – not a calculation the shopper can manage in a supermarket aisle! These dietary goals were followed by *Dietary Guidelines for Americans*, published by the Departments of Agriculture and Health, in which the corresponding recommendation in the 1995 edition[52] is headed: 'Choose a diet with plenty of grain products, vegetables and fruits'. In Australia, dietary goals were also used for statements on nutritional policy, 'Increase consumption of complex carbohydrates and dietary fibre . . .',[53] while dietary guidelines came later in a mass-produced booklet, written in less technical language for consumers: 'Eat more bread and cereals (preferably wholegrain), vegetables and fruit'.[54] Helsing[55] has suggested that recommendations are needed at three levels: (1) quantitative nutrient goals for scientists and health professionals; (2) quantitative food goals for politicians and food producers; and (3) dietary guidelines expressed as advice to individual consumers. The report *Diet, Nutrition and the Prevention of Chronic Diseases* by a WHO committee[27] defines population nutrient goals as the range in which population average intakes are judged to be consistent with a low prevalence of diet-related diseases in the population. The report sets out goals for 11 nutrients in numerical terms, e.g. total average carbohydrate for a population should be between 55 and 75% of energy. It stresses the difference between population nutrient goals and individual nutrient intakes, e.g. if the population's total carbohydrate intake is 60% of energy, individual intakes might range from 45% to 75% of energy.[56] The contrasting concept of dietary guidelines was well explained by Robbins[57] in a commentary on the first proposed nutritional guidelines for the UK: 'Guidelines express the goals in terms of foods (or combinations of foods) which are to be eaten by individuals. Guidelines need not be quantified but need to be based on goals. Many different dietary patterns can be compatible with a given set of dietary goals.' For instance, the goal of reducing total fat intake can be achieved by drinking skimmed milk, by eating less fatty meat or by reducing hard cheese and biscuits.

UK (1990, 1991)

After considerable earlier controversy,[58-60] dietary guidelines and goals are now accepted by the British establishment. In 1990 the Ministry of Agriculture published a thin book[61] for the general public (without scientific background). The eight guidelines are: (1) enjoy your food; (2) eat a variety of different foods; (3) eat the right amount to be a healthy weight; (4) eat plenty of foods rich in starch and fibre; (5) don't eat too much fat (we don't need saturates at all); (6) don't eat sugary foods too often; (7) look after the vitamins and minerals in your food; (8) if you drink, keep within sensible limits.

The next year, quantitative population goals for fats and carbohydrates were included in the new report on DRVs.[8] Of the population's average percentage of total energy (including alcohol), total fat should be 33%. Of total fatty acids, saturated fatty acids should be 10%; polyunsaturated fatty acids, 6% (not more than 10%); and *trans*-fatty acids not more than 2%. Non-starch polysaccharides should be 18–24 g/day (corresponding to around 30–35 g/day dietary fibre) and non-milk extrinsic sugars should average 60 g/day. Data in support of any specific quantified targets for non-milk extrinsic sugars were scanty.

SCIENTIFIC BASES OF GUIDELINES

The original hypotheses underlying dietary guidelines were mentioned in describing their history. After 30 years of evolution, how well are current guidelines justified by scientific knowledge? The six guidelines on which there is general agreement have clearly been reasoned by large numbers of experienced scientists, independently, in more than 20 different countries, and examined at greater length than is possible in this chapter. The following brief notes are intended to help link the six major guidelines with these scientific bases.

Eat a nutritionally adequate diet from a variety of foods

A nutritionally adequate diet means eating all (or nearly all) the RDAs of those nutrients for which there is an RDA. A varied diet, if built around the food groups of nutritional education, is a fundamental principle of nutrition, older than dietary guidelines. It maximises the probability of eating all the RDAs as well as minor nutrients that lack an RDA. At the same time, variety minimises the risk of toxins and pathogens from food and drink.

Eat less fat, particularly saturated fat

Fats in food provide more calories than any other food component, and much of this is hidden in attractive dishes and products. Reducing fat is the most important way of reducing excess energy intake. Many fatty ingredients in foods contain few other nutrients. If they are replaced by lean meat, low-fat milk and vegetable foods, the intake of essential nutrients is improved. Saturated fat raises plasma total and low-density lipoprotein cholesterol.

Adjust energy (calorie) intake to expenditure and avoid overweight and underweight

'Don't eat too much or too little'[62] is the fundamental quantitative principle of nutrition; it long antedates dietary guidelines. Mortality and morbidity are increased in people who are too thin or too fat.

Eat more food containing complex carbohydrates and fibre

The terms 'complex carbohydrates' and 'fibre' are imprecise. 'Complex carbohydrates' is presumably used here to mean starchy foods and naturally occurring sugars (as in milk and fruits). 'Fibre' presumably covers non-starch polysaccharides and resistant starch. While this heading reflected the thinking in nutrition science in the 1970s, it is now realised that foods containing complex carbohydrates and fibre very likely contain a cocktail of other potentially protective substances: carotenoids other than β-carotene, folate, flavonoids, phytoestrogens and glucosinolates.[63] The older heading is therefore being replaced by 'Choose a diet with plenty of grain products, vegetables and fruits'.[48,52]

From the preceding guidelines, these plant foods should of course be eaten in variety and without added fat. They should also be eaten as whole foods (not refined), because they are intended not only to replace fat-rich foods but also to provide generous intakes of essential nutrients and a mixture of other apparently protective substances (mentioned above).

Reduce salt intake

Reducing salt intake is recommended in an attempt to reduce the prevalence of essential hypertension and (a firmer epidemiologic index) mortality from cerebral haemorrhage.[64] The evidence may not be as strong as that for saturated fat and plasma cholesterol, but a taste for salty food is an acquired one, handed down from the era before refrigerators. Most societies consume several times more sodium than people need; no harm, and possibly some benefit, could result from limiting intakes to 50–100 mmol sodium per day (3–6 g NaCl). In explaining this guideline, it is important to stress that most sodium or salt intake comes from foods to which salt has already been added during processing or preparation.[52]

Drink alcohol in moderation, if at all

Drinking alcohol in excess causes road accidents, domestic violence, raised blood pressure, cirrhosis of the liver, fetal alcohol syndrome and many other complications.[65] While it appears that two or three standard drinks per day give some protection against coronary heart disease, this benefit is only of value in older adults and in communities with high risk of coronary heart disease. It has a smaller beneficial impact on the whole population than the adverse impact of alcohol in young people, since more person-years are lost from alcohol among people less than 35 years old than are saved in the older age group.[66]

FOOD GROUPS

In order to translate dietary guidelines into comprehensible advice for the general public, many countries have adopted pictorial impressions of the correct proportions of foods to be eaten for optimal health. Despite the wide spectrum of shapes representing food guides from around the globe, these guides use very similar methods in presenting their concepts of the ideal dietary pattern. Each of these guides gives consumers a selection of recommended food choices (food groups) as well as recommended daily amounts consumers should ingest to maintain optimum health. In essence the basis of these food group-ings is the inclusion of specific numbers of serv-ings from a number of food groups (Table 1.4.1).

Figure 1.4.1 shows a remarkable similarity in the basic food groupings of international food guide illustrations (a selection is shown here). The

Table 1.4.1 Summary of food groups

Food group	Composition of food group	Key nutrients found in group
Bread, other cereals and potatoes (6–11 servings)	All breads, cereals, including wheat, oats, barley, rice, maize, millet and rye together with products made from them, including breakfast cereals and pasta Potatoes in the form usually eaten as part of a meal (but not as a snack, e.g. crisps)	Carbohydrate NSP Vitamin-B complex Calcium Iron Recommended: Low-fat methods of cooking and sauces/dressings, spreads High-fibre varieties to maximise micronutrients
Fruit and vegetables (5–9 servings)	Fresh, frozen, chilled and canned fruit and vegetables Fruit juices Dried fruit Not included: potatoes, pulses, nuts	Vitamins C, E and carotene (antioxidant vitamins), folate Minerals; potassium, magnesium, trace minerals Carbohydrate NSP Majority are low in energy
Meat, fish and alternatives (2–3 servings)	Carcass meats, meat products (but not pastries and pies) Fish and fish products Poultry Eggs Pulses and nuts	Protein B-vitamins (especially B_{12}) Minerals; phosphorus, iron, zinc, magnesium NSP (from pulses only) Long-chain polyunsaturated fatty acids (in oily fish) Meat and its products may be significant contributors to fat intake (low-fat alternatives are available)
Milk and dairy foods (2–3 servings)	All types of milk Yogurt Cheese	Protein Calcium Fat-soluble vitamins (except in low-fat varieties) B-vitamins (riboflavin, B_{12}) Not included: butter and eggs
Fatty and sugary foods (use sparingly)	Butter, margarine, fat spreads, oils and other fats Cream Crisps and fried savoury snacks Cakes, pastries, biscuits Chocolate and sugar confectionery Sugars and preserves Ice cream Soft drinks	Energy Fat Sugar Essential fatty acids Fat-soluble vitamins

NSP, non-starch polysaccharide.
Data from Baresi ME. Human nutrition: a health perspective. London: Arnold; 1997.[1]

A US food pyramid

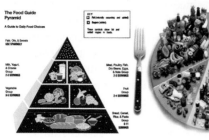

Courtesy of the US Department of Agriculture and the US Department of Health and Human Services

B UK balance of good health

Courtesy of the Health Education Authority

C Irish food pyramid

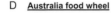

Use the Food Pyramid to plan your healthy food choices every day and watch your portion size

Courtesy of the Health Promotion Unit of the Department of Health and Children, Ireland

D Australia food wheel

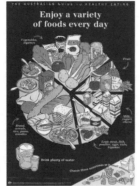

Courtesy of Public Health Division, Commonwealth Department of Health and Family Services. Copyright Commonwealth of Australia reproduced by permission.

E Chinese Food Pagoda

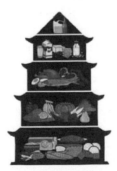

Courtesy of the Chinese Nutrition Society

Figure 1.4.1 Selection of food guides. **A**, US food pyramid. **B**, UK balance of good health. (Courtesy of the Health Education Authority.) **C**, Irish food pyramid. (Courtesy of the Department of Health and Children, Ireland.) **D**, Australian food wheel. (Copyright Commonwealth of Australia, reproduced by permission.) **E**, Chinese food pagoda. (Courtesy of the Chinese Nutrition Society.)

groups include: grains, vegetables, fruits, meats, milk and dairy products, and fats and sugars. Despite the differences in indigenous foods of each culture, along with the differences in the cultural definitions of food and what constitutes a usual dietary pattern, the fundamental classification of foods is similar in all countries.

Minor differences in food categorisation are observed in the fat and sugar group, the vegetable and fruit group, and the milk and dairy group. The existence of additional groups along with the categorisation of foods such as beans, nuts and potatoes also contributes to these differences. While most of the countries group fat and sugar as a single category, food guides for China, Sweden, Germany and Portugal do not include sugar in the group. The Chinese Nutrition Society has stated that there is no recommendation related to sugar intake in its 'food pagoda' because the current consumption of sugar by the Chinese is rather low.[67] Moreover, in some food guides, such as the Mexican food guide, the fat and sugar group is not included at all.[68] The fat and sugar group in the food guides for Canada[69] and Australia[70] is included in a brochure accompanying the illustrated guide as well as in the corner of the guide. Fruits and vegetables are grouped together in the food guides for Canada, the UK,[71] China,[67] Korea,[72] Portugal[73] and Mexico, while each of these groups appears independently in the other guides. The Philippines is the only country lacking the milk and dairy group in its food guide.[74] Since Filipinos are not milk-drinkers, and milk is not traditionally part of their diet, it is incorporated with the major protein group.[74] Mexico, on the other hand, groups it with other foods of animal origin.

An additional food group exists in the Sweden and German food circles.[68] Sweden separates potatoes and root vegetables from the essential vegetable group as they regard potatoes and root vegetables as the base food that provides the foundation for a nutritious and inexpensive diet and can remain approximately the same from day to day. It is recommended that they should be supplemented with other vegetables, which are considered foods that vary from day to day and between seasons.

Interestingly, Germany is the only country that contains a fluid group in its food guide. A separate group for beverages exists to ensure enough daily consumption of fluids. Although not classifying fluid as an independent group, Puerto Rico includes water in both its illustration and recommendations. They include water, due to their tropical climate.[75]

Most countries group potatoes in the vegetable group. However, Korea, the UK, Portugal, Germany and Mexico categorise them in the grain group. The UK places them within the grain group, yet includes other root crops such as turnips and parsnips within the fruit and vegetable group.[76] Likewise, countries have made different decisions regarding the classification of beans and legumes. While beans and legumes are usually in the meat group due to their high protein content, Sweden, Germany and Australia put them into the vegetable group in view of their high vitamin, mineral and dietary fibre content. In the case of the US Food Guide Pyramid, legumes, including kidney beans and chickpeas, are classified within the vegetable group while dry beans and nuts are grouped with meat, poultry and fish. The Chinese pagoda, on the other hand, places them in the milk and dairy products group. Nuts are also classified in different ways. Unlike, the USA, Puerto Rico and Australia, where the protein content in nuts is valued, Korea places them in the fat and oil group because of their high fat content.[72]

QUANTITATIVE RECOMMENDATIONS

For each category of food, these guides have recommended specific quantities or offered general advice emphasising suggested portions in a daily diet. The Philippines, Portugal, Mexico, Germany and Sweden avoid taking the quantitative approach in their recommendations. In the Philippines, the quantitative recommendation was perceived to be a stumbling block rather than a helpful aid, since nutritionists thought people would have a hard time interpreting serving portions.[74] As a result, the Filipino pyramid food guide uses easy-to-comprehend action words implying the proportion and frequency, instead of using specific amounts in their recommendations. The Portuguese food wheel defines the approximate proportions of food weight for only five food groups.[73] The proportion of each food category in a daily diet is expressed as a percentage. Sweden, on the other hand, prioritises variety in its recommendation. They simply recommend that individuals choose from all seven groups of food during a day.

The remainder of the food guide graphics (USA, Canada, UK, Australia, China, Korea and Germany) make quantitative recommendations based on various units such as serving sizes, portion sizes, sample sizes and grams.[68] Although Germany does not give specific amounts for each group, it provides examples. The Korean and Chinese food guide pagodas recommend a smaller number of servings for the milk group. For the remainder of the food groups, the total intake suggested for each food group does not show significant differences among countries if both the number of servings and serving sizes are considered.

Korea, for instance, recommends a relatively small number of servings for the grain group, yet has a serving size nearly three times that of others, making the actual recommendation similar to that of others. Likewise, because of the smaller serving sizes for the meat group, Korea recommends a larger number of servings in its food guide.

In summary, whether or not quantitative recommendations are presented, most countries consistently recommend a greater consumption of the grain, vegetable, and fruit groups with a lower intake of meat, milk and dairy products.

Chapter **1.5**

Digestion, absorption and transport of foods

Geraldine J Cuskelly and Ian S Young

Most foodstuffs are ingested in forms that are unavailable to the body and must be broken down into smaller molecules before they can be absorbed into the body. The gastrointestinal tract is the system that carries out the functions of digestion and absorption. The gastrointestinal tract extends from the mouth to the anus (Figure 1.5.1) and consists of a tubular structure with openings for the entry of secretions from the salivary glands, the liver and the pancreas. The gastrointestinal system includes the mouth, stomach, small intestine and large intestine, as well as accessory organs (salivary glands, pancreas, liver and gallbladder) that provide essential secretions. The major function of the gastrointestinal tract is to digest complex molecules in foods and to absorb simple nutrients, including monosaccharides, monoacylglycerols, fatty acids, amino acids, vitamins, minerals and water. It also serves as a barrier to the entry of bacteria into the body and contains specialised cells that secrete mucus, fluids, some digestive enzymes, intrinsic factor and some peptide hormones.

Digestion is defined as the chemical breakdown of food by enzymes secreted into the lumen of the gastrointestinal tract by glandular cells in the mouth, chief cells in the stomach, and the exocrine cells of the pancreas, and by enzymes in the brush-border (luminal) membrane and in the cytoplasm of mucosal cells of the small intestine. As such, digestion occurs prior to the entry of nutrients into the interstitial fluid and hence into the circulatory system by which nutrients are carried to all cells of the body.

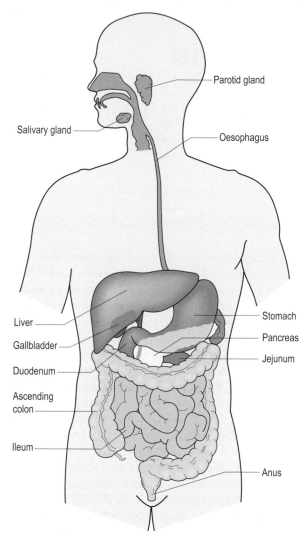

Figure 1.5.1 The human alimentary tract. (Reproduced from Tso P, Crissinger K. Overview of digestion and absorption. In: Biochemical and physiological aspects of human nutrition. Philadelphia, PA: WB Saunders; 2000, with permission.[118])

Absorption is the movement of nutrients, including water and electrolytes, across the mucosal cells into the interstitial fluid, from which they enter the blood or lymph. Processes involved in absorption include diffusion, facilitated diffusion, active transport (primary and secondary), solvent drag and endocytosis. Most substances pass from the intestinal lumen into the mucosal cells and then out of the mucosal cells to the extra-cellular fluid, and the processes responsible for movement across the luminal or brush-border membrane are often quite different from those responsible for movement across the basolateral or contraluminal cell membranes to the interstitial fluid. Once nutrients have exited from the intestinal absorptive cells into the interstitial fluid, they either enter the capillaries (into the blood) or lacteals (into the lymph). Water and some other molecules may be taken up by paracellular movement between cells.

THE MOUTH

Chewing involves the cutting as well as grinding of food by the teeth. The process of chewing not only ensures that the bolus of food is crushed into smaller particles but also allows the mixing of saliva with food. As food is mixed with saliva, salivary amylase may begin the digestion of starch, and, more importantly, the bolus of food is lubricated to facilitate swallowing.

Saliva has many functions, including digestion of nutrients, antibacterial activity (due to the presence of thiocyanate, lactoferrin and lysozyme), moistening of the mouth to facilitate speech and swallowing, and buffering. The salivary glands secrete α-amylase, which is active within the food bolus until it is inactivated by the acidic secretions of the stomach. In some species, lingual lipase is secreted by glands in the tongue, and this enzyme is most active in the acidic environment of the gastric lumen. Secretion of lingual lipase is insignificant in humans, but humans do secrete a gastric lipase that has similar acid lipase activity.[77,78] Swallowing is a highly coordinated process, and the lower oesophageal sphincter relaxes following swallowing to allow the entry of food into the stomach. Otherwise, the lower oesophageal sphincter is closed to prevent the reflux of stomach acid into the oesophagus.

THE STOMACH

The major functions of the stomach are to store food and to process the swallowed food in a preliminary fashion for delivery into the small intestine. The gastric mucosa of the stomach contains many deep glands made up of chief cells, parietal

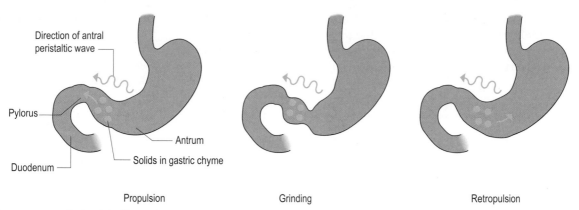

Direction of antral
peristaltic wave

Pylorus

Antrum

Solids in gastric chyme

Duodenum

Propulsion   Grinding   Retropulsion

Figure 1.5.2   Peristalsis. (Reproduced from Tso P, Crissinger K. Overview of digestion and absorption. In: Biochemical and physiological aspects of human nutrition. Philadelphia, PA: WB Saunders; 2000, with permission.[118])

cells and mucous cells. The mixed secretion of these cells is known as gastric juice. Gastric juice contains mucin, inorganic salts, hydrochloric acid (HCl) and digestive enzymes or zymogens (gastric lipase and pepsinogens/pepsins). The parietal cells are the source of gastric acid (HCl). The gastric acidity that favours the denaturation (unfolding) of proteins is necessary for activation of pepsinogen to pepsin and for the proteolytic activity of pepsin, and destroys many microorganisms that entered the gastrointestinal tract via the oral cavity. The parietal cells also secrete intrinsic factor, a glycoprotein that is required for vitamin B_{12} absorption. The neck mucous cells secrete bicarbonate and mucus. The chief cells of the gastric glands secrete pepsinogens and gastric lipase. Protein in food is a potent stimulant of gastrin release into the blood stream by endocrine cells of the stomach, but vagal stimulation, calcium ions (Ca^{2+}) and alkalinisation of the antrum of the stomach also promote gastrin release. Gastrin stimulates gastric HCl and pepsinogen secretion, and gastrin secretion is inhibited by acid within the lumen of the antrum.

Pepsins begin the process of protein digestion in the stomach by cleaving the protein into large peptide fragments and some free amino acids. Gastric lipase hydrolyses triacylglycerol in the acidic medium to form predominantly diacylglycerol and free fatty acid. Some products of fat hydrolysis may play a role in beginning the emulsification of lipids in the stomach contents.

Peristaltic contractions of the distal stomach propel the stomach contents toward the pylorus (located between the stomach and the duodenum; Figure 1.5.2). The pylorus is composed of a thickened band of circular muscle. It contracts in opposition to an approaching peristalsis. As the contractions reach the terminal antrum, the pylorus closes. This results in the grinding of solids to form finer particles. In addition, the acidic chyme (semifluid mass of partially digested food) that cannot pass forward through the opening of the pylorus will be retropelled into the body of the stomach. The retropulsion of the chyme results not only in the mixing of chyme but also in dispersion of oil droplets into very fine emulsion particles. The dispersion of oil droplets greatly facilitates the subsequent digestion of lipids in the small intestine, because pancreatic lipase acts at the water–lipid interface, and emulsification significantly increases this surface area. Only liquids and small particles in chyme are allowed to pass into the duodenum because of the small opening that results from the contraction of the pyloric sphincter. The gastrointestinal hormone that stimulates gastric motility as well as gastric acid secretion is gastrin. The neural stimulation of gastric acid secretion and gastric motility is via the vagus nerve. The stomach regulates the amount of food presented to the duodenum so as not to exceed the absorptive capacity of the small intestine. This occurs largely as a result of the actions of hormones such as gastric inhibitory peptide and cholecystokinin, which are released by the small intestine in response to the presence of digestive products and which inhibit gastric motility, gastric emptying and gastric secretion.

THE SMALL INTESTINE

Most of the digestion and uptake of nutrients takes place in the small intestine, and the small intestine is uniquely adapted to accommodate these processes. The small intestine is usually divided into three sections. The first section is the duodenum, which is about 30 cm long; this section receives the chyme from the stomach and secretions from the liver or gallbladder and the pancreas. The remainder (about 3 m) of the small intestine consists of the jejunum (the upper 40% below the duodenum) and the ileum (the lower 60%).

Anatomy

Figure 1.5.3 shows the general organisation of the intestinal wall. Four distinct strata can be identified: (1) mucosa; (2) submucosa; (3) muscularis propria; and (4) serosa. This general structural organisation is preserved throughout the gastrointestinal tract in the stomach and the large intestine, but the small intestine has some additional adaptations that greatly increase its surface area. To facilitate the surface digestion and absorption of nutrients, the small intestine is anatomically adapted to enhance greatly the epithelial digestive and absorptive surface, as illustrated in Figure 1.5.3. The small intestine has a surface area of approximately 200 m² due to folds of the mucosa, villi or finger-like projections of the mucosa, and the microvillar structure of the luminal or brush-border membrane of the absorptive cells that make up the surface layer of the villi. Altogether, these adaptations of mucosal structure increase the surface area of the small intestine to 600 times the surface area of a cylinder of the same diameter.

Digestion

Digestion in the small intestine is brought about by enzymes secreted by the pancreas, by enzymes

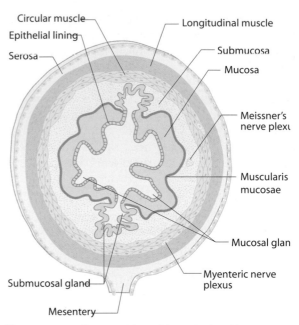

Figure 1.5.3   Cross-section of intestinal wall. (Redrawn from Guyton AC, Hall JE. Human physiology and mechanisms of disease, 6th edn. Philadelphia, PA: WB Saunders; 1997, with permission.[119])

located on the luminal membranes of the enterocytes lining the small intestine and by enzymes within the enterocytes. As the acidic chyme from the stomach enters the duodenum, the acid stimulates the enteroendocrine S cells (special endocrine cells in the duodenum) to release a gastrointestinal hormone called secretin, which stimulates the pancreatic acinar cells (cells involved in the secretion of water, electrolytes and enzymes) to secrete a bicarbonate-rich pancreatic secretion that has an alkaline pH of about 8. As expected, the highest densities of S cells are found in the duodenum and jejunum and the lowest densities are found in the ileum.

The presence of partially hydrolysed fat (fatty acids) and protein (amino acids and peptides) in the chyme that enters the duodenum, as well as the acidic pH of the chyme, stimulates enteroendocrine I cells in the small intestine to release the hormone cholecystokinin, which causes discharge of zymogen granules from the pancreatic acinar cells and the secretion of an enzyme/zymogen-rich pancreatic juice. The pancreatic secretion contains pancreatic α-amylase, lipases (pancreatic lipase and cholesterol esterase), pro-phospholipase A_2, nucleolytic enzymes (ribonuclease and deoxyribonuclease), several proenzymes for proteolytic enzymes (trypsinogen, chymotrypsinogen, proelastase and procarboxypeptidases), and a non-enzyme proprotein called procolipase. Pancreatic enzymes are most active in the neutral pH range, and the rapid neutralisation of the acid in the chyme by the bicarbonate in the pancreatic juice in the upper duodenum facilitates digestion of nutrients by pancreatic enzymes.

The liver secretes bile into the bile duct that empties into the duodenum. Bile is an alkaline solution containing electrolytes, pigments, bile salts and other substances. The pancreatic duct joins with the hepatic bile duct to form the common bile duct just prior to entering the duodenum, so the bile mixes with pancreatic secretions before they enter the duodenum. Bile salts play an important role in the normal digestion and absorption of lipids. Although the digestion of most nutrients in the small intestine is extensively carried out by enzymes secreted by the pancreas, enzymes located at the brush-border membrane of enterocytes are responsible for the completion of this process to release molecules that can be transported across the brush-border membrane.

Absorption in the gastrointestinal tract

For nutrients to be absorbed, they must move across the mucosal cells (enterocytes) that comprise a barrier between the lumen of the gastrointestinal tract and the interstitial fluid on the other side of the mucosal cell layer. Transport processes are involved in the uptake of nutrients by the brush-border or luminal membrane and also in the release of nutrients across the basolateral membrane into the extracellular fluid. The uptake of nutrients and electrolytes by the intestinal epithelial cells is usually mediated by one of four general mechanisms.

The first mechanism is mediated transport. Many compounds require a specific carrier or membrane transport protein for uptake. These carriers are located in the cell membrane. Mediated transport systems may be passive or active. Passive transport by a carrier is also called facilitated diffusion, because passive transport, like diffusion, is down the electrochemical gradient from an area of high concentration to an area of low concentration. Active mediated transport involves energy expenditure. Energy is supplied via adenosine triphosphate (ATP) hydrolysis, but the energy requirement may be primary or secondary. For example, sodium (Na^+) and potassium (K^+) concentrations in cells are maintained by Na^+,K^+-ATPase, which pumps Na^+ out of cells and K^+ into cells (against their concentration gradients) at the expense of ATP hydrolysis; this is primary active transport of Na^+ and K^+.

A second mechanism for the uptake of nutrients and electrolytes by the small intestinal epithelial cells is passive diffusion. This is especially true for water, many lipid-soluble molecules such as short-chain fatty acids, and for gases such as H_2 or CO_2 because they can diffuse through the lipid bilayer of the epithelial cell membranes. These substances diffuse across membranes in both directions, with net movement occurring down the concentration gradient. Uptake of substances by diffusion may also occur in the stomach and large intestine.

A third mechanism for uptake of some large molecules is pinocytosis. Receptor-mediated endocytosis may be responsible for uptake of some proteins as well as of any smaller molecules that are trapped within the endocytic vesicle. Similarly, molecules may be transported out of cells by exocytosis. Chylomicrons are exported from the enterocytes by exocytosis across the basolateral membrane.

The fourth mechanism for uptake of nutrients or of water and electrolytes by the small intestine is the paracellular pathway, which involves passage between cells through tight junctions. Osmolality plays an important role in the absorption of water and electrolytes by the small intestine via this process. The osmolality of the plasma is about 300 mosmol. When a hypotonic meal is ingested, water is rapidly absorbed by the duodenum and the jejunum paracellularly (between the cells) through the tight junctions. The tight junctions (pores between intestinal epithelial cells) of the duodenum and the jejunum have a larger diameter (0.8 nm) than those existing in the ileum (0.4 nm). The absorption of water facilitates the absorption of electrolytes by the small intestine (called solvent drag). When a hypertonic meal is ingested, water is drawn into the lumen. The accumulation of water in the lumen and the absorption of ions and nutrients by the small intestine bring the luminal contents to isotonicity. The proximal small intestine plays an important role in the absorption of water from a hypotonic meal, whereas the distal small intestine plays a more important role in the absorption of water and electrolytes following a hypertonic meal.

Pancreatic and biliary secretions enter the upper duodenum, and luminal digestion may occur throughout the duodenum and jejunum. Although the entire small intestine is capable of absorbing nutrients, the jejunum is by far the major site for the uptake of nutrients, and the absorption of most nutrients is complete before the chyme reaches the ileum. If nutrients are still present in the chyme that reaches the ileum, the physiological phenomenon called ileal brake may occur; this phenomenon refers to the observation that the presence of nutrients, especially long-chain fatty acids, in the ileum is a potent stimulus for slowing the emptying of chyme from the stomach as well as for reducing intestinal motility.

Bile acids and the enterohepatic circulation

The liver plays an important role in the digestion and uptake of lipids by the gastrointestinal tract because of its role in bile acid synthesis and secretion. Primary bile acids, cholic acid and chenodeoxycholic acid are synthesised from cholesterol in the liver. The liver also conjugates bile acids with either taurine or glycine to form more polar compounds. The ionisable sulfonate group of taurine or the ionisable carboxyl group of glycine has a lower pKa than the carboxyl group of the unconjugated bile acid, and conjugated bile acids exist as negatively charged sulfonate or carboxylate ions. The ratio of glycine to taurine conjugates in adult human bile is about 3:1. Because bile contains significant amounts of Na^+ and K^+ and has an alkaline pH, the bile acids and their conjugates exist in bile in a salt form and are called bile salts. The terms 'bile acid' and 'bile

salt' may be used interchangeably. The bile salts also solubilise some cholesterol in the bile and allow cholesterol to be transported from the liver to the intestine.

Conjugated bile acids exhibit detergent properties; at neutral pH values above their pKas (i.e. above pH 1.5–3.7) and at concentrations above 2–5 mmol/l, they reversibly form aggregates called micelles. Emulsification of dietary fat to increase the surface area between the lipid and aqueous phase, the digestion of cholesteryl esters, phospholipids and monoglycerides and the solubilisation and absorption of products of lipid digestion are facilitated by bile salts due to their ability to act as detergents and to form micelles.

Bile salts are recovered by the body via passive diffusion along the entire small intestine and via receptor-mediated transport in the lower ileum. The recirculation of compounds such as bile salts between the small intestine and the liver is called the enterohepatic circulation. The enterohepatic circulation of bile salts is extremely efficient, with only about 1% of the bile salts being lost via the faeces per pass through the intestine. The body pool of bile salts (about 4 g) is cycled through the intestine about 12 times per day (depending on the frequency of meal intake); a loss of 1% (0.05 g) per pass results in a loss of about 0.5 g of bile salts per day via the faeces. This loss is compensated for by daily synthesis of an equivalent amount of bile salts by the liver. Despite the synthesis of only about 0.5 g of bile salts/day by the liver, as much as 50 g of bile salts enter the small intestinal lumen each day to participate in the digestion and uptake of lipids. The loss of a small percentage of the bile salts in the faeces with each pass through the intestinal tract represents the major route for excretion of cholesterol from the body.

A portion of the primary bile acids in the intestine may be metabolised by intestinal bacteria, leading to deconjugation and 7α-dehydroxylation to produce secondary bile acids; deoxycholate is produced from cholate, and lithocholate is produced from chenodeoxycholate. These secondary bile acids, especially deoxycholate, may be reabsorbed and participate in the enterohepatic circulation along with the primary bile acids.

Metabolism of nutrients in the enterocytes

Following the uptake of digestion products into the small intestinal epithelial cells, nutrients are assimilated into either the portal blood or the lymphatic vessels for export to other parts of the body or they are used by the cells themselves. Because the small intestinal epithelial cells are metabolically very active and are continuously being renewed, nutrients supplied by the arterial circulation or taken up from the intestinal lumen are necessary to maintain the structural and functional integrity of the small intestinal mucosa.

Within the enterocytes, most of the products of fat digestion, particularly the monoacylglycerols and long-chain fatty acids, are re-esterified to form triacylglcyerols, incorporated into chylomicrons, and exported. Chylomicrons also transport cholesteryl esters, phospholipids and fat-soluble vitamins. Chylomicrons are too large to enter the pores of the capillaries, but they can pass through the large fenestrations of the lacteals and be transported by the lymphatic system. The lymphatic vessels ultimately empty into the venous circulation (by way of the thoracic duct) prior to the point where blood enters the heart.

Transport of nutrients in the circulation

Nutrients that are absorbed from the gastrointestinal tract are subsequently transported via the portal circulation or the lymphatic system. Most of the water-soluble nutrients (amino acids, monosaccharides, glycerol, short-chain fatty acids, electrolytes and water-soluble vitamins) are transported predominantly by the portal route. These nutrients enter the capillaries that feed into the portal vein, which carries the venous blood draining from the splanchnic bed to the liver. The liver is unusual in that its major blood supply is the venous portal blood, with the hepatic artery supplying only about one-quarter of the liver's blood flow. The lymphatic system in the gastrointestinal tract plays a pivotal role in the transport of lipophilic (lipid-soluble) substances. A substance transported by the lymphatic system will enter the blood just before it goes to the heart and will then circulate throughout the body in the arterial blood, whereas those substances transported in the portal blood will first pass through the liver, where they may be taken up and metabolised by the hepatocytes or returned to the venous circulation via the hepatic vein. This distinction between lymphatic versus portal transport is of great importance to the pharmaceutical industry for targeting the delivery of drugs. The lymphatic system also, of course, plays an important role in maintaining the fluid balance in the body by acting as a drainage system to return excess fluid and proteins from tissue space into the circulatory system. Although many of the molecules carried by the portal circulation can also be carried by the lymphatic circulation, the portal blood flow is many times higher than lymphatic flow, so transport by the lymphatic circulation is only of minor significance, compared with the portal circulation, for transport of most water-soluble compounds.

Regulation of digestion and absorption

The digestion and absorption of nutrients are both neurally and hormonally regulated – and this process is beyond the scope of this chapter. The regulation of digestive and absorptive processes involves a number of levels. In terms of the digestive process, regulation involves the modification of the rate of delivery of chyme to the small intestine for digestion, the release of gastric secretions, the release and composition of pancreatic secretions and the release of biliary secretions. The regulation of the absorptive process involves the absorptive surface area as well as the expression of certain transporter molecules located in the brush-border membrane.

The large intestine and the role of colonic bacteria

The residues from digestion and absorption in the small intestine pass through the ileocaecal valve into the large intestine. The colon or large intestine is larger in diameter than the small intestine; it has no villi but has colonic glands that secrete mucus. The large intestine serves two general functions: (1) the ascending colon is the location where most fermentation occurs; and (2) the descending colon provides for water and electrolyte absorption and stool formation. It takes about 4 h for the first part of a test meal to reach the upper large intestine, and all the undigested portion from a meal enters the large intestine within about 8 h of eating. In contrast, transport through the large intestine is much slower, and it may take more than a week to recover all residues from a given meal in the faeces. Carbohydrates that are not absorbed in the small intestine, as well as the carbohydrate components of mucus, are transformed into acetic, propionic and butyric acids by bacteria within the lumen of the colon.

A variety of bacteria in the colon produce hydrogen gas, methane and carbon dioxide through metabolism (fermentation) of unabsorbed polysaccharides and other food residues. Other bacteria consume gases produced by the bacterial gas producers. The degree of flatus passed is determined by the balance of bacterial gas production versus gas consumption.

Chapter **1.6**

Bioavailability of foods

Geraldine J Cuskelly and Ian S Young

The availability of vitamins from foods depends on two factors: (1) the quantity provided by a food; and (2) the amount absorbed and used by the body (the vitamins' bioavailability).[79] Nutrient quantity determination is relatively simple; researchers analyse foods to determine their vitamin contents and publish the results in tables of food composition. Determining the bioavailability of a vitamin is, however, a more complex task because it depends on many factors, including:

- efficiency of digestion and transit time through the gastrointestinal tract
- previous nutrient intake and nutrition status
- other foods consumed at the same time
- method of food preparation
- source of the nutrient (synthetic, fortified or naturally occurring).

Experts consider these factors when estimating recommended intakes.

In the context of toxicity, the bioavailability of an ingested nutrient can be defined as its accessibility to normal metabolic and physiologic processes. Bioavailability influences a nutrient's beneficial effects at physiological levels of intake and may also affect the nature and severity of toxicity due to excessive intakes. The concentration and chemical form of the nutrient, the nutrition and health of the individual, and excretory losses all affect bioavailability.

Certain B vitamins may be less rapidly absorbed when part of a meal than when taken separately. Supplemental forms of vitamins require special consideration if they have higher bioavailability and therefore may present a higher risk of producing adverse effects than does food. Folate is a very good example of a nutrient whose bioavailability has been researched extensively. In the following section, specific factors affecting bioavailability will be discussed in the context of folate nutrition.

FOLATE BIOAVAILABILITY

In pharmacokinetics, bioavailability is described as the ratio between the area under the curve derived from an oral dose, and, the area under the curve derived from an intravenous reference dose.[80] However, this definition may not be applicable with respect to nutrient bioavailability because it assumes that clearance is independent of the route of administration. This is not the case, for example, for folate.[81] As a result of the reduction and either methylation or formylation that take place in the jejunal mucosa during absorption, it is not possible to determine absolute bioavailability, but only bioavailability relative to the bioavailability of the fully oxidised monoglutamate (folic acid[82]).

The definitions of bioavailability, bioconversion and bioefficacy have developed over the years and reflect current thinking.[83] Bioefficacy is the proportion of the ingested nutrient converted to an active form of the nutrient; here the proportion of folate or folic acid converted to 5-methyltetrahydrofolate. Bioefficacy is a function of bioavailability and is often referred to as bioconversion.

However, these definitions do not include activity of ingested nutrients carrying out metabolic functions. Thus, we have introduced the term 'functional bioefficacy', which is the proportion of an ingested nutrient which carries out a certain metabolic function. Since plasma total homocysteine is a functional index of folate status, changes in plasma total homocysteine concentration in response to a given intake of folate or folic acid can be used as a measure of functional bioefficacy according to this definition. Changes in plasma folate or erythrocyte folate can be regarded as measurements of bioefficacy.

Factors influencing folate and folic acid bioavailability

de Pee & West[84] published a review on dietary carotenoids and their role in combating vitamin A deficiency. They introduced the mnemonic SLAMANGHF to order the factors influencing the bioavailability of carotenoids,[84] and the term was subsequently modified to SLAMENGHI.[85] The SLAMENGHI factors are not specific for carotenoid bioavailability, but can also be applied to the bioavailability and bioefficacy of other nutrients. The factors influencing bioavailability and bioefficacy of folate, with reference to SLAMENGHI, are *s*pecies of folate; *l*inkage at molecular level; *a*mount of folate and folic acid consumed; *m*atrix; *e*ffect modifiers; *n*utrient status; *g*enetic factors; *h*ost-related factors; and mathematical *i*nteractions between the various factors.

Species of folate

The bioefficacy of oxidised and reduced folates with or without various 1-carbon units has been investigated in a series of intervention studies with human subjects. Findings from these studies are not consistent. Perry and Chanarin[86] found a greater increase in serum folate levels after ingestion of reduced folates than after ingestion of folic acid. However, urinary excretion of folic acid was higher than that of the other monoglutamyl forms of folate. Brown et al.[87] found that the bioefficacy of other monoglutamate forms was greater than that of folic acid, except that the bioefficacy of 5-formyltetrahydrofolate was similar and that of tetrahydrofolate was less. On the basis of a study using urinary excretion of orally administered labelled folates compared with intravenously administered folic acid labelled with $^2H_4$, Gregory et al.[81] concluded that folic acid was more bioavailable than the reduced forms of the vitamin. Other studies have found no differences in bioefficacy between folic acid and the reduced forms.[88–90]

One problem with most studies investigating folate or other nutrient bioefficacy is that the variation in response between subjects can be quite substantial. Another problem is that it is not possible to determine whether these differences are caused by differences in absorption (bioavailability) or in postabsorption processes (bioconversion). In all studies, except that of Pietrzik and Remer,[89] subjects received one or more doses of folic acid for periods up to 7 days in order to presaturate the tissues with folic acid. There are no studies published investigating the effect of different species of folate on plasma total homocysteine concentrations, i.e. on functional bioefficacy.

Linkage at molecular level

Folate not only occurs as different species as discussed earlier, but also with more than one glutamate moiety (Figure 1.6.1). This section focuses on the bioefficacy of folate with different numbers (one to seven) of glutamate moieties in the side chain. Pteroylpolyglutamates are the major forms of folate in foods, and first have to be hydrolysed to monoglutamates before absorption in the small intestine can take place. A conjugase present in the jejunum is responsible for removing glutamate moieties from pteroylpolyglutamates.[91] Under normal circumstances, the activity of this folate conjugase enzyme is not rate-limiting in the absorption process.[92] Numerous studies have demonstrated this.[88,93-95] However, a well-designed study using labelled folates suggested that the bioavailability of hexaglutamate is less than that

of the monoglutamate.[96] Although the results of the studies are not unequivocal, absorption of the polyglutamates is often found to be less than that of the monoglutamate. This may imply that bioavailability of polyglutamates is less than that of monoglutamates. However, it cannot be excluded that uptake of polyglutamates takes longer, and that the net effect in the long term is similar to that of monoglutamates.

Amount of folate and folic acid consumed

Bioavailability of folate or folic acid is likely to be influenced by the amount ingested. For absorption, there are two different transport systems. In the first transport system folates are bound to membrane-associated folate-binding proteins and transported across the brush-border membrane by a carrier-mediated mechanism. However, at higher intraluminal concentrations of folate ($> 10 \, \mu mol/l$), a second non-saturable diffusion-mediated transport system plays a major role in folate absorption.[63] The effect of the amount ingested is most likely to be of significance if the saturable transport system is saturated. At physiological concentrations ($< 5 \, \mu mol/l$) of folate in the lumen, transport occurs mainly via the saturable transport system.[63] A level of intake that causes saturation of this transport system is

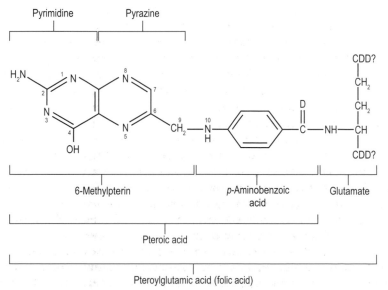

Figure 1.6.1   Structure of folic acid.

unlikely to be reached with normal intakes of natural folate from food, but could easily be reached with synthetic folic acid (from supplements or fortified food).

Matrix effects

Matrix effects on bioavailability involve both encapsulation and binding. Natural food folate can be encapsulated in plant cells or subcellular components. Generally, for folic acid added to food, binding is more important, although in food preparation encapsulation may occur. Comparison of folate bioefficacy among different foods involves not only matrix effects, but also effects of molecular linkage, species and effect modifiers. However, studies comparing folate bioefficacy among foods cannot distinguish these factors.

Effect modifiers

Effect modifiers are components in foods that influence nutrient bioavailability and bioefficacy. Adequate Zn status is known to be important for folate bioefficacy. Tamura et al.[97] showed that Zn depletion reduced the increase in serum folate concentration after supplementation with pteroylheptaglutamate by 53%, while absorption of the monoglutamate form seemed to be unaffected.[97] This finding suggested that intestinal pteroylpolyglutamate hydrolase is Zn-dependent and that Zn depletion inhibits hydrolysis of polyglutamates. Chandler et al.[98] confirmed the Zn dependency of the brush-border folate hydrolase. Tamura[99] reviewed the literature concerning the nutrient interaction of folate and Zn and concluded that, although folate conjugase is Zn-dependent, its clinical significance is not clear. Supplementation with 3.5 or 14.5 mg Zn per day in combination with folic acid for 25 days was shown to have no effect on the concentration of folate in serum, erythrocytes and urine. This finding suggests that absorption of folic acid is not influenced by Zn intake.[100] However, there are no studies investigating the effect of Zn supplementation on the bioefficacy of dietary folate.

Certain components in food may have the ability to inhibit the activity of the folate conjugase enzyme and thereby decrease the bioavailability of pteroylpolyglutamate. Tomatoes and orange juice inhibit pteroylglutamate hydrolase (folate conjugase) activity in the human intestine.[101] Furthermore, citrate, and to a lesser extent malate and formate, have been shown to affect intestinal brush-border conjugase activity in vitro.[102] This finding suggests that organic acids affect the absorption of dietary polyglutamate folate by interfering with the intestinal deconjugation of the glutamate chain.

Alcohol could be another effect modifier. Folate deficiency is prevalent among chronic alcoholic patients whose dietary intake of minerals and vitamins is often inadequate. However, alcohol may also affect folate absorption.[103]

Nutrient status

Status of the host with respect to folate, vitamin B_{12} and Zn may influence folate bioefficacy. Only a few studies have investigated the effect of folate status on folate bioavailability. Babu and Lakshmaiah[104] showed no effect of folate deficiency on jejunal conjugase activity in rats. To our knowledge, there are no studies comparing folate bioefficacy in folate-deplete and folate-replete subjects. However, the study by Bower et al.[105] showed that the increase in serum folate concentration after a pteroylpolyglutamate load (4.5 mg pteroylheptaglutamate) was higher in subjects with higher serum folate levels compared with subjects with lower baseline serum folate levels. This finding could be explained by a longer circulation time of folate in serum of replete subjects, implying that in depleted subjects' folate is rapidly transferred from serum to tissues.[105]

Genetic factors

Some genetic mutations are known to influence folate metabolism. In mice expression of the reduced folate carrier *RFC-1* gene regulates the pH-dependent folate absorption in the small intestine.[106] The organisation and structure of the human *RFC-1* gene encoding for a folate transporter have also been determined.[107] However, the significance of this gene for folate absorption needs further investigation.

Another gene that is linked to folate status is the gene encoding for methylenetetrahydrofolate reductase (MTHFR). A variant of the gene encoding for MTHFR was found to have lower specific activity and higher sensitivity to heat.[108] This thermolabile variant is caused by an alanine-to-valine missense mutation.[109] Jacques et al.[110] demonstrated that individuals homozygous for this mutation with plasma folate concentrations < 15.4 nmol/l had 24% higher fasting plasma total homocysteine concentrations than individuals with the normal genotype and similar plasma folate concentrations. No difference between genotypes was seen among individuals with plasma folate concentrations >15.4 nmol/l. They suggested that individuals homozygous for this polymorphism need more folate to regulate their plasma homocysteine concentrations.[110] This observation implies that the functional bioefficacy of folate is diminished by this polymorphism when folate status is not optimal. However, high intakes of folate or of folic acid would seem to be able to overcome the negative effects of the polymorphism.

Host–related factors

Host-related factors are factors of the host other than nutrient status and genetic factors that could influence bioavailability or bioefficacy. Examples of such factors are age, pregnancy, illness and malabsorption.

Bailey et al.[111] investigated the absorption of pteroylpolyglutamates and pteroylmonoglutamates in different age groups. They found that neither absorption nor activity of folate conjugase was affected by age. Pregnancy increases the demand for folate. This higher demand may be explained by accelerated folate breakdown.[112,113] However, Caudill et al.[114] found no differences between pregnant and non-pregnant women with respect to increase in serum folate or erythrocyte folate concentrations or in urinary excretion of 5-methyltetrahydrofolate after supplementation with 450 and 850 µg folate/day. Although the same research group suggested, from results of a controlled dietary trial, that pregnant women made more efficient use of 450 µg folic acid than of 850 µg folic acid, they found no significant difference in catabolism between pregnant and non-pregnant women.[115] Thus, it is not clear what causes the higher demand for folate during pregnancy.

Halsted[116] summarised studies from his group investigating the effect of gastrointestinal diseases on the absorption of ^{3}H-labelled folate and ^{14}C-labelled pteroylheptaglutamate. Absorption of folate and pteroylheptaglutamate was not affected by ulcerative colitis, but was diminished by tropical and coeliac sprue.

MATHEMATICAL INTERACTIONS

Mathematical interactions arise when the combined effect of two or more factors is different from that of the sum of separate effects of the factors. To our knowledge there are no reports in which this complicated problem has been addressed.

Chapter **1.7**

Measures of nutritional status

Geraldine J Cuskelly and Ian S Young

ANTHROPOMETRIC

Anthropometric indicators are basic measurements of the human body. By relating these to standards typical of the test population, any deviations indicate abnormal nutritional status. Measurements commonly used are height and weight; these can be used to calculate body mass index (BMI) (Table 1.7.1).

In children, height and weight results can be compared with standard growth curves, which indicate the rate of physical development of a child, particularly when a sequence of measurements is made. In addition, head and chest circumference measures can also be useful in children to indicate rates of growth of the brain and body.

Skinfold thickness measurements at mid-triceps, mid-biceps, subscapular and suprailiac sites using Harpenden (Figure 1.7.1A) or similar callipers give a surprisingly accurate value for body fat, when used by a skilled person. Figure 1.7.1B shows the triceps site for skinfold measurement.

Arm muscle circumference can be calculated by subtracting the thickness of the fat fold from a mid-arm circumference measurement (Figure 1.7.1B). This can indicate muscle development or wasting, and can be a useful indicator in clinical situations of change in muscle mass, for example during illness and rehabilitation.

Waist-to-hip ratio is increasingly used as an indicator of body fat distribution. The circumference of the waist at the umbilicus and of the

Table 1.7.1 Categories of body fatness based on body mass index (BMI)

BMI range	Description of category
<18.5	Underweight
18.5–24.9	Normal
>25	Overweight
25.0–29.9	Pre-obese
30.0–34.9	Obese class I
35.0–39.9	Obese class II
>40.0	Obese class III

Data from WHO (1998). Obesity: preventing and managing the global epidemic. WHO, Geneva.[117]

hips around the fattest part of the buttocks are used to calculate this ratio. A nomogram may be used, or a simple calculation performed to obtain the ratio. Values above 0.8 in women and 0.9 in men are indicative of a tendency for central fat deposition, and a possible increased health risk. Waist measurements alone have been shown to correlate well with body fatness, and may be used in future as a quick indicator of risk from over-weight. Other ratios, such as waist to height, have also been suggested to be equally useful, as they tend to be unisex and therefore a single figure can be used as a cut-off point.

Demispan is a measurement of skeletal size, which can be used as an alternative to height measurement where it is difficult to obtain an upright posture in a subject. Demispan is the distance

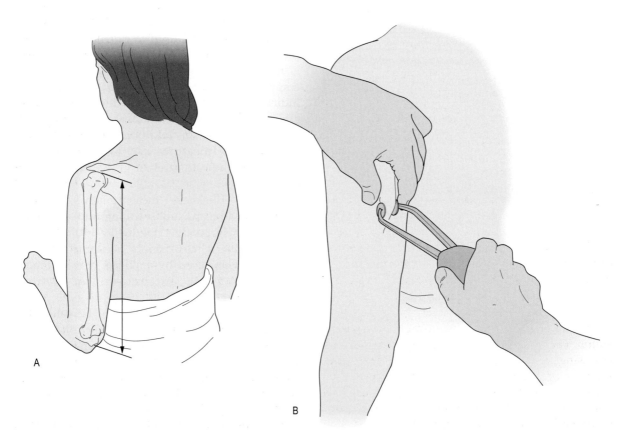

A

B

Figure 1.7.1 A&B Skinfold measurements. (Reproduced from Garrow JS. Composition of the body. In: Human nutrition and dietetics. London: Churchill Livingstone; 2000, with permission.[120])

between the sternal notch and the roots of the middle and third fingers with the arm stretched out at shoulder-height to the side of the body. It is particularly useful in elderly people, in whom height may have been lost due to vertebral collapse. The demispan value can then be used in place of 'height' in calculating BMI, substituting (demispan value)^2 in men and (demispan value) in women.

BIOCHEMICAL INDICATORS

Measurement of relevant individual analytes in body tissues, fluids or excretions – faeces, urine, sweat or expired air – provides specific, sensitive and quantitative indices of a subject's nutritional status. Such measurements are often of value in supporting, modifying or negating nutritional history and physical examination. Impaired absorption of dietary nutrients from the gut or renal tubule is a major cause of malnutrition and may be due to any one of a number of factors. To the complexity of causes of malnutrition is added the number of nutrients that may be involved singly or in combination, endpoints that result from byproducts of intestinal tract activity and/or digestive and absorptive defects, and finally the varied methodological and technical issues of analyses.

THE MATRIX TO BE ANALYSED

In assessing nutritional status, measurement of an analyte or a metabolite of a substrate is usually made in blood – whole blood, serum, plasma or erythrocytes, depending upon its normal distribution – or in urine, but other sources are often valuable. Leukocyte fractions isolated from whole blood and platelets isolated from plasma have been analysed for various nutrients to assess status. Faecal analysis is extremely important in assessing the balance of a non-metabolisable nutrient or a component, for example, nitrogen, trace metals that are excreted in bile, and components of pancreatic secretions in protein-losing enteropathy and α-antitrypsin clearance. Urine samples may be used to monitor the baseline excretion of a water-soluble nutrient, or to follow its excretion after a loading dose. Metabolites of nutrients also appear in the urine, and their levels can be monitored. Twenty-four hour urine collections can be assayed for creatinine to indicate muscle turnover rates, or for nitrogen count to check protein intakes. Analysis of expired air for a radioactively labelled metabolite – usually CO_2 or H_2 generated by bacterial action in the gut – or a stable isotope ratio (e.g. $^{13}CO_2$:$^{14}CO_2$) enables the absorption of carbohydrates or fat to be determined. Labelled expired air is also analysed for O_2 or CO_2 by indirect or direct calorimetry and more recently by isotope dilution methods using $^2H_2^{18}O$ to determine resting energy expenditure.

Analysis of bone includes bone marrow biopsies which will show the blood-forming cells, and radiographic examination, which can detect stages of bone development or rarefaction in ageing. Bone densitometry can provide an essential measure of the density of the skeleton. It is also possible to measure the levels of some trace elements in the hair, although the scientific accuracy of these assays is not proven, and therefore they should not be relied upon.

While depletion of a nutrient is often detected by its low concentrations, depletion may be indicated by increased concentration of a related metabolite occurring because of altered intermediary metabolism, for example, high homocysteine levels in the absence of the folate or vitamin B_{12} coenzyme required for its conversion to methionine.

An alternative to measuring the concentration of a specific mineral, trace element or vitamin in blood or urine uses a test that indicates the function of a related component in the body; for example, enzymatic activities in erythrocytes for which thiamin pyrophosphate, pyridoxal-5-phosphate, or flavin adenine dinucleotide (FAD) are the coenzymes of the vitamins thiamin, pyridoxine and riboflavin, respectively. If the cofactor raises the respective in vitro enzyme activity more than 20% above its initial value, a deficiency of the vitamin in vivo is indicated.

In summary, biochemical indicators can include assessment of blood and urine samples for a variety of nutrients and/or their byproducts or for levels of nutrient-linked enzyme activities. In addition, analysis can be performed on samples of hair or bone marrow.

Blood (plasma, cells, or serum) can provide a great deal of information. Analysis can be used to determine:

- actual levels of a nutrient in relation to expected levels (e.g. vitamin B_{12}, folate, carotenes, vitamin C in white blood cells)
- the activity of a nutrient-dependent enzyme (e.g. transketolase for thiamin)
- the activity of a nutrient-related enzyme (e.g. alkaline phosphatase for vitamin D)
- the rate of a nutrient-dependent reaction (e.g. clotting time for vitamin K)
- the presence of a nutrient carrier or its saturation level (e.g. retinal-binding protein, transferrin (iron))
- levels of nutrient-related products (e.g. lipoprotein levels).

CLINICAL INDICATORS

Clinical indicators are used to detect changes in the external appearance of the body. A number of nutritional deficiencies may cause alterations in superficial structures, although many are non-specific. In addition, changes in appearance may also be unrelated to nutritional state. Signs occur most rapidly in those parts of the body where cell turnover is frequent, such as hair, skin and digestive tract (including mouth and tongue). Therefore, a clinical examination may include the hair, face, eye, mouth, tongue, teeth, gums, glands (such as the thyroid), skin and nails, subcutaneous tissues (to detect fat thickness, oedema) and the musculoskeletal system (to note bone deformities, ability to walk, muscle-wasting). Some internal organs, like the liver, may be felt to denote any enlargement. Reflex tests may be performed to test nerve pathways and muscle function. A trained observer will be able to detect many changes in appearance; generally these are followed up with more specific tests of nutritional status.

References to Section 1

1. Baresi ME. Human nutrition: a health perspective. London: Arnold; 1997.
2. Barbosa-Canovas GV, Rodriguez JJ. Update on non-thermal food processing technologies: pulsed electric field, high hydrostatic pressure, irradiation and ultrasound. Food Aust 2002; 54:513–520.
3. British Nutrition Foundation (BNF). Vegetarianism. London: British Nutrition Foundation; 1995.
4. Department of Health. Report on health and social subjects 46. Nutritional aspects of cardiovascular disease. Committee on Medical Aspects of Food Policy. London; HMSO; 1994.
5. Department of Health. Report on health and social subjects 48. Nutritional aspects of the development of cancer. Committee on Medical Aspects of Food Policy. London; HMSO; 1998.
6. Garrow JS. Obesity. In: Human nutrition and dietetics. London: Churchill Livingstone; 2000.
7. Schoeller DA, Vansanten E. Measurement of energy-expenditure in humans by doubly labeled water method. J Appl Physiol 1982; 53:955–959.
8. Department of Health. Report on health and social subjects 41. Dietary reference values for food energy and nutrients for the United Kingdom. Committee on Medical Aspects of Food Policy. London: HMSO; 1991.
9. Eichholzer M, Luthy J, Gutzwiller F, Stahelin HB. The role of folate, antioxidant vitamins and other constituents in fruit and vegetables in the prevention of cardiovascular disease: the epidemiological evidence. Int J Vitamin Nutr Res 2001; 71:5–17.
10. Van Straten M, Josling P. Preventing the common cold with a vitamin C supplement: a double-blind, placebo-controlled survey. Adv Ther 2002; 19:151–159.
11. Southgate DAT. Food composition tables and nutritional databases. In: Human nutrition and dietetics. London: Churchill Livingstone; 2000.
12. Wild CP, Andersson C, O'Brien NM et al. A critical evaluation of the application of biomarkers in epidemiological studies on diet and health. Br J Nutr 2001; 86 (Suppl. 1):S37–S53.
13. Department of Health and Social Security. Reports on health and social subjects 15. Recommended daily amounts of food energy and nutrients for groups of people in the United Kingdom. London: HMSO; 1979.
14. FAO/WHO/UNU. Report of a joint FAO/WHO/UNU expert consultation. Technical report series 724. Energy and protein requirements. Geneva: World Health Organization (WHO); 1985.
15. National Research Council, Food and Nutrition Board, Commission on Life Sciences. Recommended dietary allowances, 10th edn. Washington, DC: National Academy Press; 1989.
16. Institute of Medicine (USA). Dietary reference in-takes. Calcium, phosphorus, magnesium, vitamin D and fluoride. National Academy Press, Washington, DC; 1997.
17. Food and Nutrition Board – Institute of Medicine. Dietary reference intakes for calcium, phosphorus, magnesium, vitamin D, and fluoride. Washington, DC: National Academy Press; 1997.
18. Food and Nutrition Board – Institute of Medicine. Dietary reference intakes for thiamin, riboflavin, niacin, vitamin B_6, folate, vitamin B_{12}, pantothenic acid, biotin, and choline. Washington, DC: National Academy Press; 1998.
19. Food and Nutrition Board – Institute of Medicine. Dietary reference intakes for vitamin C, vitamin E, selenium, and carotenoids. Washington, DC: National Academy Press; 2000.
20. Food and Nutrition Board – Institute of Medicine. Dietary reference intakes for vitamin A, vitamin K, arsenic, boron, chromium, copper, iodine, iron, manganese, molybdenum, nickel, silicon, vanadium, and zinc. Washington, DC: National Academy Press; 2001.
21. Food and Nutrition Board – Institute of Medicine. Dietary reference intakes for energy, carbohydrate, fiber, fat, fatty acids, cholesterol, protein, and amino acids. Washington, DC: National Academy Press; 2002.

22. Food and Nutrition Board – Institute of Medicine. Dietary reference intakes for electrolytes and water. Washington, DC: National Academy Press; 2004.

23. Food and Nutrition Board – National Research Council. Recommended dietary allowances, 10th edn. Washington, DC: National Academy Press; 1989.

24. EC Scientific Committee for Food Report. Nutrient and energy intakes for the European Community, 31st series. Luxembourg; Directorate-General, Industry; 1993.

25. James WPT. Healthy nutrition. Preventing nutrition-related diseases in Europe. WHO regional publications, European series no 24. Copenhagen: WHO; 1988.

26. WHO. Handbook on human nutritional requirements. Monograph series no 61. Geneva: WHO; 1974.

27. WHO. Diet, nutrition, and the prevention of chronic diseases. Technical report series 797. Geneva: WHO; 1990.

28. WHO. Trace elements in human nutrition and health. Geneva: WHO, in collaboration with FAO, AEA; 1996.

29. WHO/FAO. α-Tocopherol. In: Toxicological evaluation of certain food additives and contaminants. WHO food additives series 21. Cambridge: WHO/FAO; 1987:55–69.

30. FAO/WHO. Report of a joint FAO/WHO expert consultation. Requirements for vitamin A, iron, folate and vitamin B_{12}. Food and nutrition series. Rome: Food and Agriculture Organization (FAO); 1988.

31. Oltersdorf U, Schlettwein-Gsell D, Winkler G. Assessing eating patterns – an emerging research topic in nutritional sciences: Introduction to the symposium. Appetite 1999; 32:1–7.

32. Blundell JE, Halford JCG. Regulation of nutrient supply – the brain and appetite control. Proc Nutr Soc 1994; 53:407–418.

33. Godwin SL, Chambers E, Cleveland L. Accuracy of reporting dietary intake using various portion-size aids in-person and via telephone. J Am Diet Assoc 2004; 104:585–594.

34. Nelson M, Atkinson M, Meyer J. Food portion sizes: a photographic atlas. London: MAFF; 1997.

35. Sackett DL, Rosenberg WMC, Gray JAM et al. Evidence based medicine: what it is and what it isn't – it's about integrating individual clinical expertise and the best external evidence. Br Med J 1996; 312:71–72.

36. Dickersin K, Berlin JA. Meta-analysis – state-of-the-science. Epidemiol Rev 1992; 14:154–176.

37. Cannon G. Food and health: the experts agree. An analysis of 100 authoritative scientific reports on food, nutrition and public health published throughout the world in 30 years, between 1961 and 1991. London: Consumers' Association; 1992.

38. World Health Organization and Food and Agriculture Organization of the United Nations. Preparation and use of food-based dietary guidelines. Report of a joint FAO/WHO consultation, Nicosia, Cyprus. WHO/Nut/96.6. Geneva: WHO Nutrition Programme; 1996.

39. James WPT, Ferro-Luzzi A, Isaksson B et al. Healthy nutrition. Preventing nutrition-related diseases in Europe. Copenhagen: WHO Regional Office for Europe; 1988.

40. Surgeon General's Report on Nutrition and Health. US Department of Health and Human Services publ. PHS 88-50210. Washington, DC: US Government Printing Office; 1988.

41. World Health Organization Nutrition Programme. Highlights from the second WHO symposium on health issues for the 21st century: nutrition and quality of life (November 1993, Kobe, Japan). Geneva: WHO; 1994.

42. New Zealand Department of Health. Food and nutrition guidelines for infants and toddlers. Wellington, New Zealand: Department of Health; 1994.

43. Reid J, George J, Pears R. Food and nutrition guidelines for children aged 2 to 12 years. Wellington, New Zealand: Department of Health; 1992.

44. Public Health Commission. Food and nutrition guidelines for New Zealand adolescents. Wellington, New Zealand: Public Health Commission; 1993.

45. Report of the Nutrition Taskforce. Food for health. Wellington, New Zealand: Department of Health; 1991.

46. New Zealand Public Health Commission. Guidelines for healthy pregnant women. A background paper. Wellington, New Zealand: PHC; 1995.

47. New Zealand Ministry of Health. Guidelines for healthy older people. A background paper, 2nd edn. Wellington, New Zealand: Ministry of Health; 1996.

48. National Health Medical Research Council. Dietary guidelines for Australians, 2nd edn. Canberra: Australian Government Publishing Service; 1992.

49. National Health and Medical Research Council. Dietary guidelines for children and adolescents. Canberra: Australian Government Publishing Service; 1995.

50. Joint working group of the Canadian Paediatric Society and Health Canada. Nutr Rev 1995; 53:367–375.

51. Select Committee on Human Needs, US Senate. Dietary goals for the United States. Washington, DC: US Government Printing Office; 1977.

52. US Department of Agriculture and US Department of Health and Human Services. Dietary guidelines for Americans, 4th edn. Home and garden bulletin no. 232. Washington, DC: US Government Publishing Office; 1995.

53. Langsford WA. Food and nutrition notes and reviews (Australian Commonwealth Department of Health) 1979; 36:100–103.

54. Commonwealth Department of Health. Dietary guidelines for Australians. Canberra: Australian Government Publishing Service; 1982.

55. Helsing E (rapporteur). Nutrition targets in the EEC. In: Important components for a food and nutrition policy in the EEC (Corfu, Greece, 6–8 October 1988). Report of a workshop. Athens: School of Public Health, Department of Nutrition and Biochemistry; 1988:15.

56. Bloch AS, Shils ME. Appendix contents (Appendix Table II-A-9). In: Modern nutrition in health and disease, 9th edn. Baltimore, Maryland: Williams & Wilkins; 1999.

57. Robbins C. Implementing the NACNE report. 1. National dietary goals – a confused debate. Lancet 1983; 2:1351–1353.

58. Walker C, Cannon G. The food scandal. London: Century Publishing; 1984.

59. Passmore R. Food propagandists – the new puritans. J R Coll Gen Pract 1985; 35:387–389.

60. Anderson D. (ed.) A diet of reason. London: The Social Affairs Unit Board, National Research Council Symposium. Washington, DC: National Academy Press; 1986:126–140.

61. Ministry of Agriculture, Fisheries and Food. Eight guidelines for a healthy diet. Advice for healthy eating from HM government. London: Food Sense; 1990.

62. Leitzmann C. Ten guidelines for sensible nutrition. Frankfurt am Main: Deutsche Gesellschaft fur Ernahrung; 1985.

63. Mason JB. Intestinal transport of monoglutamyl folates in mammalian systems. In: Picciano MF, Stokstad ELR, Gregory JF III, eds. Folic acid metabolism in health and disease. New York: Wiley-Liss; 1990:47–64.

64. Truswell AS. Protective plant foods: new opportunities for health and nutrition. Food Aust 1997; 49:40–43.

65. Feinman L, Lieber CS. Nutrition and diet in alcoholism. In: Modern nutrition in health and disease, 9th edn. Baltimore, Maryland: Williams & Wilkins; 1999.

66. Scragg R. A quantification of alcohol-related mortality in New Zealand. Aust NZ J Med 1995; 25:5–11.

67. Chinese Nutrition Society. Dietary guidelines and the food pagoda. J Am Diet Assoc 2000; 100:886–887.

68. Painter J, Rah JH, Lee YK. Comparison of international food guide pictorial representations. J Am Diet Assoc 2002; 102:483–489.

69. Minister of Public Works (MPW) and Government Services Canada. Canada's guide to healthy eating. H39-252/1992E. Ottawa, Ontario: Health Canada; 1997.

70. Commonwealth Department of Health. Australian guide to healthy eating. Canberra, Australia: Commonwealth Department of Health and Aged Care; 1998.

71. Health Education Authority. The balance of good health. UK: HEA; 1994.

72. Korean Nutrition Society. Recommended dietary allowances for Koreans, 7th edn. Seoul, Korea: Jung-Ang; 2000.

73. GraAa P. Dietary guidelines and food nutrient intakes in Portugal. Br J Nutr 1999; 81 (Suppl. 2):S99–S103.

74. Orbeta SS. The Filipino pyramid food guide. Nutr Today 1998; 33:210–216.

75. Macpherson-Sanchez AE. A food guide pyramid for Puerto Rico. Nutr Today 1998; 33:198–209.

76. Gatenby SJ, Hunt P, Rayner M. The national food guide: development of dietetic criteria and nutritional characteristics. J Hum Nutr Diet 1995; 8:323–334.

77. Abrams CK, Hamosh M, Lee TC et al. Gastric lipase – localization in the human stomach. Gastroenterology 1988; 95:1460–1464.

78. Moreau H, Laugier R, Gargouri Y et al. Human preduodenal lipase is entirely of gastric fundic origin. Gastroenterology 1988; 95:1221–1226.

79. Sauberlich HE. Bioavailability of vitamins. Progr Food Nutr Sci 1985; 9:1–33.

80. Rowland M, Tozer TN. Clinical pharmacokinetics: concepts and applications. Philadelphia, PA: Lea & Febiger; 1989.

81. Gregory JF, Bhandari SD, Bailey LB et al. Relative bioavailability of deuterium-labeled monoglutamyl tetrahydrofolates and folic acid in human subjects. Am J Clin Nutr 1992; 55:1147–1153.

82. Rogers LM, Pfeiffer CM, Bailey LB, Gregory JF. A dual-label stable-isotopic protocol is suitable for determination of folate bioavailability in humans: evaluation of urinary excretion and plasma folate kinetics of intravenous and oral doses of $[^{13}C_5]$ and $[^2H_2]$folic acid. J Nutr 1997; 127:2321–2327.

83. van Lieshout M, West CE, Muhilal PD et al. Bioefficacy of beta-carotene dissolved in oil studied in children in Indonesia. Am J Clin Nutr 2001; 73:949–958.

84. dePee S, West CE. Dietary carotenoids and their role in combating vitamin A deficiency: a review of the literature. Eur J Clin Nutr 1996; 50:S38–S53.

85. Castenmiller JJM, West CE. Bioavailability and bioconversion of carotenoids. Annu Rev Nutr 1998; 18:19–38.

86. Perry J, Chanarin I. Intestinal absorption of reduced folate compounds in man. Br J Haematol 1970; 18:329–339.

87. Brown JP, Scott JM, Foster FG, Weir DG. Ingestion and absorption of naturally occurring pteroylmonoglutamates (folates) in man. Gastroenterology 1973; 64:223–232.

88. Tamura T, Stokstad ELR. The availability of food folate in man. Br J Haematol 1973; 25:513–532.

89. Pietrzik K, Remer T. Zur Bioverfugbarkeitsprufung von Mikronahrstoffen (Bioavailability study of micro-nutrients). ZeitschriftfiirErnahrungswissenschaft 1989; 15:130–141.

90. Bhandari SD, Gregory JF. Folic-acid, 5-methyl-tetrahydrofolate and 5-formyl-tetrahydrofolate exhibit equivalent intestinal-absorption, metabolism and in vivo kinetics in rats. J Nutr 1992; 122:1847–1854.

91. Reisenauer AM, Krumdieck CL, Halsted CH. Folate conjugase: two separate activities in human jejunum. Science 1977; 198:196–197.

92. Reisenauer A, Halsted C. Human folate requirements. J Nutr 1987; 117:600–602.

93. Rosenberg IH, Godwin HA. The digestion and absorption of dietary folate. Gastroenterology 1971; 60:445–463.

94. Godwin HA, Rosenberg IH. Comparative studies of the intestinal absorption of $[^3H]$pteroylmonoglutamate and $[^3H]$pteroylheptaglutamate in man. Gastroenterology 1975; 69:364–373.

95. Bailey LB, Barton LE, Hillier SE, Cerda JJ. Bioavailability of mono and polyglutamyl folate in human subjects. Nutr Rep Int 1988; 38:509–518.

96. Gregory JF, Bhandari SD, Bailey LB et al. Relative bioavailability of deuterium-labeled monoglutamyl and hexaglutamyl folates in human subjects. Am J Clin Nutr 1991; 53:736–740.

97. Tamura T, Shane B, Baer MT et al. Absorption of mono- and polyglutamyl folates in zinc-depleted man. Am J Clin Nutr 1978; 31:1984–1987.

98. Chandler CJ, Wang TTY, Halsted CH. Pteroylpolyglutamate hydrolase from human jejunal brush-borders – purification and characterization. J Biol Chem 1986; 261:928–933.

99. Tamura T. Nutrient interaction of folate and zinc. In: Bailey LB, ed. Folate in health and disease. New York: Marcel Dekker; 1995:287–312.

100. Kauwell GPA, Bailey LB, Gregory JF et al. Zinc status is not adversely affected by folic acid supplementation and zinc does not impair folate utilization in human subjects. J Nutr 1995; 125:66–72.

101. Bhandari SD, Gregory JF. Inhibition by selected food components of human and porcine intestinal pteroyl-polyglutamate hydrolase activity. Am J Clin Nutr 1990; 51:87–94.

102. Wei MM, Gregory JF. Organic acids in selected foods inhibit intestinal brush border pteroylpolyglutamate hydrolase in vitro: potential mechanism affecting the bioavailability of dietary polyglutamyl folate. J Agric Food Chem 1998; 46:211–219.

103. Halsted CH. Alcohol and folate interactions: clinical implications. In: Bailey LB, ed. Folate in health and disease. New York: Marcel Dekker; 1995.

104. Babu S, Lakshmaiah N. Availability of food folate by liver folate repletion in rats. Nutr Rep Int 1987; 35:831–836.

105. Bower C, Stanley FJ, Croft M et al. Absorption of pteroylpolyglutamates in mothers of infants with neural-tube defects. Br J Nutr 1993; 69:827–834.

106. Chiao JH, Roy K, Tolner B et al. RFC-1 gene expression regulates folate absorption in mouse small intestine. J Biol Chem 1997; 272:11165–11170.

107. Tolner B, Roy K, Sirotnak FM. Structural analysis of the human *RFC-1* gene encoding a folate transporter reveals multiple promoters and alternatively spliced transcripts with 5' end heterogeneity. Gene 1998; 211:331–341.

108. Kang S-S, Zhou J, Wong PWK et al. Intermediate homocysteinemia: a thermolabile variant of methylen-etetrahydrofolate reductase. Am J Hum Genet 1988; 43:414–421.

109. Goyette P, Simmer JS, Milos R et al. Human methylene-tetrahydrofolate reductase: isolation of cDNA, mapping and mutation identification. Nature Genet 1994; 7:195–200.

110. Jacques PF, Bostom AG, Williams RR et al. Relation between folate status, a common mutation in methylenetetrahydrofolate reductase, and plasma homocysteine concentrations. Circulation 1996; 93:7–9.

111. Bailey LB, Cerda JJ, Bloch BS et al. Effect of age on polyglutamyl and monoglutamyl folacin absorption in human subjects. J Nutr 1984; 114:1770–1776.

112. Kownacki Brown PA, Wang C, Bailey LB et al. Urinary excretion of deuterium-labeled folate and the metabolite *p*-aminobenzoylguitainate in humans. J Nutr 1993; 123:1101–1108.

113. McPartlin JM, Halligan A, Scott JM et al. Accelerated folate breakdown in pregnancy. Lancet 1993; 341:148–149.

114. Caudill MA, Cruz AC, Gregory JF et al. Folate status response to controlled folate intake in pregnant women. J Nutr 1997; 127:2363–2370.

115. Caudill MA, Gregory JF, Hutson AD, Bailey LB. Folate catabolism in pregnant and nonpregnant women with controlled folate intakes. J Nutr 1998; 128:204–208.

116. Halsted CH. Intestinal absorption of dietary folates. In: Picciano MF, Stokstad ELR, Gregory JF, eds. Folic acid metabolism in health and disease. New York: Wiley-Liss; 1990:23–45.

117. WHO (1998). Obesity: preventing and managing the global epidemic. WHO, Geneva.

118. Tso P, Crissinger K. Overview of digestion and absorption. In: Biochemical and physiological aspects of human nutrition. Philadelphia, PA: WB Saunders; 2000.

119. Guyton AC, Hall JE. Human physiology and mechanisms of disease, 6th edn. Philadelphia, PA: WB Saunders; 1997.

120. Garrow JS. Composition of the body. In: Human nutrition and dietetics. London: Churchill Livingstone; 2000.

SECTION 2

Nutrients and nutrient derivatives relevant to ocular health

Chapter **2.1**

Proteins

Orla O'Donovan

INTRODUCTION

The proteins dealt with in this part include retinal rhodopsin and lens crystallins. Other important structural collagenous proteins do exist in the vitreous and cornea, in combination with carbohydrate, and are dealt with later in this chapter.

RETINAL RHODOPSIN

Light-sensitive pigments, distinguished by their spectral properties, found in the retina include the rod pigment, rhodopsin (required for night vision) and three cone pigments responsible for normal daylight vision and colour discrimination. Retinal rod pigments are more abundant and stable than cone pigments.

All visual pigments consist of an apoprotein, opsin, to which a chromophore is attached. The spectral properties of these visual pigments are largely determined by the retinene chain of the chromophore. Rhodopsin, the rod pigment, is the most studied and contains the chromophore 11-*cis*-retinal, an aldehyde derivative of vitamin A with a peak sensitivity/absorption (λ_{max}) of 498 nm. The cone pigments consist of blue-sensitive cones (λ_{max} = 419 nm), green-sensitive cones (λ_{max} = 531 nm) and red-sensitive cones (λ_{max} = 558 nm).[1–5]

Vision involves the conversion of light into electrochemical signals that are processed by the retina, and subsequently sent to and interpreted by the brain. Rhodopsin, which enables us to see in dim light, is located in the disc membranes of

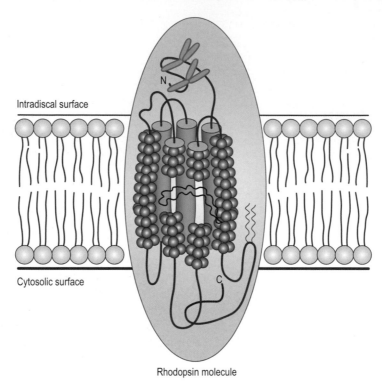

Intradiscal surface

Cytosolic surface

Rhodopsin molecule

Figure 2.1.1   Structure of rhodopsin molecule, containing seven transmembrane domains, to which the 11–cis retinal chromophore is attached.

the rod outer segments (ROS) of the photoreceptor cells of the retina, where it comprises 80% of the total protein with the other proteins present all involved in the phototransduction cascade.[6] It catalyses the only light-sensitive step in vision. A chromophore, 11-*cis*-retinal, lies in a pocket of the protein, which is isomerised to all-*trans*-retinal when light is absorbed.

G-protein-coupled receptors (GPCRs) are a large structurally related class of cell receptors and rhodopsin is probably the best-studied GPCR. The isomerisation of the chromophore in the internal hydrophobic pocket leads to a conformational change which is propagated to the cytoplasmic surface of the receptor, enabling binding and activation of visual G protein (transducin). This initiates a cascade of reactions leading to a nerve impulse, which is transmitted to the brain by the optical nerve (Figure 2.1.1).[7,8]

Rhodopsin activation (the bleaching pathway)

Retinal rhodopsin undergoes a change in colour (bleaching) on exposure to light. The 11-*cis*-retinal chromophore of rhodopsin is the light-absorbing moiety of the molecule.[9] Its concentration in human rods is 0.1 mmol/l and, with up to 1000 discs, the number of molecules is approximately 10 million. A rod could be stimulated by one of these molecules absorbing a quantum; however, more than one rod may have to be stimulated for a perception of light to be generated.[10,11]

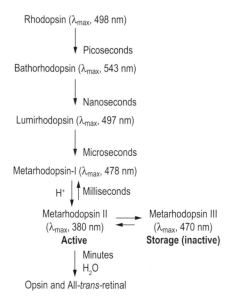

Rhodopsin (λ_{max}, 498 nm)

↓ Picoseconds

Bathorhodopsin (λ_{max}, 543 nm)

↓ Nanoseconds

Lumirhodopsin (λ_{max}, 497 nm)

↓ Microseconds

Metarhodopsin-I (λ_{max}, 478 nm)

H^+ ↓↑ Milliseconds

Metarhodopsin II ⟶ Metarhodopsin III
(λ_{max}, 380 nm) ⟵ (λ_{max}, 470 nm)
Active   **Storage (inactive)**

↓ Minutes
↓ H_2O

Opsin and All-*trans*-retinal

Figure 2.1.2   The stages in the bleaching pathway of rhodopsin with the appropriate decay times of intermediates at physiological temperatures. Wavelengths are absorption maxima of the intermediates.

Rhodopsin absorbs radiations of wavelengths in or near the visible part of the electromagnetic spectrum and absorption is necessary for visual response. Its spatial configuration changes following the capture of a quantum, leading to changes in its spectral absorption and a series of thermally driven reactions which can occur in the absence of irradiation and hence referred to as dark reactions; however, they may occur in the presence of light. These reactions give rise to photoproducts with varying lifetimes.[4,12]

The bleaching pathway (Figure 2.1.2) involves the isomerisation of the chromophore 11-*cis*-retinal around the $C_{11}\!=\!C_{12}$ double bond to form all-*trans*-retinal. The first reaction, which involves the conversion of rhodopsin to bathorhodopsin, occurs in picoseconds and is the only reaction involving light. Resonance Raman spectroscopic studies have demonstrated that the bound chromophore present in bathorhodopsin is all-*trans*-retinal.[12–14]

Following absorption of a quantum, the link between 11-*cis*-retinaldehyde is altered. Activation of rhodopsin causes conformational changes at the cytoplasmic surface of rhodopsin, leading to the initiation of the phototransduction cascade.

The final reaction in the bleaching process involves hydrolysis and dissociation to all-*trans*-retinaldehyde and the apoprotein opsin, a requirement for full deactivation of light-stimulated photoreceptor cells. 11-*cis*-retinal is then regenerated and supplied to opsin by the visual cycle to restore the dark pigment.

LENS CRYSTALLINE PROTEINS

The main function of the lens is to refract light entering the eye through the pupil and focus it on the retina. In order to carry out this function the lens must maintain its own clarity, provide refractive power and absorb ultraviolet (UV).

The lens is quite a distinct tissue in that it is avascular and its protein concentration is the highest of any organ.[15] In the centre of a human lens this concentration reaches a value of 450 mg/ml.[16] The lens proteins are uniformly packed in high density within the fibre cells, which minimises light-scattering and contributes to the transparency of the lens.[17]

Lens fibre cells are derived from epithelial cells, and during cell differentiation high concentrations of proteins are synthesised and the cells lose their nuclei, ribosomes and other organelles. The lens is a growing tissue in which concentric layers of fibre cells continuously overlay their predecessors. The outer younger part of the lens is called the cortex and the older core or inner part is called the nucleus.[18] The lens has a unique growth pattern, in that there is no protein turnover in the differentiated fibre cells and no diffusion of proteins between cells. Therefore, proteins synthesised during embryogenesis are still present in fibre cells located in the core of an aged lens.[19,20]

The soluble proteins of the vertebrate lens consist mainly of the structural proteins crystallins which are classified into α, β and γ; however, they also contain enzymatic proteins, including glyceraldehyde-3P dehydrogenase, glucose-6P dehydrogenase and enolase. The crystallins, which account for 90% of total lens proteins, maintain the refractive properties of the lens.[21,22]

In the centre of the lens (nucleus), older proteins begin to unfold and denature with age. Once denatured, the hydrophobic core is exposed; this tends to interact with exposed hydrophobic regions of other denatured proteins, leading to the formation of insoluble aggregates. Such insoluble protein aggregates cause light-scattering which interferes with lens transparency and, hence, with vision (cataract).

UV radiation from sunlight is known to cause structural and functional alterations to lens macromolecules and is one of the major risk factors in the aetiology of human cataract formation.[23,24] The lens fibre cells contain a group of UV filter compounds. These compounds absorb harmful radiation (295–400 nm), preventing it reaching the retina, thus increasing visual acuity.[25,26]

Paradoxically, some UV filters can over time form reactive substances[27,28] which bind to the crystallin proteins in human lens, leading to coloration, fluorescence and ultimately cataract formation.

However, the α-crystallins appear to maintain lens transparency in a twofold manner: (1) structurally, by packaging in symmetrical oligomeric assemblies; and (2) functionally by acting as molecular chaperones, preventing denatured lens proteins forming insoluble precipitated aggregates which would cause light-scattering (see Chapter 4.5).

SUMMARY

The lens is a unique tissue in that it contains differentiated cells with very high protein content and no organelles. The absence of organelles, which would cause light-scattering, contributes to lens transparency; however, the lack of ribosomes means that no protein synthesis can occur in these cells.

The soluble α-, β- and γ-crystallin proteins comprise 90% of the lens proteins. The individual protein structures and their interaction with each other are important in providing the refractive power and visual acuity of the lens. Much knowledge of the structure of these proteins has been gained; however, a large gap remains, reflected in the lack of a tertiary and quaternary structure of α-crystallin.

Age-related cataract is one of the leading causes of blindness in humans. The pathogenesis of this condition involves lens opacification, leading to loss of vision. Although the mechanisms of cataractogenesis are not fully understood, protein denaturation and aggregation (leading to loss of solubility) are associated with cataract formation in humans. α-Crystallin has been shown to function as a molecular chaperone by combining with unfolding proteins and preventing their precipitation. However, α-, β- and γ-crystallins themselves are subject to in vivo aggregation and precipitation, contributing to lens opacification.

References

1. Wald G. The receptors of human color vision. Science 1964; 145:1007.
2. Brown PK, Wald G. Visual pigments in single rods and cones of the human retina. Science 1964; 144:45.
3. Wald G, Brown PK. Human color vision and color blindness. Cold Spring Harbor Symp Quant Biol 1965; 30:345.
4. Wald G. The molecular basis of visual excitation. Nature 1968; 219:800–807.
5. Dartnall HJA, Bowmaker JK, Mollon JD. Micro-spectrophotometry of human photoreceptors. In: Mollon JD, Sharpe LT, eds. Colour vision. London: Academic Press; 1983:69–80.
6. Kuhn H. Interactions between photoexcited rhodopsin and light-activated enzymes in rods. Progr Retinal Res 1984; 3:123–156.
7. Sakamar TP. Structure of rhodopsin and the superfamily of seven-helical receptors: the same and not the same. Curr Opin Cell Biol 2002; 14:189–195.
8. Karnik SS, Gogonea C, Patil S et al. Activation of G-protein-coupled receptors: a common molecular mechanism. Trends Endocrinol Metab 2003; 14:431–437.
9. Ostroy SE. Rhodopsin and the visual process. Biochem Biophys Acta 1977; 463:91–125.
10. Baylor DA, Lamb TD, Yau K-W. The membrane current of a single rod outer segments. J Physiol (Lond) 1979; 288:589–611.
11. Baylor DA, Lamb TD, Yau K-W. Responses of retinal rods to single photons. J Physiol (Lond) 1979; 288:613–634.

12. Yoshizawa T, Wald G. Pre-luminrhodopsin and the bleaching of visual pigments. Nature 1963; 197:1279–1286.

13. Eyring G, Curry B, Mathies R et al. Interpretation of the resonance raman spectrum of bathorhodopsin based on visual pigment analogues. Biochem 1980; 19:2410–2418.

14. Schoenlein RW, Peteanu LA, Mathies RA, Shank CV. The first step in vision: femtosecond isomerization of rhodopsin. Science 1991; 254:412–415.

15. Ingolia TD, Craig EA. Four small *Drosophila* heat shock proteins are related to each other and to mammalian alpha-crystallin. Proc Natl Acad Sci USA 1982; 79:2360–2364.

16. Arrigo A-P, Suhan JP, Welch WJ. Dynamic changes in the structure and intracellular locale of the mammalian low-molecular weight heat shock protein. Mol Cell Biol 1988; 8:5059–5071.

17. Kim KK, Kim R, Kim SH. Crystal structure of small heat shock protein. Nature 1998; 394:595–599.

18. Ellis J. Proteins as molecular chaperones. Nature 1987; 328:378–379.

19. Wistow G. Domain structure and evolution in alpha-crystallins and small heat-shock proteins. FEBS Lett 1985; 181:1–6.

20. De Jong WW, Caspers GJ, Lwunissen JAM. Genealogy of the alpha-crystallin-small heat shock protein superfamily. Int J Biol Macromol 1998; 22:151–162.

21. Horwitz J. Alpha-crystallin can function as a molecular chaperone. Proc Natl Acad Sci USA 1992; 89:10449–10453.

22. Jakob U, Gaestel M, Engel K, Buchner J. Small heat-shock proteins are molecular chaperones. J Biol Chem 1993; 268:1517–1520.

23. Brady JP, Garland D, Duglas-Tabor Y et al. Targeted disruption of the mouse alpha A-crystallin gene induces cataract and cytoplasmic inclusion bodies containing the small heat shock protein alpha B-crystallin. Proc Natl Acad Sci USA 1997; 94:884–889.

24. Brady JP, Garland D, Green DE et al. Alpha B crystallin in lens development and muscle integrity: a gene knockout approach. Invest Ophthalmol Vis Sci 2001; 42:2924–2934.

25. Iwaki T, Wisniewski T, Iwaki A et al. Accumulation of alphaB-crystallin in central nervous system glia and neurons in pathological conditions. Am J Pathol 1992; 140:345–356.

26. Lowe J, Landon M, Pike I et al. Dementia with beta-amyloid deposition: involvement of alphaB-crystallin supports two main diseases. Lancet 1990; 336:515–516.

27. Renkawek K, Voorter CEM, Bosman GJGM et al. Expression of alpha B-crystallin in Alzheimer disease. Acta Neuropathol 1994; 87:155–160.

28. Van den Oetelaar PJ, Clauwaert J, Van Laethem M, Hoenders HJ. The influence of isolation conditions on the molecular weight of bovine alpha crystallin. J Biol Chem 1985; 260:14030–14034.

29. Palczewski K, Kumasaka T, Hori T et al. Crystal structure of rhodopsin: a G-protein-coupled receptor. Science 2000; 289:739–745.

Chapter **2.2**

Lipids

Orla O'Donovan

INTRODUCTION

The major role of lipids in ocular tissue is as key components of membrane structure. Membrane lipids comprise the matrix that gives form and structure to membranes, and in which membrane proteins are embedded. The membrane is an important structural component of all cells; it is especially important in ocular and brain tissue. In ocular tissue, the disc membranes of the outer segments of the photoreceptor cells of the retina play an important role in the vision process (see Chapter 2.1).

All membranes contain amphipathic lipids – phospholipids, glycolipids (sphingolipids) and cholesterol. The main feature of these lipids is that they have hydrophobic and hydrophilic functions, the former oriented towards the centre, and the latter to the exterior, of the membrane. The hydrophobic fatty acid residues contained within the membrane lipids determine the rigidity/fluidity of the structure. The length of the fatty acid chains and the degree of unsaturation contribute favourably towards the fluidity of the membrane. Conversely, short-chain saturated fatty acids allow for dense packaging and favour the rigid state. The structural lipids of the membranes of the photoreceptor disc membranes are unique in their composition, with phospholipids accounting for 80–90% and cholesterol for only 8–10%,[1] and this large proportion of phospholipids contributes to the very high fluidity of these membranes.[2,3]

PHOSPHOLIPIDS

The major phospholipids of membranes are phosphoglycerolipids (Figure 2.2.1).

Phospholipids are amphipathic molecules containing a highly polar head group (the alcohol) and non-polar hydrocarbon chains of fatty acids. The alcohol moiety found in the phospholipids can vary; however, the most common alcohols found in membranes are choline, ethanolamine, serine and inositol.

Fatty acids

A fatty acid is classified according to the number of its carbon atoms, the number of its double bonds (if present) and the proximity of the first double bond to the methyl (Ω) terminus of the acyl chain, which is also used in the abbreviation of the chemical structure. Linolenic acid, C18:3 Ω-3, has an 18-carbon chain with three double bonds and the first double bond is located at carbon 3, while docosahexaenoic acid (DHA), C22:6 Ω-3, has a 22-carbon chain with six double bonds and the first double bond is at carbon 3 (Figure 2.2.2).

Many fatty acids can be synthesised in the body while others, referred to as essential fatty acids (EFAs), cannot be synthesised, and must be provided in the diet. EFAs are classified into two families; omega-3 (Ω-3) and omega-6 (Ω-6).

Long-chain polyunsaturated fatty acids (LCPUFAs) contain a hydrophilic carboxyl head group and a hydrophobic long even-numbered carbon chain ($\geq$ 18 carbons) with two or more double (unsaturated) bonds. LCPUFAs are provided by the diet or can be synthesised in vivo from dietary EFAs of shorter chain length, and hence can also be classified as Ω-3 and Ω-6.

The dietary LCPUFAs are predominantly found in triacylglycerols (triglycerides) (Figure 2.2.3), and they are transported through the body in this form. The LCPUFAs in membranes are present in phospholipids.

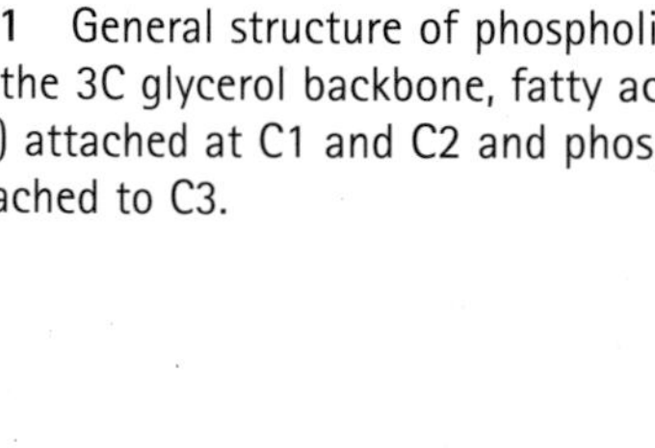

Docosahexaenoic acid, C22:6 Ω-3

DHA, C22:6 Ω-3, is found in high concentrations in a few select mammalian tissues[4,5] such as the brain synaptosomes,[6] sperm[7] and the retinal ROS.[8] The highest body concentrations of DHA is located in the retinal ROS.[4,5]

DHA can be synthesised from the EFA linolenic acid (C18:3 Ω-3); however, despite the necessity of DHA for its cell function, the retina is limited in the capacity to synthesise this PUFA from its precursor EFA.[9] The liver plays an essential role in synthesising DHA from its precursor and for packaging the newly synthesised, or dietary, DHA into lipoproteins for export to the retina and other tissues.[10]

Dietary intake and digestion of EFA and DHA

The diet is the sole source of the EFA linolenic acid, a precursor of DHA, and EFA linolenic acid is found in high concentrations in vegetable oils such as linseed, soybean and canola oils. DHA is

O
‖
R1—C—O—CH$_2$

O
‖
R2—C—O—CH

H$_2$C—O—PO^{3-}—Alcohol

Figure 2.2.1   General structure of phospholipids, containing the 3C glycerol backbone, fatty acyl chains (R1 and R2) attached at C1 and C2 and phosphoryl-alcohol attached to C3.

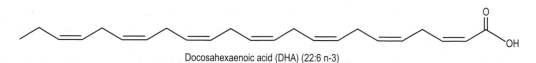

Docosahexaenoic acid (DHA) (22:6 n-3)

Figure 2.2.2   Structure of docosahexaenoic acid.

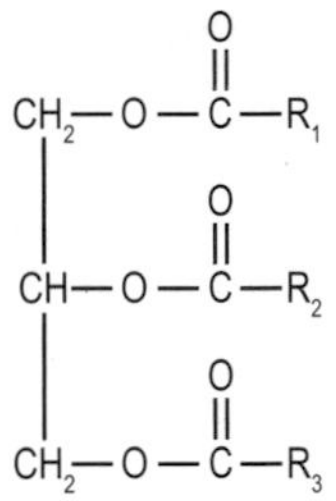

O
||
CH₂—O—C—R₁

O
||
CH—O—C—R₂

O
||
CH₂—O—C—R₃

Figure 2.2.3 Triacylglycerol (or triglyceride) structure: 3-carbon glycerol backbone with three fatty acyl chains R_1, R_2, R_3 attached.

also available from dietary sources of fish, or fish and marine mammal oil, and eggs.

Synthesis of DHA from EFA linolenic acid in the liver

The liver plays an important role in the homeostasis of DHA (C22:6 Ω-3) by synthesising this PUFA from its precursor EFA linolenic acid (C18:3 Ω-3).[10]

DHA accumulation in the retina

The choriocapillaries supply the nutrients to the retinal pigment epithelial (RPE) cells, which delivers them to the interphotoreceptor matrix.[11] Low-density lipoprotein (LDL) is the main carrier of DHA, and since the RPE cells contain LDL receptors[12] it is likely that the uptake and delivery of DHA to the photoreceptor cells are receptor-mediated with subsequent release of DHA phospholipids, or free DHA, into the interphotoreceptor matrix.[13]

Fatty acid-binding proteins (FABPs) present in the interphotoreceptor matrix bind DHA, and are believed to be involved in the transport of DHA to the photoreceptor cells.[14–16]

Once delivered to the photoreceptors, free DHA is activated by fatty acyl coenzyme A in the inner segment and rapidly becomes incorporated into phospholipids. The DHA-containing phospholipids are assembled into new photoreceptor disc membranes where they remain unmetabolised, which results in concentration of DHA (~90%) in the disc membrane, leading to an uneven distribution of this fatty acid within the retina.[17–20] This distribution demonstrates the selective accumulation of DHA into this specific location within retinal tissue.

DHA conservation in the retina

Disc membranes are assembled at the inner segment, and form discs at the base of the outer segment. These membranes have a short lifetime, and are replaced every 9–14 days. The discs move outward toward the tip apical region where they are shed into the adjacent RPE, phagocytosed and digested by the lysosomal system. However, the retina conserves its DHA by retrieving it from the phagosomal membranes within the RPE and recycling it for incorporation into newly forming disc membranes.[13,20] The recycling mechanism is not fully understood, but it has been postulated to occur via one of the two following mechanisms: (1) by returning the DHA from the RPE back to the photoreceptors (short-loop); or (2) by entry of DHA into the systemic circulation, where it follows a similar pathway to cellular and dietary DHA via the liver, and reuptake by the RPE cells, with delivery to photoreceptor cells for new disc formation (long-loop).[13,21] This selective retention of lipid is unique to the photoreceptor cells.

DHA and retinal oxidative stress

DHA, owing to its high degree of unsaturation, is susceptible to oxidation within the photoreceptor disc membranes. This is compounded by the retina's exposure to light, high oxygen tension and high concentrations of photosensitising retinoids.[22] However, there are effective mechanisms present within this tissue to protect against oxidative damage, such as the membrane-stabilising substances, vitamin E and taurine, along with the retinal antioxidants, vitamin C, carotenoids, superoxide dismutase and glutathione (and its associated enzymes)[23–25] (see Chapter 2.7).

Therefore, once DHA is delivered to the retinal tissue, it is conserved and protected from oxidative damage. However, due to this tissue's high oxidative stress, a constant cellular and dietary supply is required to maintain the disc membranes. The supply of DHA is especially important during fetal and infant development, and several studies have demonstrated that depletion of DHA from the developing retina leads to abnormalities in electroretinogram (ERG) and visual evoked potential (VEP), resulting in reduced visual function.[26–28]

Role of DHA in the structure and function of the photoreceptor disc membranes

DHA affects the membrane structure by altering its permeability, fluidity, thickness and lipid-phase properties while increasing the rate of rhodopsin activation (and hence the phototransduction cascade).

While phospholipids diffuse easily among discs,[29,30] DHA-rich phospholipids behave like rhodopsin and, once incorporated into a disc, remain with that disc from root to tip, indicating its close association (non-covalently) with the rhodopsin protein.[17] DHA surrounds rhodopsin (approximately 60 molecules of phospholipid for each rhodopsin), excluding cholesterol from creating a fluid microenvironment within the rod outer-segment membranes.[31,32]

The phototransduction cascade involves the activation of three proteins, with an amplification of the signal at each stage. Rhodopsin is activated by the capture of a photon of light, leading to the formation of metarhodopsin II (MII). MII interacts with, and activates, a second type of disc membrane protein, transducin. Once activated, transducin and MII dissociate, and MII activates further transducin molecules leading to an amplification (or cascade) of the signal. The activated transducin in turn activates a third type of membrane protein, phosphodiesterase (PDE), and again these proteins dissociate and transducin activates further PDE proteins, it comes into contact with the disc membrane, leading to further amplification of the signal.

Therefore, membrane fluidity is an important biophysical factor of the disc membranes, and this fluidity is brought about by the presence of DHA and other PUFAs on the constituent phospholipids. The membrane's fluid state allows Brownian movement of the protein components within the plane of the disc membrane, enabling transduction and amplification of the signal,

which occurs on a millisecond timescale.[2,3,33,34] Studies investigating disc membrane phospholipids have shown that membranes containing DHA have higher MII formation,[35] MII–transducin interaction and activation[36] and, finally, PDE activation.[37] Therefore, DHA and PUFAs confer properties on the disc membranes which maximise the efficiency and gain of the phototransduction cascade.

Dietary deficiency of DHA and visual function

Extensive studies carried out with rats deprived of dietary EFA have demonstrated alterations to retinal function, which ultimately led to the discovery of the importance of DHA in the visual process.[38–40] The ERGs of both the a- and b-waves were altered; however, the effect on the a-wave was larger and more persistent, indicating that perturbations were occurring at the photoreceptor level.[26,38,39]

Similar results were found in human studies, where diets low in Ω-3 fatty acids led to impaired visual acuity and ERGs.[41,42] The retinal dysfunction occurs due to inadequate disc membrane DHA phospholipids to support rhodopsin in light capture, and hence MII formation.[43]

Cells will compensate for depletion of Ω-3 fatty acids, by elongating and desaturating Ω-6 EFA linoleic acid (18:2 Ω-6) to docosapentaenoic acid (22:5 Ω-6), which only differs from DHA by one single bond; however, this PUFA is unable to support rhodopsin as efficiently as DHA.[27,39,44,45]

DHA deficiency studies in ocular tissue, caused by diets low in Ω-3 fatty acids, have focused on fetal and infant subjects to determine the effect during growth and development; while some effects of DHA deficiency appear to be transitionary, others are long-lasting and irreversible.[5] The ERG amplitudes have been shown to return to normal in some studies, even when the low-Ω-3 diet is maintained.[46,47] However, even where the retinal abnormalities are reversible, the responsiveness of the visual cortex, and the higher cortical centres involved in visual function, appear long-lasting and irreversible.[5]

DHA supplementation is used to combat dietary deficiency, especially in premature human infants. However, supplementation should be approached with caution as these infants have low retinal levels of vitamin E, and are often exposed to high levels of constant light and oxygen in neonatal intensive care units.[48] Too little DHA has certainly been demonstrated to be harmful during this period of development; however, supplementation in an attempt to increase retinal DHA concentration could increase their susceptibility to retinal oxidative damage, a factor thought to be involved in the aetiology of retinopathy of prematurity.[49]

Inherited retinal degenerations and DHA

Systemic alterations in plasma DNA and circulating lipoproteins are frequently displayed with inherited progressive retinal degenerations.

Indeed, low levels of plasma DHA have been reported for members of families with retinitis pigmentosa[50,51] and Usher's syndrome.[52,53]

Therefore, inherited progressive retinal degenerations may be associated with abnormalities of DHA metabolism in tissues other than the retina, such as the liver, or with problems influencing delivery of the PUFA on circulating lipoproteins.

SUMMARY

Dietary intake of EFAs and DHA is essential to maintain ocular health. The liver plays a central role in the homeostasis of DHA in retinal tissue by synthesising DHA from its precursor EFA, and packaging this Ω-3 fatty acid into LDLs for delivery to the retina. Once incorporated into the disc membranes of the photoreceptor cells, DHA phospholipids associate with rhodopsin and enable its activation, and hence facilitate visual transduction.

References

1. Daemen F. Vertebrate rod outer segment membranes. Biochim Biophys Acta 1973; 300:255.
2. Fleisler SJ, Anderson RE. Chemistry and metabolism of lipids in the vertebrate retina. Prof Lipid Res 1983; 22:79.
3. Poo M, Cone CA. Lateral diffusion of rhodopsin in the photorecptor membrane. Nature 1974; 247:438.
4. Salem N Jr, Kim H-Y, Yergey JA. Docosahexaenoic acid. membrane function and metabolism. In: Simopolous AP, Kifer RR, Martin RE, eds. Health effects of polyunsaturated fatty acids in seafoods. New York: Academic Press; 1986:319–351.
5. Neuringer M. The relationship of fatty acid composition to function in the retina and visual system. Paper presented at: Lipids, learning and the brain: fats in infant formulas, 103rd Ross Conference on Pediatric Research, Adelaide, South Australia; 1993.
6. Breckenridge WC, Gombos G, Morgan IG. The lipid composition of adult rat brain synaptosomal membranes. Biochim Biophys Acta 1972; 266:695–707.
7. Neill AR, Masters CJ. Metabolism of fatty acids by ovine spermatozoa. J Reprod Fertil 1973; 34:279–287.
8. Weigand RD, Anderson RE. Phospholipid molecular species of frog rod outer segment membranes. Exp Eye Res 1983; 37:159–173.
9. Wetzel MG, Li J, Alvarez RA et al. Metabolism of linolenic acid and docosahexaenoic acid in rat retinas and rod outer segments. Exp Eye Res 1991; 53:437–446.
10. Scott BL, Bazan NG. Membrane docosahexaenoate is supplied to the developing brain and retina by the liver. Proc Natl Acad Sci USA 1989; 86:2903–2907.
11. Rodriquez de Turco EB, Gordon WC, Bazan NG. Rapid and selective uptake, metabolism and differential distribution of docosahexaenoic acid among rod and cone photoreceptor cells in the frog retina. J Neurosci Res 1991; 11:3667.
12. Hayes KC, Lindsey S, Stephan ZF, Brecker D. Retinal pigment epithelium possesses both LDL and scavenger receptor activity. Invest Ophthalmol Vis Sci 1989; 20:225.
13. Bazan NG, Rodriguez de Turco EB, Gordon WB. Supply, uptake and retention of docosahexanoic acid by the developing and mature retina and brain. Paper presented at: Lipids, learning and the brain: fats in infant formulas, 103rd Ross Conference on Pediatric Research, Adelaide, South Australia; 1993.
14. Bazan NG, Reddy TS, Redmond TM et al. Endogenous fatty acids are covalently and non convalently bound to interphotoreceptor retinoid-binding protein in the monkey retina. J Biol Chem 1985; 260:13677–13680.
15. Chen Y, Saari JC, Noy N. Interactions of all-trans retinal and long-chain fatty acids with interphotoreceptor retinoid-binding protein. Biochem 1993; 32:11311–11318.
16. Lee J, Jiao X, Gentleman S et al. Soluble-binding proteins for docosahexaenoic acid are present in neural retina. Invest Ophthalmol Vis Sci 1995; 36:2032–2039.
17. Gordon WC, Bazan NG. Docosahexaenoic acid utilization during rod photoreceptor cell renewal. J Neurosci 1990; 10:2190.
18. Bazan NG, Gordon WC, Rodriguez de Turco EB. Delivery of docosahexaenoic acid (^{3}H-22:6) by the liver

to the retina in the frog. Invest Ophthalmol Vis Sci 1991; 32 (suppl):701.

19. Rodriguez de Turco EB, Gordon WC, Peyman GA, Bazan NG. Preferential uptake and metabolism of docosahexaenoic acid in membrane phospholipids from rod and cone photoreceptor cells of human and monkey retinas. J Neurosci Res 1990; 27:522.

20. Gordon WC, Rodriguez de Turco EB, Bazan NG. Retinal pigment epithelial cells play a central role in the conservation of docosahexaenoic acid by photoreceptor cells after shedding and phagocytosis. Curr Eye Res 1992; 11:73.

21. Bazan NG. The identification of a new biochemical alteration early in the differentiation of visual cells in inherited retinal degeneration. In: La Vail MM, Anderson RE, Hollyfield JG, eds. Inherited and environmentally induced retinal degenerations. New York: Alan R Liss; 1989:191–2125.

22. Mittag T. Role of oxygen radicals in ocular inflammation and cellular damage. Exp Eye Res 1984; 39:759–769.

23. Katz ML, Robinson WG. Light and ageing effects on vitamin E in the retina and retinal pigment epithelium. Vision Res 1987; 27:1875–1879.

24. Eldred GE. Vitamins A and E in RPE lipofuscin formation and implications for age-related macular degenerations. Progr Clin Biol Res 1989; 314:113–129.

25. Armstrong D, Hiramitsu T. Studies of experimentally induced retinal degenerations: 2. Early morphological changes produced by lipid peroxides in the albino rat. Jpn J Ophthalmol 1990; 34:158–173.

26. Wheeler TG, Benolken RM, Anderson RE. Visual membranes: specificity of fatty acid precursors for the electrical response to illumination. Science 1975; 188:1312.

27. Neuringer M, Connor WE, Lin DS et al. Biochemical and functional effects of prenatal and postnatal omega-3 deficiency on retina and brain in rhesus monkeys. Proc Natl Acad Sci USA 1986; 83:4021–4025.

28. Innis SM. Essential fatty acids in growth and development. Progr Lipid Res 1991; 30:39–103.

29. Bibb C, Young RW. Renewal of fatty acids in the membranes of visual cell outer segments. J Cell Biol 1974; 61:327.

30. Fliesler SJ, Basinger SF. Monensin stimulates glycerol incorporation into rod outer segment membranes. J Biol Chem 1987; 262:17516.

31. Van Blitterswijk WJ, van der Meer B, Hilkmann H. Quantitative contributions of cholesterol and the individual classes of phospholipids and their degree of fatty acyl (un)saturation to membrane fluidity measured by fluorescence polarization. Biochemistry 1987; 26:1746.

32. Lynch DV, Thompson GA. Retailored lipid molecular species: a tactical mechanism for modulating membrane properties. Trends Biochem Sci 1984; 9:442.

33. Liebman PA. Lateral diffusion of visual pigment in photoreceptor disk membranes. Science 1974; 185:457–459.

34. Baylor DA, Lamb TD, Yau K-W. Response of retinal rods to single photons. J Physiol 1979; 288: 613–634.

35. Litman BJ, Mitchell DC. A role for phospholipid polyunsaturation in modulating membrane protein function. Lipids 1996; 31 (suppl):S193–S197.

36. Salem N Jr, Liman B, Kim HY, Gawrisch K. Mechanisms of action of docosahexaenoic acid in the nervous system. Lipids 2001; 36:945–959.

37. Litman BJ, Niu SL, Polozova A, Mitchell DC. The role of docosahexaenoic acid containing phospholipids in modulating G protein-coupled signalling pathways: visual transduction. J Mol Neurosci 2001; 16:237–242 (discussion 279–284).

38. Benolken RM, Anderson RE, Wheeler TG. Membrane fatty acids associated with the electrical response in visual excitation. Science 1973; 182:1253.

39. Bourre JM, Francois M, Youyou A et al. The effects of dietary alpha-linolenic acid on the composition of nerve membranes, enzymatic activity, amplitude of electrophysiological parameters, resistance to poisons and performance of learning tasks in rats. J Nutr 1989; 11:1880–1892.

40. Lamptey MS, Walker BL. A possible essential role for dietary linolenic acid in the development of the young rat. J Nutr 1976; 106:86.

41. Bjerver KS. Omega3 fatty acid deficiency in man: implications for the requirement of alpha-linolenic acid and long-chain omega-3 fatty acids. World Rev Nutr Diet 1991; 66:133.

42. Uauy RD, Birch DG, Birch EE et al. Effect of dietary omega-3 fatty acids on retinal function of very-low-birth-weight neonates. Pediatr Res 1990; 28:485-492.

43. Bush RA, Reme C, Malnoe A. The effect of dietary deprivation of Ω-3 fatty acids on acute structural alterations. Exp Eye Res 1991; 53:741.

44. Bazan NG. The metabolism of omega-3 polyunsaturated fatty acids in the eye: possible role of docosahexaenoic acid and docosanoids in retinal physiology and ocular pathology. Progr Clin Biol Res 1989; 312:95–112.

45. Bazan NG. The metabolism of omega-3 polyunsaturated fatty acids in the eye: the possible role of docosahexaenoic acid and docosanoids in retinal physiology and ocular pathology. In: Bito LZ, Stjernschantz J, eds. The ocular effects of prostaglandins and other eicosanoids. New York: Alan R Liss; 1989:95–112.

46. Birch DG, Birch EE, Hoffman DR, Uauy R. Retinal development in very-low-birth-weight infants fed diets differing in omega-3 fatty acids. Invest Ophthalmol Vis Sci 1992; 33:2365.

47. Uauy R, Birch DG, Birch EE et al. Visual and brain development in infants as a function of essential fatty acid supply provided by the early diet. Paper presented at: Lipids, learning and the brain: fats in infant formulas, 103rd Ross Conference on Pediatric Research, Adelaide, South Australia; 1993.

48. Nielsen JC, Naash MI, Anderson RE. The regional distribution of vitamins E and C in mature and

premature human retinas. Invest Ophthalmol Vis Sci 1988; 29:22.

49. Johnson L, Quinn GE, Abbasi S et al. Effect of sustained phamacologic vitamin E levels on incidence and severity of retinopathy of prematurity: a controlled clinical trial. J Pediatr 1989; 114:827–838.

50. Anderson RE, Maude MB, Lewis RA et al. Abnormal plasma levels of polyunsaturated fatty acid in autosomal dominant retinitis pigmentosa. Exp Eye Res 1987; 44:155–159.

51. Voaden MJ, Polkinghorne PJ, Belin J, Smith AD. Studies on blood from patients with dominantly inherited retinitis pigmentosa. In: LaVail MM, Anderson RE, Hollyfield JG, eds. Progress in clinical and biological research: inherited and environmentally induced retinal degeneration. New York: Alan R Liss; 1989:57–68.

52. Bazan NG, Scott BL, Reddy TS, Pelias MZ. Decreased content of docosahexaenoate and arachidonate in plasma phospholipids in Usher's syndrome. Biochem Biophys Res Commun 1986; 141:600.

53. Williams LL, Horrocks L, Leguire LE, Shannon BT. Serum fatty acid proportions in retinitis pigmentosa may be affected by a number of factors. In: LaVail MM, Anderson RE, Hollyfield JG, eds. Inherited and environmentally induced retinal degeneration. New York: Alan R Liss; 1989:49–56.

Chapter **2.3**

Carbohydrates

Orla O'Donovan

CHAPTER CONTENTS

INTRODUCTION

The aqueous, lens, cornea and vitreous are all transparent tissues comprising the optical elements in the mammalian visual system. The aqueous is a fluid which is secreted from the ciliary processes. The lens, however, contains a large concentration of proteins which one would expect to produce intense scattering of light; however, their uniform packing in high density minimises light-scattering and contributes to the transparency of the lens (see Chapter 2.1).

The cornea and vitreous contain a macromolecular structure composed of collagen proteins, which form fibres (with diameters which are thinner than half the wavelength of light) and interfibrillar spaces filled with polysaccharides known as glycosaminoglycans (GAGs), at intervals which reduce the effects of diffraction.[1] By virtue of the interlinking protein and carbohydrate in these tissue structures, both molecules will be described in this chapter. Although they have similar macromolecular structures, the respective functions of the two tissues differ in that the cornea forms a fibrous protective capsule for the eye, whereas the vitreous provides a space-filling gel-like cushion inside the eye.[2,3]

The major protein component in these tissues is collagen (Figure 2.3.1). Collagens are fibrous proteins (Table 2.3.1).

Collagen is found in extracellular matrices, where it forms tissue-specific scaffolds. Carbohydrate, proteoglycans, glycoproteins and non-collagenous proteins are associated with the

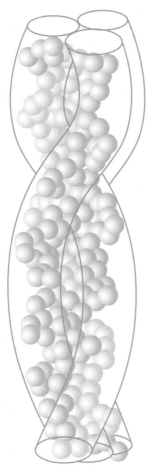

Figure 2.3.1 Collagen molecule (triple helix): three right-handed helical polypeptide chains which wrap around each other in a left-handed helical array.

Table 2.3.1 The vertebrate collagen family

Fibril-forming collagens:	
I, II, III, V, XI	
Fibril-associated collagens (FACITs)	
IX, XII, XIV, XVI	
Non-fibrillar collagens	
Short-chain collagens:	IV, VIII, X
Basement membrane collagen:	IV
Anchoring fibrils:	VII
Microfibrillar:	VI
BP-antigen	XVII

Reproduced from Ihanamaki T, Pelliniemi LJ, Vuorio E. Collagens and collagen-related matrix components in the human and mouse eye. Progr Retinal Eye Res 2004; 23:403–434;[4] and Robert L, Legeais JM, Robert AM, Renard G. Corneal collagens. Pathol Biol 2001; 49:353–363.[123]

Proteoglycans (mucoproteins) are proteins which contain one or more GAG covalently linked to it, and are classified by the structure of the core protein.[8] While these proteins are usually non-collagenous proteins, some GAGs have been found to be linked to certain collagen types and are referred to as 'part-time' proteoglycans. The proteoglycans in ocular matrices interact with collagen in a functional manner which regulates collagen fibril diameter, and maintains the fibril distance in the collagen network.[8–10]

THE CORNEA

The cornea consists of five layers: (1) epithelium; (2) Bowman's layer; (3) stroma; (4) Descemet's membrane; and (5) endothelium. The stroma constitutes the largest part of this tissue, and its macromolecular structure is the most studied.

Corneal stroma

This central connective tissue layer forms 90% of the cornea, and by weight it is 78% water, 1% salts and 21% biological macromolecules. The macromolecules are composed primarily of collagen fibres (80%), ground substance (15%) and stromal cells (5%).[11]

collagen scaffold, which builds a large macromolecular structure, each characteristic of its tissue origin and location.[4–6]

The carbohydrates present in these ocular tissues are GAGs, previously referred to as mucopolysaccharides. These polysaccharides consist of repeating disaccharide units forming long polysaccharide chains. The major GAG of the vitreous is hyaluronic acid, containing the disaccharide unit of glucuronate and N-acetyl glucosamine.[7] The cornea contains four different types of GAG: (1) keratan sulphate; (2) chondroitin; (3) chondroitin sulphate; and (4) dermatan sulphate.[4]

Collagen

Collagen, which is stable, was long regarded as metabolically inert;[12] however, protein turnover, although relatively slow, has been demonstrated.[13] Keratocytes, the predominant cell of the stroma, maintain the collagen and extracellular matrix.[14,15]

The collagen architecture is unique, and has been studied with regard to its contribution to transparency of the tissue. The collagen fibrils are 25–35 nm in diameter,[16,17] and are axially staggered with a typical 64–66 nm periodicity of collagen.[18,19] The collagen fibrils are laid down in lamellae that lie roughly parallel to the surface of the globe.[20]

Maurice[21] attributed transparency of the corneal stroma to the organised lattice structure of the collagen fibrils and its consequential destructive interference, where light scattered by neighbouring fibrils in predictable and opposing directions cancels each other out, except in the primary visual axis. However, it is now believed that fibril size and interfibrillar space play important roles in maintaining transparency of this tissue. Light-scattering occurs when the regional fluctuation in refractive index exceeds the dimension equal to one-half the wavelength of light (200 nm).[22,23] During corneal swelling, the interfibrillar spaces can increase to greater than 200 nm and corneal opacity develops.[24]

The stromal collagen is composed of types I (~60%), V (~10%) and VI (~30%).[12,25–27] Type III collagen may be present in low concentrations, but it is mainly associated with fetal cornea or post corneal injury.[26,28]

The proteoglycans are responsible for maintaining the relative positions of the fibrils,[29–31] and for restricting fibril lateral growth, thereby controlling fibril diameter,[32,33] which both play an important role in ensuring correct fibrillogenesis and corneal transparency.[8–10]

MACROMOLECULAR STRUCTURE

The corneal macromolecular structure incorporates two main components: (1) the collagen network; and (2) the GAG-containing proteoglycans. Collagen plays an important role in this tissue at a macroscopic level by conferring shape and strength to the cornea, and at a microscopic level by maintaining tissue transparency. GAGs and proteoglycans play an important role in fibrillogenesis and matrix assembly. Therefore, both components appear to be functional in maintaining the structure and transparency of the cornea.

THE VITREOUS

The vitreous is a clear mass located in a posterior cavity between the ciliary body and retina. It is composed of a hydrogel structure, which is virtually acellular, highly hydrated (> 98% water) and transmits 90% of visible light.[34] The gel structure is maintained by a network of thin unbranched collagen fibrils with GAGs (principally hyaluronan) filling the spaces of the network. This protein/carbohydrate structure excludes cells and large molecules from the central vitreous in order to maintain transparency.[35]

The peripheral or cortical vitreous contains hyalocyte cells, which are similar to macrophages and are believed to originate from blood macrophages.[36–38] The hyalocytes are secretory cells responsible for the synthesis of hyaluronan and collagen which then move toward the central vitreous for matrix assembly.[39–44]

The concentration of adult vitreous hyaluronan has been estimated between 65 and 400 µg/ml.[45] However, hyaluronan is not uniformly distributed throughout the vitreous, and is subject to age-dependent concentration changes, involving an initial increase in the first 20 years followed by a relatively constant concentration up to 70 years of age and then a further increase.[46,47]

Hyaluronan has special physicochemical properties such as viscoelasticity, exceptionally high hydration volume and important biological roles. Its high molecular mass and numerous mutually repelling anionic groups give rise to a highly hydrated viscous matrix. Hyaluronan chains do not form strong stable intermolecular associations;[48] however, at high concentrations they form hydrodynamic interactions which give rise to networks which can act as a molecular sieve, excluding cells and large molecules, thereby contributing to vitreous transparency.[49,50] These space-filling networks can interact with collagen, thus forming a stable macromolecular vitreous structure.[4]

MOLECULAR ORGANISATION OF THE VITREOUS GEL

The collagen–hyaluronan network is responsible for the molecular structure, distribution of cells, volume and transparency of the vitreous.[51] In humans, the vitreous is normally present as a gel-like structure where the two macromolecules interact in a stabilising manner: the crossed protein fibrils providing an elastic collagen network, in which the hyaluronan carbohydrate is entwined and providing viscosity. Models have been proposed where the highly hydrated hyaluronan plays a pivotal role in maintaining the network spacing and stabilising the gel structure;[52,53] however, entirely removing the hyaluronan meshwork (by digestion with hyaluronan lyase) does not destroy the gel structure,[54] indicating that this GAG is not essential for gel structure, although it is likely that it increases the gel's mechanical stability.

The collagen fibrillar network is crucial in maintaining the vitreal gel structure. Other molecules present in the vitreous, such as those associated with the collagen fibril surface, could indirectly link the collagen fibrils together and stabilise the network.[55] In summary, maintenance of the vitreous matrix structure involves interactions between all its macromolecular components: collagens, hyaluronan, proteoglycans and glycoproteins.[52,56,57]

AGE–RELATED CHANGES IN VITREAL CONNECTIVE TISSUE

The human vitreous is subject to age-related changes, and morphologically two distinct but simultaneous structural alterations occur: (1) collapse of the collagen network (syneresis); and (2) formation of collagen free, liquid-filled spaces (synchysis). Clinically, these alterations are important, as they lead to posterior vitreous detachment.

The vitreous undergoes liquefaction with age, initially occurring in pockets which then coalesce.[58] The liquefaction is due to a decrease in gel volume, believed to occur by syneresis (contraction) of the collagen fibrillar network. The collagen fibrils aggregate into large bundles and the rheology of the vitreous body is therefore modified.[59] These structural changes occur by the time the eye has reached adult size; 14–15 years (20% liquefied), progressing steadily after the age of 40–50 years, and by 80–90 years ~50% of the vitreous is liquefied.[47,60]

With syneresis, the collagen fibrils separate away from the gel and interact together, forming precipitates, which produce symptoms recognised as floaters.[58] The posterior border of the vitreous base separates from the retina as the gel-like structure of the vitreous collapses, leading to posterior vitreous detachment (PVD).[61–63] PVD is common with ageing, and usually makes a clean break away from the retina. However, the vitreous adheres tightly to the retina in certain places and a small, horseshoe-shaped tear in the retina can result from persistent tugging by the vitreous, leading to retinal detachment.[64]

Some recent studies have shown that collagen fibril degradation (most likely enzymatic), rather than aggregation, is central to the pathogenesis of age-related vitreous liquefaction, prompting future studies re-evaluating the mechanism of degradation of the collagen network.[65]

GLUCOSE METABOLISM

Glucose is an important metabolite which is present in all tissues of the eye. Its presence in tears and aqueous humour arises from plasma, and provides a source of glucose to intraocular avascular eye structures. The vitreous glucose is utilised by the hyalocytes to form glucosamine, and ultimately hyaluronic acid; however, much of the glucose is utilised by the adjoining retina.

Glucose metabolism giving rise to energy in the form of adenosine triphosphate (ATP) occurs in the cornea, lens and retina. All of these tissues are capable of storing limited glucose as glycogen for additional energy requirements; however, these tissues depend on the continuous supply of essential glucose to maintain the integrity of the tissue.[66,67]

There are various pathways utilised in metabolising glucose in ocular tissue, including glycolysis (yielding 2 ATP) which occurs under aerobic and anaerobic conditions; the tricarboxylic acid (TCA) cycle produces a further 36 ATP, but only occurs under aerobic conditions; under anaerobic conditions, lactate is produced from pyruvate, the end-product of glycolysis. The hexose monophosphate or pentose phosphate shunt utilises glucose-6-phosphate with no ATP production; however, its products ribose-5-phosphate and reduced nicotinamide adenine dinucleotide phosphate (NADPH) are important metabolites. At high glucose concentration glucose can be converted to sorbitol by auto-oxidation, or enzymaticaly utilising NADPH, with no net ATP production (Figure 2.3.1).

CORNEAL GLUCOSE METABOLISM

The cornea is bathed in tears to the exterior, and by the aqueous humour to the interior, providing nutrients including glucose, its major metabolic fuel supplying energy for maintenance of transparency.[68,69] Aerobic metabolism of glucose to CO_2 and H_2O, through glycolysis and Krebs (TCA) cycle, yields 38 ATP per glucose molecule.[66,70] However, much of the glucose is metabolised by the hexose monophosphate pathway (the pentose shunt) with no production of ATP. The products are ribose-5-phosphate, a metabolite for nucleic acid synthesis and NADPH (×2), an important reducing cofactor.[71–73]

The corneal epithelium is permeable to oxygen, and therefore oxidising reactions giving rise to reactive oxygen species (which oxidise the sulfhydryl (-SH) groups of proteins) occur. Reduced glutathione (GSH) present in the cornea reduces reactive oxygen species, and during the reaction GSH becomes oxidised to glutathione disulfide (GSSG). Auto-oxidation of GSH itself can also give rise to GSSG. The enzyme GSH reductase functions to regenerate GSH via the following reaction:

$$GSSG + NADPH + H^+ \rightarrow 2GSH + NADP^+$$

The NADPH required for this reaction is provided by the hexose monophosphate pathway, and therefore this metabolic pathway and GSH reductase play an important role in protecting the corneal tissue against oxidative stress.[74,75] Conversely, the restriction of oxygen access to the corneal epithelium by tight contact lenses worn for long periods of time, or the replacement of air with N_2 in goggles, leads to anaerobic lactic

acid production from pyruvate (the end-product of glycolysis), leading to corneal swelling and opacity.[76]

LENS GLUCOSE METABOLISM

The lens receives glucose from the aqueous and vitreous humour, where it is rapidly metabolised through three main pathways: (1) glycolysis (80–85%); (2) TCA (Krebs) cycle (~5%); and (3) hexose monophosphate (pentose shunt) (10–15%).[77,78] The entry of glucose appears to occur by facilitated diffusion.[69,79] Glycolysis yields 2 ATP per glucose molecule, and under anaerobic conditions the end-product pyruvate is converted to lactic acid, which diffuses into the aqueous and is eliminated via the circulation. During aerobic conditions, the pyruvate is further metabolised via the TCA cycle to CO_2 and H_2O, yielding a further 36 ATP molecules.[80]

The maintenance of the lens structural integrity requires: (1) osmotic balance provided by Na^+,K^+-ATPase; (2) redox balance provided by glutathione (and GSH reductase); and (3) protein synthesis necessary for growth and maintenance of the tissue. The ATP generated by glycolysis and Krebs cycle is utilised in active ion and amino acid transport, and in continuous protein and GSH synthesis.[81]

The lens proteins (crystallins) are important in maintaining lens transparency (see Chapter 2.1), and the GSH plays a role in maintaining the native unaggregated state of these proteins by reducing or reversing oxidative damage by ultraviolet radiation. The hexose monophosphate pathway in the lens provides the NADPH required by GSH reductase, which is important in maintaining GSH and redox balance.[78]

Glucose can be converted to sorbitol by auto-oxidation,[82,83] or enzymatically by aldose reductase,[84] which utilises NADPH supplied by the hexose monophosphate pathway.[80,85] Sorbitol can be converted to fructose by sorbitol dehydrogenase; however, the ratio of the two enzymes in the human lens favours sorbitol production.[86] Less than 5% of glucose is converted to sorbitol under normal conditions, and it slowly diffuses out to the aqueous humour and therefore does not accumulate in the lens. However, high external glucose concentrations lead to increased lens glucose, which saturates the normal metabolic pathways, leading to increased sorbitol synthesis.[86,87] Sorbitol accumulation leads to increased osmolarity of the lens, which affects the structural organisation of crystallins and promotes denaturation and aggregation, leading to increased scattering of light and possibly cataract.[80,88]

Due to ease of diffusion from aqueous, the lens is rarely glucose-deficient; however, infantile hypoglycemia, a group of diseases with low glucose levels, leads to a decrease in lens and cataract development.[89,90]

RETINAL GLUCOSE METABOLISM

The retina is one of the most metabolically active tissues and, like the brain, it derives most of its energy from glycolysis.[91,92] Hence, the glucose supply to the photoreceptors is very important.[93] The retinal capillaries supply glucose and oxygen to the inner layers, while the choroidal circulation supplies them to the retinal pigment epithelium and the photoreceptor cells. The blood–retinal barrier is overcome by carrier-mediated facilitated diffusion through specific plasma membrane glycoproteins, the glucose transporters GLUT 1 and GLUT 3.[94–97]

The glucose from the choriocapillaris is converted to glycose-6-phosphate by hexokinase enzyme in the pigment epithelium, which then diffuses to the ellipsoid of the photoreceptor cells, which contains the cytoplasmic glycolytic and mitochondrial TCA cycle enzymes capable of converting glucose to pyruvate and then to CO_2 and H_2O.[98]

Even though glucose metabolism occurs under aerobic conditions, there is a large accumulation of lactate in retina, indicating that the rate of glycolysis far exceeds the TCA cycle.[99–103] This lactate accumulation under aerobic conditions is also seen in brain, embryonic tissue and leukocytes.

Most of the in vitro respiration and lactate production in the retina is attributable to the photoreceptor cells.[102,104–108] ATP requirements here are high for the maintenance of Na^+,K^+ ATPase, which is active during steady dark current.[102,105,108–110] However, ATP also provides energy during illumination for axonal transport (neuronal signal-

processing), outer segment renewal and biosynthesis of cell membranes.[108,111]

Glucose metabolism is the primary source of ATP in this tissue, but in the absence of glucose (hypoglycemia, aglycemia) the retina can metabolise exogenous lactate or pyruvate, protecting the tissue from the toxic effects of glucose deprivation.[112,113]

The hexose monophosphate pathway (HMP) is also active in the retina. In the rod and cone nuclei, this pathway provides ribose for DNA and RNA synthesis. The provision of NADPH by this pathway in the retina is used for the maintenance of GSH, like other ocular tissues. Although the retinal HMP activity is low, it is upregulated during conditions of oxidative stress.[93,114]

The polyol pathway converts glucose to fructose via a sorbitol intermediate. Aldose reductase catalyses the conversion of glucose to sorbitol utilising NADPH as its reducing cofactor, and the second reaction is catalysed by sorbitol dehydrogenase, which utilises NAD^+ cofactor to transform sorbitol to fructose.[115,116] During hyperglycaemia, the production and accumulation of sorbitol occur in the retina along with the cornea and lens. The increased metabolism of glucose via the polyol pathway, and hence raised intracellular sorbitol concentration, has been linked to the onset and severity of diabetes-associated pathology of these ocular tissues such as retinopathy and cataract.[117–120] Many studies are investigating inhibition of aldose reductase, and hence sorbitol, formation as a pharmacological treatment for ocular diabetic complications.[117,121]

SUMMARY

Glucose is a very important ocular metabolite, and its supply is of utmost importance in the cornea, lens and retina where metabolism via glycolysis and TCA cycle produces ATP, an important cellular energy supply. The alternative HMP generates no ATP but does provide ribose-5-phosphate needed for nucleic acid synthesis and the reducing cofactor NADPH. The NADPH supplied by the HMP is used by GSH reductase to regenerate glutathione, which combats reactive oxygen species and oxidative stress. The polyol pathway has little activity under normal physiological conditions; however, in an environment of high glucose concentrations an increase of glucose is metabolised through this pathway, possibly contributing to the pathology of some ocular diseases. In other words, excess glucose can have very toxic effects, consistent with the production of advanced glycation end-products and Maillard products. This has serious implications for macromolecular structure, and hence tissue transparency.[122]

References

1. Forrester JV, Dick AD, McMenamin P, Lee WR. The eye. Basic sciences in practice. London: WB Saunders; 1996.
2. Freeman IL. The eye. In: Weiss JB, Jayson MIV, eds. Collagen in health and disease. Edinburgh: Churchill Livingstone; 1982:388–403.
3. Foulds WS. Is your vitreous really necessary? The role of the vitreous in the eye with particular reference to retinal attachment, detachment and the mode of action of vitreous substitutes. Eye 1987; 1:641–664.
4. Ihanamaki T, Pelliniemi LJ, Vuorio E. Collagens and collagen-related matrix components in the human and mouse eye. Progr Retinal Eye Res 2004; 23:403–434.
5. Engel J, Dfimov VP, Maurer P. Domain organisations of extracellular matrix proteins and their evolution. Development Supplement 1994; 35–42.
6. Rubin K, Ahlen K, Reed RK. Dynamic interactions between cells and the extracellular matrix. In: Reed RK, Rubin K, eds. Connective tissue biology: integration and reductionism. London: Portland Press; 1998:17–25.
7. Allen WS, Ottenbein EC, Wardi AH. Isolation and characterization of the sulphated glycosaminoglycans of the vitreous body. Biochim Biophys Acta 1977; 498:167–175.
8. Iozzo RV. The biology of the small leucine-rich proteoglycans. Functional network of interactive proteins. J Biol Chem 1999; 274:18843–18846.
9. Hedbom E, Heingard D. Interaction of a 59kDa connective tissue matrix protein with collagen I and collagen II. J Biol Chem 1989; 264:6898–6905.
10. Schonherr E, Witsch-Prehn P, Harrach B et al. Interaction of biglycan with type I collagen. J Biol Chem 1995; 270:2776–2783.
11. Chakravarti S. The cornea through the eyes of knockout mice. Exp Eye Res 2001; 73:411–419.
12. Smelser GK, Pollack FM, Ozaniks V. Persistence of donor collagen in corneal transplants. Exp Eye Res 1965; 4:349.
13. Kern P, Menasche M, Robert L. Relative rates of biosynthesis of collagen type I, type V and type VI in calf cornea. Biochem J 1991; 274:615–617.
14. Moller-Pederson T, Ledet T, Ehlers N. The keratocyte density of human donor corneas. Curr Eye Res 1994; 13:163.
15. Kuwabara T. Current concepts in anatomy and histology of the cornea. Contact intraocular lens. Med J 1978; 4:101.
16. Craig AS, Robertson JG, Parry DA. Preservation of corneal fibril structure using low temperature procedures for electron microscopy. J Ultrastructure Mol Struct 1986; 96:172–175.
17. Komai Y, Ushiki T. The three-dimensional organization of collagen fibrils in the human cornea and sclera. Invest Ophthalmol Vis Sci 1991; 32:2244.
18. Jakus M. The fine structure of the human cornea. In: Smelser G, ed. The structure of the eye. New York: Academic Press; 1961:344.
19. Meek KM, Holmes DF. Interpretation of the electron microscopical appearance of collagen fibrils from corneal stroma. Int J Biol Macromol 1983; 5:17–25.
20. Meek KM, Fullwood NJ. Corneal and scleral collagens – a microscopist perspective. Micron 2001; 32:261–274.
21. Maurice DM. The structure and transparency of the cornea. J Physiol 1957; 136:263–286.
22. Hart RW, Farrel RA. Light scattering in the cornea. J Opt Soc Am 1969; 59:766–774.
23. Farrel RA, McCalley RL. Corneal transparency. In: Albert DN, Jakobiec FA, eds. Principles and practice of ophthalmology. Philadelphia, PA: WB Saunders; 2000:629–644.
24. Goldman JN, Benedek GB, Dohlman CH, Kravitt B. Structural alterations affecting corneal transparency in swollen human corneas. Invest Ophthalmol 1968; 7:501–519.
25. Doane KJ, Yang G, Birk DE. Corneal cell–matrix interactions: type IV collagen promotes adhesion and spreading of corneal fibroblasts. Exp Cell Res 1992; 200:490.
26. Freeman IL. Collagen polymorphism in mature rabbit cornea. Invest Ophthalmol Vis Sci 1978; 17:171.
27. Meek KM, Boote C. The organization of collagen in the corneal stroma. Exp Eye Res 2004; 78:503–512.
28. Ihanamaki T, Salminen H, Saamanen A-M et al. Age-dependent changes in the expression of matrix components in the mouse eye. Exp Eye Res 2001; 72:423–431.
29. Borcherding MS, Blacik IJ, Sittig RA et al. Proteoglycans and collagen fibre organisation in human corneoscleral tissue. Exp Eye Res 1975; 21:59–70.
30. Scott JE. Proteoglycan: collagen interactions and corneal ultrastructure. Biochem Eye 1991; 19:877.
31. Scott JE, Thomlinson AM. The structure of interfibrillar protein bridges (shape modules) in extracellular matrix of fibrous connective tissues and their stability in various chemical environments. J Anat 1998; 192:391–405.

32. Rada JA, Cornuet PK, Hassell JH. Regulation of corneal collagen fibrillogenesis in vitro by corneal keratan sulfate proteoglycan (lumican) and decorin core proteins. Exp Eye Res 1993; 56:635–648.

33. Scott JE, Orford CR. Dermatan sulphate-rich proteoglycan associates with rat tail tendon at the d-band in the gap region. Biochem J 1981; 197:213–216.

34. Bottner EA, Wolter JR. Transmission of the ocular media. Invest Ophthalmol 1962; 1:776.

35. Fatti I. Hydraulic flow conductivity of the vitreous gel. Invest Ophthalmol Vis Sci 1977; 16:565–568.

36. Balazs EA, Toth LZJ, Eckl EA, Mitchell AP. Studies on the structure of the vitreous body. XII. Cytological and histochemical studies on the cortical tissue layer. Exp Eye Res 1964; 3:57–71.

37. Balazs EA, Toth LZ, Ozanics V. Cytological studies on the developing vitreous as related to the hyaloid vascular vessel system. Graefes Arch Clin Exp Opthalmol 1980; 213:71–85.

38. Balazs EA, Ozanics V. Functional anatomy of the vitreous. In: Jakobiec FA, ed. Ocular anatomy, embryology and teratology. Philadelphia: Harper & Row; 1982:425–440.

39. Osterlin SE, Jacobson B. The synthesis of hyaluronic acid in vitreous. I. Soluble and particulate transferases in hyalocytes. Exp Eye Res 1968; 7:497–510.

40. Osterlin SE, Jacobson B. The synthesis of hyaluronic acid in vitreous. II. The presence of soluble transferase and nucleotide sugar in the acellular vitreous gel. Exp Eye Res 1968; 7:511–523.

41. Jacobson B. Biosynthesis of hyaluronic acid in the vitreous: V. Studies on a particulate hyalocytes glycosyl transferase. Exp Eye Res 1978; 27:247–258.

42. Newsome DA, Linsenmayer TF, Trelstad RL. Vitreous body collagen. Evidence for a dual origin from the neural retinal and hyalocytes. J Cell Biol 1976; 71:59–67.

43. Bleckman H. Glycosaminoglycan metabolism of cultured fibroblasts from bovine vitreous. Graefes Arch Clin Exp Ophthalmol 1984; 222:90–94.

44. Osterlin SE. The synthesis of hyaluronic acid in vitreous. III. In vivo metabolism in the owl monkey. Exp Eye Res 1968; 7:524–533.

45. Grimshaw J, Kane A, Trocha-Grimshaw J et al. Quantitative analysis of hyaluronan in vitreous humor using capillary zone electrophoresis. Electrophoresis 1994; 15:936–940.

46. Balazs EA, Laurent TC, Laurent UBG. Studies on the structure of the vitreous body. VI. Biochemical changes during development. J Biol Chem 1959; 234:422.

47. Balazs EA, Denlinger JL. Aging changes in the vitreous. In: Dismikes N, Sekular R, eds. Aging and human visual function. New York: Alan R Liss; 1982:45–57.

48. Almond A, Brass A, Sheehan JK. Deducing polymeric structure from aqueous molecular dynamics simulations of oligosaccharides: predictions from simulations of hyaluronan tetrasaccharides compared with hydrodynamic and X-ray fibre diffraction data. J Mol Biol 1998; 284:1425–1437.

49. Ushi T, Amano S, Oshika T et al. Expression, regulation of hyaluronan synthase in corneal endothelial cells. Invest Ophthalmol Vis Sci 2000; 41:3261–3267.

50. Bishop PN. Structural macromolecules and supramolecular organisation of the vitreous gel. Progr Retin Eye Res 2000; 19:323–344.

51. Balazs EA. The molecular biology of the vitreous. In: McPherson A, ed. New and controversial aspects of retinal detachment. New York: Harper & Row; 1968:3–15.

52. Scott JE. The chemical morphology of the vitreous. Eye 1992; 6:553–555.

53. Mayne R, Brewton RG, Ren Z-H. Vitreous body and zonular apparatus. In: Harding JJ, ed. Biochemistry of the eye. London: Chapman & Hall; 1997:135–143.

54. Bishop PN, McLeod D, Reardon A. The role of glycosaminoglycans in the structural organisation of mammalian vitreous. Invest Ophthalmol Vis Sci 1999; 40:2173–2178.

55. Bishop PN. Structural macromolecules and supramolecular organisation of the vitreous gel. Prog Retin Eye Res 2000; 19:323–344.

56. Balazs EA. Molecular morphology of the vitreous body. In: Smelser GK, ed. The structure of the eye. New York: Academic Press; 1961:293–310.

57. Balazs EA. The vitreous. Int Ophthalmol Clin 1973; 13:169–187.

58. Sebag J. Age-related changes in human vitreous structure. Graefes Arch Clin Exp Ophthalmol 1987; 225:89–93.

59. Sebag J. The vitreous: structure, function and pathobiology. New York: Springer-Verlag; 1989:73–95.

60. O'Malley C. The pattern of vitreous syneresis – a study of 800 autopsy eyes. In: Irvine AR, O'Malley C, eds. Advances in vitreous surgery. Springfield, IL: C Thomas; 1976:17–33.

61. Foos RY, Wheeler NC. Vitreoretinal juncture: synchysis senelis and posterior vitreous detachment. Opthalmologica 1982; 12:1502–1512.

62. Larsson L, Osterlin S. Posterior vitreous detachment. A combined clinical and physiochemical study. Graefes Arch Clin Exp Ophthalmol 1985; 223:92–95.

63. Wang J, McLeod D, Henson DB, Bishop PN. Age-dependent changes in the basal retinovitreous adhesion. Invest Ophthalmol Vis Sci 2003; 44:1793–1800.

64. McLeod D, Leaver PK. Trampolines and triangles. The surgical pathology of the vitreous. Trans Ophthalmol Soc UK 1977; 97:225–231.

65. Los LI, van der Worp RJ, van Luyn MJA, Hooymans JMM. Age-related liquefaction of the human vitreous body: LM and TEM evaluation of the role of proteoglycans and collagen. Invest Ophthalmol Vis Sci 2003; 44:2328–2333.

66. de Roeth A. Glycolytic activity of the cornea. Arch Ophthalmol 1951; 45:1239.

67. Kuwabara T, Cogan D. Retinal glycogen. Arch Ophthalmol 1961; 66:680.

68. Thoft RA, Friend J, Dohlam CH. Corneal glucose flux. Arch Ophthalmol 1971; 86:685.

69. di Mattio J. In vivo entry of glucose analogs into lens and cornea of the rat. Invest Ophthalmol Vis Sci 1984; 25:160–165.

70. Langham M. Utilization of oxygen by the component layers of the living cornea. J Physiol 1952; 117:461.

71. Kinoshita JH, Masurat T. Aerobic pathways of glucose metabolism in bovine corneal epithelium. Am J Ophthalmol 1959; 48:47.

72. Geroski DH, Edelhauser H, O Brien WJ. Hexose-monophosphate shunt response to diamide in the component layers of the cornea. Exp Eye Res 1978; 26:611–619.

73. Masterson E, Whitehart DR, Chader GJ. Glucose oxidation in the chick cornea: effect of diamide on the pentose shunt. Invest Ophthalmol Vis Sci 1978; 17:449–454.

74. Ng MC, Rilley MV. Relation of intracellular levels and redox state of glutathione to endothelial function in the rabbit cornea. Exp Eye Res 1980; 30:511–517.

75. Rilley MV. A role for glutathione and glutathione reductase in control of corneal hydration. Exp Eye Res 1984; 39:751–758.

76. Kaufman HE, Gasset AR. Clinical experience with the epikeratoprosthesis. Am J Ophthalmol 1969; 67:38.

77. Chylack LT, Cheng H. Sugar metabolism in the crystalline lens. Surv Ophthalmol 1978; 23:26.

78. Harding JJ, Crabbe MJC. The lens: development, proteins, metabolism and cataract. In: Davson H, ed. The eye, vol. II. New York: Academic Press; 1984:207–492.

79. Elbrink J, Bihler I. Characteristics of the membrane transport of sugars in the lens of the eye. Biochem Biophys Acta 1972; 282:337.

80. Kinoshita JH. Pathways of glucose metabolism in the lens. Invest Ophthalmol 1965; 4:786.

81. Kinoshita JH, Merola LA, Kern H. Factors affecting the cation transport of calf lens. Biochem Biophys Acta 1961; 47:458.

82. Wolff SP, Crabbe MJC, Thornalley PJ. The autooxidation of glyceraldehydes and other simple monosaccharides. Experientia 1984; 40:244.

83. Wolff SP, Crabbe MJC. Low apparent aldose reductase activity produced by monosaccharide auto-oxidation. Biochem J 1985; 226:625–630.

84. Varma SD. Aldose reductase and the etiology of diabetic cataracts. Curr Top Eye Res 1970; 2:95.

85. Giblin FJ, Nies DE, Reddy VN. Stimulation of the hexose monophosphate shunt in rabbit lens in response to the oxidation of glutathione. Exp Eye Res 1981; 33:289.

86. Kuck JFR. The formation of fructose in the ocular lens. Arch Ophthalmol 1961; 65:840.

87. Clark R, Zigman S, Lerman S. Studies on the structural proteins of the human lens. Exp Eye Res 1969; 8:172.

88. Kuriyama H, Sasaki K, Fukuda M. Studies on diabetic cataract in rats induced by streptozotocin. Ophthalmol Res 1983; 15:191.

89. Chlack LT. Mechanism of 'hypoglycaemic' cataract formation in the rat lens. I. The role of hexokinase instability. Invest Ophthalmol 1971; 10:887.

90. Merlin S, Crawford JS. Hypoglycemia and infantile cataract. Arch Ophthalmol 1971; 86:495.

91. Krebs HA. The Pasteur effect and the relations between respiration and fermentation. Essays Biochem 1972; 8:1–35.

92. Sokoloff L. Circulation and energy metabolism of the brain. In: Siegel GJ, Albers RW, Katzman R, Agranoff B, eds. Basic neurochemistry, 3rd edn. Boston: Little, Brown, 1981:471–495.

93. Miceli MV, Newsome DA, Schriver GW. Glucose uptake, hexose monophosphate shunt activity and oxygen consumption in cultured human retinal pigment epithelial cells. Invest Ophthalmol Vis Sci 1990; 31:277–283.

94. Takata K, Kasahara T, Kasahara M et al. Ultracytochemical localization of the erythrocyte/HepG2-type glucose transporter (GLUT 1) in cells of the blood–retinal barrier in the rat. Invest Ophthalmol Vis Sci 1992; 33:377–383.

95. Olson AL, Pessin JE. Structure, function and regulation of the mammaliam facilitative glucose transporter gene family. Annu Rev Nutr 1996; 16:235–256.

96. Knott RM, Robertson M, Forrester JV. Regulation of glucose transporter (GLUT 3) and aldose reductase mRNA in bovine retinal endothelial cells and retinal pericytes in high glucose and high galactose culture. Diabetologia 1993; 36:808–812.

97. Knott RM, Robertson M, Muckersie E, Forrester JV. Regulation of glucose transporters (GLUT-1 and GLUT-3) in human retinal endothelial cells. Biochem J 1996; 318:313–317.

98. Lowry O, Roberts N, Lewis C. The quantitative histochemistry of the retina. J Biol Chem 1956; 220:879.

99. Warburg O. Uber die Klassifizierung tierischer Gewebe nach ihrem Stoffwechsel. Biochem Z 1927; 184:484.

100. Cohen LH, Noell WK. Relationships between visual function and metabolism. In: Graymore C, ed. Biochemistry of the eye. London: Academic Press; 1965:36–50.

101. Winkler BS. Glycolytic and oxidative metabolism in relation to retinal function. J Gen Physiol 1981; 77:667–692.

102. Winkler BS. A quantitative assessment of glucose metabolism in the isolated rat retina. In: Christen Y, Doly CY, Droy-LeFaix MT, eds. Les seminaries opthalmologiques dIPSEN: vision et adaptation. Amsterdam: Elsevier; 1995:78–96.

103. Winkler BS, Arnold MA, Brassell MA, Puro DG. Energy metabolism in human retinal Muller (glial) cells. Invest Ophthalmol Vis Sci 2000; 41:3183–3190.

104. Cohen LH, Noell WK. Glucose metabolism of rabbit retina before and after development of visual function. J Neurochem 1960; 5:253–276.

105. Ames A III, Li Y-Y, Heber EC, Kimble CR. Energy metabolism of rabbit retina is related to function: high cost of Na⁺ transport. J Neurosci 1992; 12:840–853.

106. Ahmed J, Braun RD, Dunn R, Lisenmeier RA. Oxygen distribution in the macaque retina. Invest Ophthalmol Vis Sci 1993; 34:516–521.

107. Wang L, Kondo M, Bill A. Glucose metabolism in cat outer retina. Invest Ophthalmol Vis Sci 1997; 38:48–55.

108. Wang L, Tornquist P, Bill A. Glucose metabolism in pig outer retina in light and darkness. Acta Physiol Scand 1997; 160:75–81.

109. Sillman AJ, Ito H, Tomita T. Studies of the major receptor potential of the isolated frog retina. Vision Res 1969; 9:1435.

110. Hagins WA. The visual process: excitatory mechanisms in the primary receptor cells. Ann Rev Biophys Bioeng 1972; 1:131.

111. Sickel W. Retinal metabolism in dark and light. In: Fuortes MGF, ed. Handbook of sensory physiology, vol 7/2. Heidelberg: Springer-Verlag; 1972:667.

112. Zeevalk GD, Nicklas WJ. Lactate prevents the alterations in tissue amino acids, decline in ATP and cell damage due to aglycemia in retina. J Neurochem 2000; 75:1027–1034.

113. Winkler BS, Starnes CA, Sauer MW et al. Cultured retinal neuronal cells and Muller cells both show net production of lactate. Neurochem Int 2004; 45:311–320.

114. Winkler BS, Giblin FJ. Glutathione oxidation in retina: effects on biochemical and electrical activities. Exp Eye Res 1982; 36:287–297.

115. Kinoshita JH, Nishimura C. The involvement of aldose reductase in diabetic complications. Diabetes Metab Rev 1998; 4:323–337.

116. Yabe-Nishimura C. Aldose reductase in glucose toxicity: a potential target for the prevention of diabetic complications. Pharmacol Rev 1998; 50:21–33.

117. Kern TS, Engerman RL. Microvascular metabolism in diabetes. Metabolism 1986; 35:24–27.

118. Pugliese G, Tilton RG, Speedy A et al. Modulation of hemodynamic and vascular filtration changes in diabetic rats by dietary myo-inositol. Diabetes 1990; 39:312–322.

119. Pugliese G, Tilton RG, Speedy A et al. Vascular filtration function in galactose-fed versus diabetic rats: the role of polyol pathway activity. Metabolism 1990; 39:690–697.

120. Lee AYW, Chuang SSM. Contribution of polyol pathway to oxidative stress in diabetic cataract. FASEB J 1999; 13:23–30.

121. Ao S, Kikuchi C, Ono T, Notsu Y. Effect of instillation of aldose reductase inhibitor FR74366 on diabetic cataract. Invest Ophthalmol Vis Sci 1991; 32:3078–3083.

122. Paget C, Lecomte M, Ruggiero D et al. Modification of enzymatic antioxidants in retinal microvascular cells by glucose or advanced glycation end products. Free Radicals Biol Med 1998; 25:121–129.

123. Robert L, Legeais JM, Robert AM, Renard G. Corneal collagens. Pathol Biol 2001; 49:353–363.

Chapter **2.4**

Vitamins

Kumari Neelam and John Nolan

INTRODUCTION

Vitamins are organic micronutrients, which protect cells and tissues from detrimental effect of physical, chemical and microbial agents. The protective action of vitamins is attributable to maintenance and/or augmentation of the body's existing defence systems. Vitamins form an essential component of a balanced diet, as they cannot be synthesised de novo in humans.

The human body needs 13 different vitamins. Of these, four are fat-soluble (A, D, E and K) and nine are water-soluble vitamins (C and B-group). Fat-soluble vitamins differ from water-soluble vitamins in several respects. Water-soluble vitamins are readily absorbed from the diet, and do not require transport proteins in the plasma. Also, fat-soluble vitamins are stored in liver and adipose tissue, and therefore can be mobilised during periods of deprivation. In contrast, deficiency states of water-soluble vitamins can occur after a relatively short period of deprivation.

Some vitamins, such as A, C and E, serve as antioxidants, and protect cells against free radical damage. Free radicals are ubiquitous in the human body, and disrupt the physiological functioning at a cellular level. The antioxidant vitamins act synergistically with antioxidant enzymes in scavenging free radicals, and their site of action can be intracellular or extracellular.

Evidence is accumulating that oxidative damage may contribute to the pathogenesis of various age-related eye diseases, such as cataract and age-related macular degeneration (AMD).

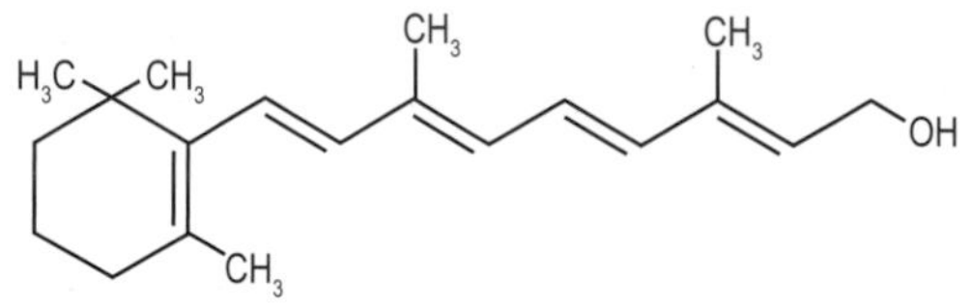

Figure 2.4.1   Biochemical structure of retinol.

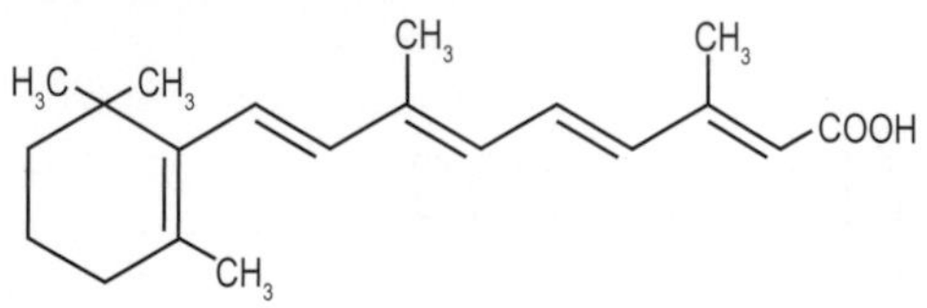

Figure 2.4.2   Biochemical structure of retinoic acid.

Antioxidant vitamins protect the eye against oxidative damage and may, therefore, prevent the development of these diseases. However, it is very difficult to isolate the influence of a specific vitamin in this process for two reasons. Firstly, the age-related eye diseases progress gradually with time, and, secondly, a multitude of factors (genetic and environmental) affect the development and progression of these conditions.

VITAMIN A

Vitamin A earned its name from the fact that it was the first vitamin to be discovered. It is a generic term for a large number of related compounds, and can be categorised into two main groups: preformed vitamin A (retinoids) and provitamin A (carotenoids).

Retinoids

Retinoids include retinol, retinal, retinoic acid and related compounds, and are found entirely in food sources of animal origin. Retinol is primarily an alcohol containing a β-ionone ring with an unsaturated side chain (Figure 2.4.1). It is the most reduced form of vitamin A, and satisfies the requirement for all known functions of vitamin A. Retinol may be reversibly oxidised to retinal, the active form for visual functions involving rods and cones of the retina. Retinol can also be irreversibly oxidised to retinoic acid (Figure 2.4.2), which cannot be converted to retinol and retinal.

Carotenoids

Carotenoids include β-carotene and related compounds, and are limited to food sources of plant origin where they are closely associated with chlorophyll. Of the approximately 600 carotenoids that occur in nature, only 10% are precursors of vitamin A.[1] One molecule of β-carotene gives rise to two molecules of retinal; however, in vivo this reaction is inefficient because the intestinal mucosal enzyme is readily saturated, and, as a result, a considerable amount is absorbed as carotenes. In addition to provitamin A activity, carotenoids have antioxidant properties.

Digestion, absorption and transport

Vitamin A is heat-stable, with 70–90% retention during cooking over a wide range of temperatures. Vitamin A is a fat-soluble vitamin, and hence it must be incorporated into micelles in a bile-dependent reaction before its absorption. Consequently, dietary fat must be consumed with sources of vitamin A to ensure adequate absorption. Very low fat intake (<15% of total energy) reduces bioavailability of vitamin A.

In the diet, vitamin A in the form of retinyl esters is hydrolysed in the intestinal mucosa, releasing retinol and free fatty acids. The β-carotenes, provitamin A compounds, are first cleaved by dioxygenase to yield retinal, which is subsequently reduced to retinol by retinaldehyde reductase before absorption.

Retinol is esterified to palmitic acid, incorporated into chylomicrons and delivered to the blood. The uptake of chylomicron remnants by the liver results in storage of vitamin A as lipid ester within lipocytes. Transport of retinol from liver to the other tissues, including the outer retina, occurs by binding of the hydrolysed retinol to retinol-binding protein (RBP), the stability of which is enhanced by the incorporation of albumin.

On reaching the basal side of the RPE in the retina, the complex attaches to specific membrane-binding sites, followed by cleavage of RBP and albumin from the retinol. The retinol then passes into the RPE cell, and is stored as retinyl esters or bound to cellular RBP and transported to the apical RPE cell membrane. In the apical membrane, the cellular RBP detaches, and the retinol passes into the subretinal space where it binds to interphotoreceptor retinol-binding protein (IRBP). It is finally conveyed to the photoreceptor cells where retinol gives rise to visual pigment rhodopsin, and is used in the visual cycle.

Much of the retinol produced during the photobleaching process diffuses out of the photoreceptor outer segments, and is esterified within the RPE. Esterification of retinol within the RPE appears to facilitate the retention of retinol within the eye. This may also act indirectly by protecting the retina from sustained exposure to high concentrations of retinol, which is well known to affect the stability of photoreceptor membranes. Furthermore, the RPE also serves as the site where reoxidation of retinol to retinal takes place.

Functions

Since its discovery, vitamin A has been shown to be pivotal in several bodily functions. One such function is related to vision, where it is intimately involved in visual transduction. The photoreceptor pigment of rod cells is called visual purple or rhodopsin, a complex between a protein opsin and 11-*cis*-retinal form of vitamin A. When exposed to light, 11-*cis*-retinal triggers a series of conformational changes on the way to conversion to the all-*trans*-retinal form. The altered form of opsin interacts with other proteins, activating the second messenger system, which results in the transmission of a nerve impulse and the perception of light. The all-*trans*-retinal is oxidised to retinol, then slowly converted to 11-*cis*-retinal for the reformation of rhodopsin (Figure 2.4.3).

Zinc deficiency interferes with vitamin A metabolism in several ways. Firstly, there is a decrease in synthesis of RBP, which transports retinol through the circulation to retina and other tissues. Secondly, there is decreased activity of the enzyme that releases retinol from its storage form, retinyl palmitate, in the liver. Thirdly, there is decreased conversion of retinol to retinal.[2]

Sources

Yellow and orange vegetables and fruits are good sources of β-carotenes and other carotenoids. Green vegetables also contain carotenoids, though they are masked by the presence of green pigment chlorophyll. The richest sources of retinol are beef and chicken liver. Other sources include whole milk, butter, cheese and other dairy products. Substances that adversely affect vitamin A availability include high doses of ferrous sulphate (iron supplement), tannic acid (black tea), aspirin and nitrates from processed meats.

Requirement

Although vitamin A requirements are given in mg of retinol equivalents (RE), vitamin A content of foods appears on the label in international units (IU). The conversion of IU to RE is made using conversion factors that depend on the source. One RE = 1 µg of retinol, 6 µg of β-carotene, or 12 µg of other carotenoids (6 µg of β-carotene = 1 µg retinol; 12 µg other carotene = 1 µg retinol). The recommended daily allowance (RDA) is 1000 RE for men and 800 RE for women.

Supplements

The principal forms of preformed vitamin A in supplements are retinyl palmitate and retinyl acetate. β-Carotene is also a common source of vitamin A in supplements, alone or in combination with retinol. If the total percentage of vitamin A content comes from β-carotene, then this information is included in the supplement facts label under vitamin A. Fortification of food products such as cereals, skim milk and margarine is done by addition of retinyl palmitate or other retinyl esters.

VITAMIN E

Vitamin E is recognised as one of the most important chain-breaking antioxidants of cellular membranes. It consists of eight tocopherols, the four

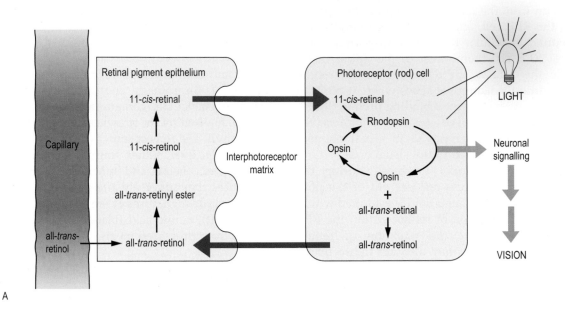

Figure 2.4.3   **A**, Role of vitamin A in vision; **B**, structure of 11-*cis*-retinal; **C**, structure of all-*trans*-retinal.

most common being α-tocopherol (TP), β-tocopherol, γ-tocopherol and δ-tocopherol. Of these, TP (Figure 2.4.4) is the most active and effective scavenger of free radicals, and the most predominant tocopherol in blood and tissues, including retina. In addition, this form appears to have the greatest nutritional significance, and meets the latest RDA for vitamin E. For these reasons, vitamin E intake is often expressed in terms of milligrams of TP equivalent.

Vitamin E is absorbed from the intestines packaged in chylomicrons. It is delivered to the tissues

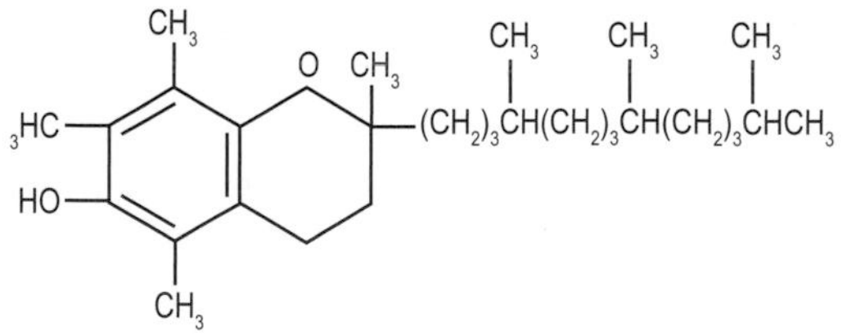

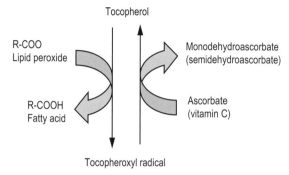

Figure 2.4.4　Biochemical structure of α-tocopherol.

Tocopherol

R-COO·
Lipid peroxide

Monodehydroascorbate
(semidehydroascorbate)

R-COOH
Fatty acid

Ascorbate
(vitamin C)

Tocopheroxyl radical

Figure 2.4.5　Interaction of vitamin E with lipid peroxides in cellular membranes.

via chylomicron, and then remnants of chylomicrons are taken up by liver that can export vitamin E in very-low-density lipoproteins. Due to its lipophilic nature, vitamin E accumulates in cellular membranes, fat deposits and other circulating lipoproteins. The major site of vitamin E storage is adipose tissue.

The vitamin E content of RPE is 4–7 times that in neurosensory retina (in the rod outer segments) and rises with increasing age, probably in response to an increase in oxidative stress. Further, the concentrations within these tissues are very sensitive to dietary intake of the vitamin.

Functions

Vitamin E is known to be a physiological antioxidant that protects biological membranes from auto-oxidation. It is uniquely suited to intercept the peroxidation of polyunsaturated fatty acids existing in cellular and subcellular membranes, thereby preventing them from establishing a chain reaction in the membrane (Figure 2.4.5). Apart from maintaining the integrity of cellular membranes, vitamin E also protects the lipids in low-density lipoproteins from oxidation. In addition, in the retina, vitamin E is believed to protect vitamin A from oxidative degeneration. Selenium, a micronutrient, complements the antioxidant function of vitamin E.

When a molecule of vitamin E quenches a free radical, it results in the formation of a vitamin E radical, which loses its antioxidant potential. However, vitamin C is capable of regenerating the active form of vitamin E and yields a vitamin C radical. Vitamin C radical, unlike vitamin E, is not a reactive specie because its unpaired electron is stable. The vitamin C radical is then converted back to vitamin C by glutathione.

Sources

Dietary sources of vitamin E, except for fish, are largely limited to the food sources rich in fat. Major sources of TP in the diet include vegetable oils (olive, sunflower, safflower oils), nuts, whole-grain and green leafy vegetables. It is advisable to take vitamin E supplements rather than increase high-fat foods in diet. Dietary intake of vitamin E is very difficult to estimate, because the long-term consumption of oils, in which the TP concentration varies considerably, is difficult to determine by questionnaire.

Requirement

RDA = 10 mg for men and 8 mg for women. Requirement increases as intake of polyunsaturated fatty acids increases.

Supplements

Synthetic TP does not have the same biological potency as the naturally occurring compound. In the naturally occurring compound, all three centres of asymmetry have the R-configuration, and therefore naturally occurring tocopherol is known as all-R- or RRR-TP. The bioavailability of this isomer is highest in the body. However, when it is synthesised chemically, the result is a mixture of the various isomers with less bioavailability and reduced potency.

TP supplements are available in the ester forms, TP succinate and tocopherol acetate. γ-Tocopherol and mixed tocopherol supplements are also commercially available.

VITAMIN C

Ascorbic acid, more commonly known as vitamin C, is a major water-soluble antioxidant in the body. In primates, the enzyme L-gulonolactone oxidase, responsible for the conversion of gulono-lactone to ascorbic acid, is absent, thus making vitamin C essential to the human diet. It is highly concentrated in all ocular tissues, with significant levels in aqueous. The active form of vitamin C is ascorbate acid itself (Figure 2.4.6). The primary causes of vitamin C deficiency are a decrease in dietary intake, or an increased requirement by tissues as a result of severe stress or trauma.

Functions

The most clearly established role of vitamin C is in collagen synthesis, where it acts as cofactor in the hydroxylation of proline and lysine residues. Hence, it is required for the maintenance of normal connective tissue, as well as for wound-healing.

Vitamin C is also a highly effective antioxidant. It reacts with, and inactivates, free radicals in cytosole, plasma and extracellular fluid. It is an ideal scavenger because of its water-solubility, stability, and the fact that it can be transported, reabsorbed and recycled. Vitamins C and E are interrelated in their antioxidant capabilities. Vitamin C may regenerate the active form of vitamin E following scavenging of free radical.[3]

Sources

Citric fruits such as strawberries, oranges and grapefruits are rich sources of vitamin C. Among vegetables, sweet red pepper and tomatoes are also good sources. Past studies have shown that the bioavailability of vitamin C from vegetables is similar to that from a supplement, as release of vitamin C from the food matrix is not a limiting step during its absorption.[4]

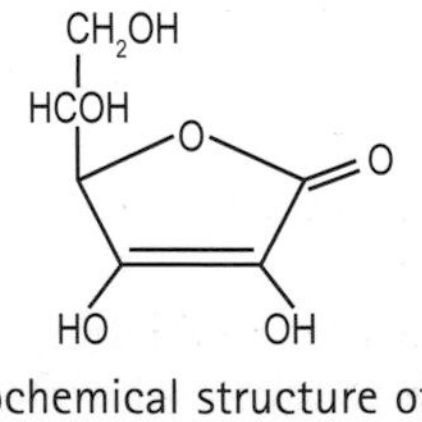

Requirement

The requirement for vitamin C to prevent clinical scurvy is less than 10 mg/day, and for optimum wound-healing an intake of 20 mg/day is required. This illustrates extremely well how different criteria of adequacy, and different interpretations of experimental evidence, can lead to different estimates of requirements.

Supplementation

The major factor predicting the plasma response of vitamin C following supplementation depends on the previous status existing in the volunteers, because saturation of plasma occurs at about 80 µmol/l.[5] Natural and synthetic L-ascorbic acids are chemically identical, and there are no known differences in their biological activities or bioavailability. Of the various supplements of vitamin C (L-ascorbic acid) available, there is little scientific evidence that any one form is better absorbed or more effective than another.

VITAMINS AND EYE DISEASES

Vitamin A deficiency

Vitamin A deficiency is the leading preventable cause of blindness among children in South-East Asian countries.[2] In the USA, night blindness is mainly encountered in the context of chronic alcoholism or malabsorption. The term 'xerophthalmia' refers to a constellation of classic signs and symptoms of vitamin A deficiency. Night blindness is the earliest and most common symptom of vitamin A deficiency, and is characterised by an increase in visual threshold, making it difficult to see in dim light. The effect on visual adaptation may be magnified when associated with Zn deficiency. The earliest sign is Bitot spots,

Figure 2.4.6 Biochemical structure of ascorbic acid.

which are seen as bilateral triangular foamy lesions at the temporal limbus.

Severe deficiency of vitamin A leads to keratomalacia (melting of cornea), resulting in scarring and irreversible blindness.[6] With the exception of Bitot spots and corneal scar formation from keratomalacia, the various forms of xerophthalmia are rapidly reversible with timely treatment. See Chapter 3.1 for more details on vitamin A deficiency.

Age-related macular degeneration

AMD is the leading cause of irreversible blindness in the western world. Studies in animal models indicate a possible role of cumulative oxidative damage in the aetiopathogenesis of AMD. In the retina, reactive oxygen species can promote lipid peroxidation of photoreceptor outer-segment membranes that are rich in polyunsaturated fatty acids. Thus, the hypothesis that vitamins with antioxidant properties might defend the retina against this damage seems biologically plausible. Supplementation with antioxidant vitamins does prevent retinal damage in several species.[7,8] However, epidemiological evidence for a beneficial effect of antioxidant vitamins against AMD in humans has been conflicting.[9,10] See Chapter 4.6 for more details on AMD.

Cataract

Currently, age-related cataract is the leading cause of visual impairment in the elderly population worldwide. It is proposed that, within the lens, reactive species of oxygen, generated through photo-oxidation and metabolic processes, can damage various components, including crystalline proteins, lens fibre membranes and enzymes, thus contributing to cataractogenesis.[9,11,12]

There is a growing interest in the possibility that a diet rich in antioxidant vitamins might reduce the risk of cataract by protecting lens proteins from oxidative injury. Indeed, in vitro animal research has suggested that the presence of antioxidant vitamins A, C and E may prevent cataractogenesis.[13,14] However, epidemiological studies in humans have shown inconsistent results.[15,16] See Chapter 4.5 for more details on cataract.

Retinitis pigmentosa

Retinitis pigmentosa (RP) is a group of hereditary retinal disorders characterised by progressive night blindness, waxy disc pallor and arteriolar attenuation. In a randomised double-masked trial, Berson et al. observed a significant retardation in the decline of cone electroretinogram with vitamin A supplementation (15 000 IU/day) in 601 patients with RP.[17] However, there was no statistically significant effect on the rate of decline in visual acuity and visual field.

Bassen–Kornzweig syndrome/hereditary abetalipoproteinemia is a variant of RP characterised by the inability to synthesise chylomicrons. The underlying defect seems to be an inability to secrete apolipoproteins B-100 and B-48. This results in malabsorption of fat and fat-soluble vitamins, including vitamins A and E. It has been observed that vitamin A and E treatment in the initial phase of this disease can prevent retinal degeneration and reversal of night blindness.[18,19] See Chapter 3.4 for more details on RP.

Gyrate atrophy

Gyrate atrophy occurs due to a mutation in the enzyme ornithine keto-acid aminotransferase, resulting in increased ornithine levels in serum and tissue. It is characterised by night blindness, myopia and scalloped areas of peripheral chorioretinal atrophy. Oral supplementation with vitamin B_6 (300–500 mg/day) results in a 30–50% decrease in plasma ornithine levels in a subset of patients with this disorder.[20,21]

Retinopathy of prematurity

Retinopathy of prematurity (ROP) is a vitreoretinopathy that occurs in premature infants with high ambience of oxygen. Premature infants have abnormally low levels of plasma vitamin E levels, and the levels can decrease rapidly because of lack of adipose tissue, the storage site for vitamin E.[22] Furthermore, vitamin E may prevent lipid peroxidation of the plasma membranes of the spindle cells in the developing retina.[23]

Several clinical trials have observed a decrease in the rate of development, or severity, of ROP in infants supplemented with vitamin E.[24–26]

Subsequently, a large randomised trial of vitamin E therapy for ROP has failed to demonstrate a consistent effect of vitamin E on the incidence, severity and blinding sequelae of ROP.[27] However, meta-analyses of existing data continue to indicate a beneficial effect of vitamin E therapy in ROP infants.[28]

Nutritional amblyopia

Nutritional amblyopia is associated with chronic alcoholism and heavy smoking. The main cause is poor nutrition, and a diet deficient in thiamin. It is characterised by a visual field defect in and around the point of fixation, resulting in centro-caecal scotoma. Vitamin supplementation may prevent further damage, but fail to reverse the existing degenerative changes.[28]

Chemical burns of the cornea

Vitamin C may play a role in the promotion of corneal healing in alkali burns by enhancing the production of collagens by keratocytes, and increasing the growth of keratocytes themselves. Experiments in animal models support this finding; however, data from humans are lacking.[29,30]

Vitamin C deficiency

The most significant ocular changes due to vitamin C deficiency include haemorrhage in the lids, conjunctiva, anterior chamber and/or retina.[31] In scorbutic infants, subperiosteal haemorrhage can result in significant proptosis of the eyeball.[32] The haemorrhagic tendency in various tissues in response to vitamin C deficiency occurs because of unstable vascular walls.

Riboflavin deficiency

Early symptoms of riboflavin deficiency in the eye include photophobia, tearing, burning and itching of the eyes. In late stages, ocular involvement can occur in the form of corneal neovascularisation. Riboflavin deficiency has also been implicated in cataractogenesis.

Nicotinic deficiency

Ocular involvement in nicotinic deficiency is rare, but optic neuritis or retinitis may develop.

References

1. Groff JL. Advanced nutrition and human metabolism, 2nd edn. St Paul: West Publishing; 1995.
2. Underwood BA, Arthur P. The contribution of vitamin A to public health. FASEB J 1996; 10:1040–1048.
3. Carr AC, Frei B. Toward a new recommended dietary allowance for vitamin C based on antioxidant and health effects in humans. Am J Clin Nutr 1999; 69:1086–1107.
4. Mangels AR, Block G, Frey CM et al. The bioavailability to humans of ascorbic acid from oranges, orange juice and cooked broccoli is similar to that of synthetic ascorbic acid. J Nutr 1993; 123:1054–1061.
5. Levine M, Conry-Cantilena C, Wang Y et al. Vitamin C pharmacokinetics in healthy volunteers: evidence for a recommended dietary allowance. Proc Natl Acad Sci USA 1996; 93:3704–3709.
6. Semba RD. Impact of vitamin A on immunity and infection in developing countries. In: Bendich A, Decklebaum RJ, eds. Preventive nutrition: the comprehensive guide for health professionals, 2nd edn. Totowa: Humana Press; 2001:329–346.
7. Snodderly DM. Evidence for protection against age-related macular degeneration by carotenoids and antioxidant vitamins. Am J Clin Nutr 1995; 62 (suppl):1448S–1461S.
8. Organisciak DT, Wang H, Li ZY, Tso MOM. The protective effect of ascorbate in retinal light damage of rats. Invest Ophthalmol Vis Sci 1985; 26:1580–1588.
9. Taylor A, Jacques PF, Dorey CK. Oxidation and aging: impact on vision. Toxicol Ind Health 1993; 9:349–371.
10. Christen WG. Antioxidant vitamins and age-related eye disease. Proc Assoc Am Phys 1999; 111:16–21.
11. Lerman S. Free radical damage and defence mechanisms in the ocular lens. Lens Eye Toxicity Res 1992; 9:9–24.
12. Anderson RE, Kretzer FL, Rapp LM. Free radicals and ocular disease. Adv Exp Med Biol 1994; 366:73–86.
13. Delamere N. Ascorbic acid and the eye. Subcell Biochem 1996; 25:313–329.
14. Fryer MJ. Evidence for the photoprotective effects of vitamin E. Photochem Photobiol 1993; 58:304–312.
15. Taylor A, Jacques PF, Epstein EM. Relations among aging, antioxidant status, and cataract. Am J Clin Nutr 1995; 62 (suppl):1439S–1447S.

16. Bunce GE, Kinoshita J, Horwitz J. Nutritional factors in cataract. Annu Rev Nutr 1990; 10:233–254.

17. Berson EL, Rosner B, Sandberg MA et al. A randomised trial of vitamin A and vitamin E supplementation for retinitis pigmentosa. Arch Ophthalmol 1993; 111:761–772.

18. Gouras P, Carr RE, Gunkel RD. Retinitis pigmentosa in abetalipoproteinemia: effects of vitamin A. Invest Ophthalmol Vis Sci 1971; 10:784–793.

19. Bishara S, Merin S, Cooper M. Combined vitamin A and E therapy prevents retinal electrophysiological deterioration in abetalipoproteinemia. Br J Ophthalmol 1982; 66:767–770.

20. Weleber RG, Kennaway NG. Clinical trial of vitamin B_6 for gyrate atrophy of the choroid and retina. Ophthalmology 1981; 88:316–324.

21. Kaiser-Kupfer MI, Caruso RC, Valle D. Gyrate atrophy of the choroid and retina, long-term reduction of ornithine slows retinal degeneration. Arch Ophthalmol 1991; 109:1539–1548.

22. Haga P, Ek J, Kran S. Plasma tocopherol levels and vitamin E/β-lipoprotein relationship during pregnancy and in cord blood. Am J Clin Nutr 1982; 36:1200–1204.

23. Kretzer FL, Mehta RS, Johnson AT et al. Vitamin E protects against retinopathy of prematurity through action on spindle cells. Nature 1984; 309:793–795.

24. Hittner HM, Godio LB, Rudolph AJ et al. Retrolental fibroplasia: efficacy of vitamin E in a double blind clinical study of pre-term infants. N Engl J Med 1981; 305:1365–1371.

25. Hittner HM, Rudolph AJ, Kretzer FL. Suppression of severe retinopathy of prematurity with vitamin E supplementation. Ultrastructural mechanism of clinical efficacy. Ophthalmology 1984; 91:1512–1523.

26. Finer NN, Schindler RF, Peters KL, Grant GD. Vitamin E and retrolental fibroplasia: improved visual outcome with early vitamin E. Ophthalmology 1983; 90:428–435.

27. Johnson L, Quinn GE, Abbasi S et al. Effect of sustained pharmacologic vitamin E levels on incidence and severity of retinopathy of prematurity: a controlled clinical trial. J Pediatr 1989; 114:827–838.

28. Coles WH. Ophthalmology: a diagnostic text. Baltimore, MD: Williams & Wilkins; 1989:326.

29. Pfister RR, Haddox JL, Lank KM. Citrate or ascorbate/citrate treatment of established corneal ulcers in the alkali-injured rabbit eye. Invest Ophthalmol Vis Sci 1988; 29:1110–1115.

30. Saika S, Uenoyama K, Hiroi K et al. Ascorbic acid phosphate ester and wound healing in rabbit alkali burns: epithelial basement membrane and stroma. Graefes Arch Clin Exp Ophthalmol 1993; 231:221–227.

31. Hoyt CS. Vitamin metabolism and therapy in ophthalmology. Surv Ophthalmol 1979, 24.177–190.

32. Dunnington J. Exophthalmos in infantile scurvy. Arch Ophthalmol 1931; 6:731–739.

Chapter **2.5**

Minerals and trace elements

Kumari Neelam and John Nolan

INTRODUCTION

Minerals and trace elements are inorganic substances, which are essential for the maintenance of haemostasis and physiological functioning of the human body. Each mineral is required in specific amounts, ranging from micrograms to grams per day, and the optimum balance is crucial for the survival of every cell in an organism. It has been estimated that about 20 different minerals are required in the human diet; of these, only seven have a well-established biological role.

Minerals, often known as micronutrients, are needed in very minute quantities, and can be categorised into one of the two following groups based on the daily requirement: (1) macrominerals; and (2) microminerals.

The daily requirement of macrominerals (minerals) exceeds 100 mg, and includes calcium, magnesium and phosphorus. The daily requirement of microminerals (trace elements) is less than 100 mg, and includes zinc (Zn), iron, copper (Cu), manganese (Mn), chromium, selenium (Se) and iodine.

Mineral and trace element deficiency is more common than vitamin deficiency. Those at increased risk include elderly people because of reduced dietary intake.[1] Moreover, a reduction in the stomach acid in the elderly further reduces the release of trace elements from ingested foodstuffs, and hence decreases their absorption. Deficient intake in association with reduced gastrointestinal absorption of minerals and trace elements inevitably results in inadequate bioavailability of these compounds.

Table 2.5.1   Trace elements in relation to the antioxidant enzymes/compounds that depend on them

	Antioxidant enzyme	Location	Mineral
1	Superoxide dismutase	Photoreceptors	Zn, Cu, Fe, Mn
2	Glutathione peroxidase	Retina, RPE, lens	Zn, Se, Cu, Fe
3	Catalase	RPE, lens	Zn, Cu, Fe
4	Retinal reductase	Retina	Zn
5	Metallothionein	RPE	Zn

RPE, retinal pigment epithelium; Zn, zinc; Cu, copper; Fe, iron; Mn, manganese; Se, selenium.

With ageing, there is a general decline in the antioxidant defences of many organ systems, including the eye.[2,3] The antioxidant system is dependent on a variety of nutritionally derived cofactors (Table 2.5.1). Indeed, oxidative stress has been proposed as the underlying mechanism for many age-related eye diseases such as cataract and age-related macular degeneration (AMD). Thus, it is reasonable to hypothesise that a declining bioavailability of trace elements could exacerbate the overall age-related reduction in antioxidant capability, and contribute to the onset of various age-related eye diseases.

ZINC (Zn)

Zn is the second most abundant trace element in the human body: total body content is approximately 2 g.[4,5] It is an essential trace element, and is believed to play a role in maintaining the health of the eye by protecting ocular tissues from age-related wear and tear.

Tauber and Krauss, in 1943, first demonstrated the existence of Zn in the human eye.[6] Later, Galin et al. observed high concentrations of Zn in the retina–choroid complex: 463 mg/kg body weight of the dried tissue.[7] Recent studies have shown that maximum concentration of Zn is present in melanin-containing tissues of the eye, most notably the retinal pigment epithelium (RPE). Other ocular tissues that contain Zn, in descending order of concentration, include: (1) iris; (2) choroid; (3) sclera; (4) vitreous; (5) lens; (6) cornea; and (7) retina.[8]

According to Newsome et al., Zn is mainly contained in the pigment granules of RPE (macular; 93.7%, peripheral; 92.4%). Therefore, the total concentration of Zn in RPE is greater at the macula, as opposed to the periphery, due to the presence of more pigment granules at the macular RPE. However, the amount of Zn per granule in RPE does not differ significantly between macular and peripheral regions of the retina. In contrast to the granular fraction, the concentration of the soluble fraction of Zn is higher in the peripheral RPE.[3]

The essential nature of Zn is related to its role with several metalloenzymes, as it acts as a cofactor for regulating the activity of specific Zn-dependent enzyme systems. Zn is also involved in membrane stabilisation and DNA and RNA synthesis. In recent years, its role in maintaining an intact immune system has become increasingly recognised. In the eye, its functions have been predominantly studied in the retina and RPE. The ocular functions of Zn which deserve special mention are as follows.

Vitamin A metabolism

Zn plays an important role in the transport and metabolism of vitamin A. In the retina, the conversion of retinol (circulating form) to retinal (active form) is mediated by a Zn metalloenzyme (retinol reductase), an alcohol dehydrogenase enzyme. Retinal is then utilised for the synthesis of rhodopsin, a visual pigment found in the rod photoreceptors, which is responsible for scotopic vision. Further, Zn also affects the synthesis and/or release of retinol-binding protein in liver. Vitamin A is bound to the retinol-binding protein in the plasma, and this complex transports vitamin A from liver to the retina.

Antioxidant properties

Zn plays a fundamental role in the antioxidant activity within cells, by several mechanisms. Firstly, it stabilises the cellular membranes, thus protecting the cell against lipid peroxidation. This process is particularly important in tissues such as retina, where high oxidative conditions prevail.[9] Therefore, loss of Zn from biological cell membranes, especially photoreceptors, increases their susceptibility to oxidative damage and impairs their ability to function properly. Secondly, Zn induces the formation of metallothionein (MT), and combines with the thiol group present on MT to form Zn–MT complexes.[10,11] When exposed to reactive oxygen intermediates (ROI), these complexes release Zn molecules, which protect membranes and other cellular organelles against oxidative damage.[12] Thirdly, Zn, with its high affinity for protein-sulfhydryl (SH) groups, may inhibit ROI from interacting with these proteins at these SH sites.[13] The binding of Zn with protein-SH groups results in displacement of Fe^{2+} and Cu^{2+} (ROI generators), which could interact with H_2O_2 in a Fenton-type reaction with consequential generation of highly reactive hydroxyl molecules.[14] Fourthly, Zn protects cells against oxidative damage indirectly through its action on several enzymes involved in the generation of ROI (e.g. reduced nicotinamide adenine dinucleotide phosphate (NADPH)-oxidases), and through its interaction with peptidases and hydrolases, which are crucial to the metabolism of ingested ROI.[15] Zn also participates in the regulation of the antioxidant system through its effect on catalase, the activity of which has been shown to decline in experimental animals with Zn deficiency, in an organ-specific manner.[16] Finally, Zn stabilises the structure of antioxidant enzymes such as superoxide dismutase (SOD), which seems to protect

aerobic cells against the detrimental effect of the superoxide radical. SOD occurs in several different compartments of the cell; however, Zn is only associated with the cytosolic and extracellular components.

Taurine and Zn work synergistically in the protection of cell membranes from free radical damage, by entrapping hydroxyl radicals. Recently, Zn has been found to play a role in apoptosis, or programmed cell death. Apoptosis can be triggered by oxidative stress, and has been implicated in many age-related eye diseases such as AMD, retinitis pigmentosa and low-tension glaucoma.

Sources

Zn is found in a wide variety of foods, and oysters contain the highest mole concentration of Zn, followed by shellfish and red meat. Nuts and legumes are relatively good plant sources. Of note, vegetarians need 50% more Zn than non-vegetarians, as a diet rich in plant proteins has high concentrations of phytates, which decrease Zn absorption from the digestive tract. A number of Zn supplements are commercially available, including Zn acetate, gluconate, picolinate and sulphate. Zn picolinate has been promoted as the most absorbable form of Zn, but there are few scientific data to support this claim. Tannins, present in red wines, chelate metal cations in the digestive tract, resulting in insufficient absorption of Zn. Large quantities of Zn in the diet can interfere with the bioavailability of Cu, through its induction of MT, a Cu-binding protein, which traps Cu within intestinal cells and prevents its systemic absorption.

Zinc and age–related macular degeneration

AMD, a degenerative disease of the macula, is the leading cause of blindness in western countries, and investigators have hypothesised that Zn plays a role in the pathogenesis of AMD. The rationale for such a hypothesis rests on the observed age-related alterations in Zn-dependent functions. Indeed, Newsome et al. have demonstrated an age-related decline of total Zn in human RPE, with the greatest decline in the soluble fraction of macular RPE, and in eyes with signs of AMD. This decline, in turn, results in a reduction in MT and catalase antioxidant activity, thus rendering RPE cells vulnerable to oxidative damage.[3]

A subsequent randomised, placebo-controlled trial provoked further interest, when it was found that a dietary supplement of 200 mg/day of Zn decreased the incidence of visual loss in patients with AMD.[17] Later, observational studies, as well as randomised trials, did not show a consistent association between dietary Zn intake and risk for AMD and/or its progression. However, the Age-Related Eye Disease Study (AREDS), a large randomised controlled trial of daily antioxidant supplements and high-dose Zn (80 mg), found that supplemental Zn in combination with antioxidants significantly reduced the risk of advanced AMD.[18] See Chapter 5.1 for more details on AREDS.

Zinc and cataract

Zn is important in maintaining the health of the crystalline lens in the eye, and is thought to reduce the risk for cataract formation by protecting the lens proteins from oxidative damage. Indeed, Zn deficiency has been associated with cataractogenesis in experimental animals.[19] However, the results from various observational studies in humans show conflicting results.

Zinc and night blindness

Deficiency of Zn reduces the levels of plasma retinol-binding protein, and retinol reductase,[20] with resultant low levels of vitamin A in the retina. This is consistent with the work of several investigators demonstrating that Zn deficiency can result in alteration of dark adaptation and/or night blindness, and that such changes can be reversed by supplementation of Zn.[21]

Zinc and retinitis pigmentosa

Retinitis pigmentosa (RP) is a heterogeneous group of hereditary retinal degenerations characterised by gradual progressive loss of photoreceptors. Currently, apoptosis appears to represent a common final pathway in the pathogenesis of RP, as suggested by human cases and animal models. Zn inhibits photoreceptor apoptosis through scavenging of intracellular ROI, establishing oxidative stress as a possible mediator of photoreceptor apoptosis in RP.[22]

Zinc and optic nerve diseases

A deficiency of Zn may play a role in the pathogenesis of certain toxic and nutritional optic neuropathies. In animal studies, Zn stabilises microtubules, which are necessary for axonal transport in neural tissue. In vitro, rapid axonal transport is affected by Zn deficiency, and may suggest a causative role in diseases of the optic nerve.[23] Indeed, an association between Zn deficiency and optic nerve disease is observed in acrodermatitis enteropathica, an autosomal recessive defect in intestinal Zn absorption. The ocular findings include development of optic atrophy, and gaze aversion due to cone abnormalities.[24] Further evidence for the role of Zn in optic nerve disease is seen in ethambutol-induced optic neuritis, as this antituberculosis medication is known to cause Zn deficiency.

Zinc and cornea

Although the existing knowledge of Zn metabolism in the cornea is not extensive, experimental studies have shown that Zn may play a role in the corneal repair process. The data from past studies indicate that epithelial and stromal corneal wound-healing is markedly delayed in Zn-deficient animals, as measured by tensile strength of the wound.[25] However, data from well-designed human studies are lacking.

SELENIUM

Se is an essential trace element with important antioxidant properties, and is the metal element in the antioxidant enzyme GSH.

Function

GSH is an Se-dependent enzyme, consisting of four identical subunits with an atom of Se, proba-

Figure 2.5.1 Glutathione peroxidase-selenium and antioxidation. GSSG, oxidised glutathione peroxidase; GSH, reduced glutathione peroxidase; NADP, nicotinamide adenine dinucleotide phosphate; NADPH, reduced NADP.

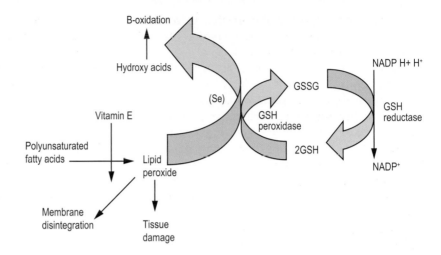

bly present as seleno-cysteine, at each active site. This natural sulphur-bearing peptide, found in the cytosole and mitochondria, acts in conjunction with vitamin E to protect cells against free radical damage by preventing lipid peroxidation (Figure 2.5.1).

Sources

The most concentrated food source for Se is the Brazil nut: a single nut contains 120 µg of Se. Other natural sources include seafood, meats, cereals (oat and brown rice), dairy products, fruit and vegetables (in descending order of importance). The concentration of Se in food sources depends on the level of Se in the soil in which the plant has been grown, as the distribution of Se on the Earth's crust is uneven. Due to decreased soil content of Se, there is widespread deficiency in many parts of China, the USA and Finland. Further, there is great concern about the declining levels of Se in the soil, possibly due to acid rain and heavy use of artificial fertilisers. Indeed, fertiliser is often fortified with Se in order to augment Se intake of the population. The reference nutrient intake of Se, given in a range rather than a fixed level due to lack of consensus on the ideal requirement, is 60–75 µg/day.[26] Of note, Se is possibly harmful if taken in excess.

Selenium and cataract

There is a very high concentration of GSH in the lens, where it acts as an antioxidant and is a key protective factor against intra- and extralenticular toxins. It has been proposed that a lack of Se to activate GSH impedes the destruction of peroxides/free radicals in the lens, leading to accumulation of free radicals, and consequential cataract formation. GSH is found to be markedly low in virtually all cases of cataract, and the activity of GSH in lens is significantly reduced in Se-deficient animals.[27]

Selenium and age-related macular degeneration

Although the aetiopathogenesis of AMD remains unclear, evidence is accumulating that oxidative damage may play an important role. GSH forms part of the complex antioxidant system of photoreceptors and RPE that protects the retina from oxidative damage. Further, there is a strong positive correlation between the dietary intake of Se and tissue GSH activity.[28] In laboratory animals, experimental Se deficiency is associated with increased lipid peroxidation.[29,30] This finding is consistent with the view that the age-related decline in plasma Se levels, established by previous investigators, would result in increased retinal oxidative injury (presumably related to reduced GSH activity in the retina), and thereby contribute to the development of AMD.

MANGANESE

The trace mineral Mn functions primarily as a component of the antioxidant enzyme superoxide dismutase (SOD), which limits the damaging effects of the superoxide free radical from destroying cellular components. Mn, therefore, may prevent cataract formation via its antioxidant properties, as development of age-related cataract is ultimately related to oxidative damage. Indeed, past studies have observed that SOD has a protective effect in the antioxidant defence of cultured lens epithelial cells.

COPPER

Although Cu is present in SOD, the role of Cu (and, indeed, other trace elements) in the ocular tissues remains poorly understood, and warrants further study.

References

1. Carroll MD, Abraham S, Dresser CM. Dietary intake source data: United States. Vital Health Stat 1983; 11:1–483.
2. Liles MR, Newsome DA, Oliver PD. Antioxidant enzymes in the ageing human retinal pigment epithelium. Arch Ophthalmol 1991; 109:1285–1288.
3. Newsome DA, Miceli MV, Tate DJ et al. Zinc content of human retinal pigment epithelium decreases with age and macular degeneration, but superoxide dismutase activity increases. J Trace Elements Exp Med 1995; 8:193–199.
4. Hsu JM. Biochemistry and metabolism of zinc. In: Karcioglu ZA, Sarper MR, eds. Zinc and copper in medicine. Springfield, IL: Charles C Thomas; 1980: 66–93.
5. Halsted JA, Smith JC Jr, Irwin MJ. A conspectus of research on zinc requirements of man. J Nutr 1974; 104:345.
6. Tauber FW, Krauss AC. The role of iron, copper, zinc, and manganese in the metabolism of ocular tissues with special reference to the lens. Am J Ophthalmol 1943; 26:260–266.
7. Galin MA, Nano HD, Hall T. Ocular zinc concentration. Invest Ophthalmol 1962; 1:142–148.
8. Eckhert CD. Elemental concentrations in ocular tissues of various species. Exp Eye Res 1983; 37:639–647.
9. Bray TM, Bettger WJ. The physiological role of zinc as an antioxidant. Free Radic Biol Med 1990; 8:281–291.
10. Hidalgo J, Campmany L, Borras M et al. Metallothionein response to stress in rats: role of free radical scavenging. Am J Physiol 1988; 254:E71–E78.
11. Thornally PJ, Vasak M. Possible role for metallothionein in protection against oxidative stress. Kinetics and mechanisms of its reaction with superoxide and hydroxyl radicals. Biochem Biophys Acta 1985; 827:36–44.
12. Fliss H, Menard M. Oxidant-induced mobilization of zinc from metallothionein. Arch Biochem Biophys 1992; 293:195–199.
13. Gibbs PNB, Gore MG, Jordan PM. Investigation of the effect of metal ions on the reactivity of thiol groups in human D-aminolevulinic dehydratase. Biochem J 1985; 225:573–580.
14. Stadtman ER. Metal ion-catalyzed oxidation of proteins: biochemical mechanisms and biological consequences. Free Radic Biol Med 1990; 9:315–325.
15. Ludwig JC, Misiorowski RL, Chvapil M, Seymor MD. Interaction of zinc ions with electron carrying coenzymes NADPH and NADH. Chem Biol Interact 1980; 30:25–34.
16. Taylor C, Bettger W, Bray T. Effect of dietary zinc or copper deficiency on the primary free radical defence system in rats. J Nutr 1988; 118:613–621.
17. Newsome DA, Swartz M, Leone NC et al. Oral zinc in macular degeneration. Arch Ophthalmol 1998; 106:192–198.
18. Age-related Eye Disease Research Group. A randomised, placebo controlled, clinical trial of high dose supplementation with vitamins C and E, beta carotene, and zinc for age related macular degeneration and vision loss. Arch Ophthalmol 2001; 119:1417–1436.
19. Barash H, Poston HA, Rumsey GL. Differentiation of soluble proteins in cataracts caused by deficiencies of methionine, riboflavin or zinc diets fed to Atlantic salmon, Salmo salar, rainbow trout, Salmo gairdneri, and lake trout, Salvelinus namaycush. Cornell Vet 1982; 72:361–371.
20. Huber AM, Gershoff SN. Effects of zinc deficiency on the oxidation of retinol and ethanol in rats. J Nutr 1975; 105:1486–1490.
21. McClain C, Kasarskis E, Allen J. Functional consequences of zinc deficiency. Progr Food Nutr Sci 1985; 9:185–226.
22. Carmody RJ, McGowan AJ, Cotter TG. Reactive oxygen species as mediators of photoreceptor apoptosis in vitro. Exp Eye Res 1999; 248:520–530.
23. Solomons NW, Russell RM. The interaction of vitamin A and zinc: implications for human nutrition. Am J Clin Nutr 1980; 33:2031–2040.
24. Karcioglu ZA. Zinc in the eye. Surv Ophthalmol 1982; 27:114–122.

25. Anderson AR, Kastl PR, Karcioglu ZA. Comparison of aqueous humour and serum zinc levels in humans. Br J Ophthalmol 1987; 71:212–214.

26. Department of Health. Dietary reference values for food energy and nutrients for the UK. London: HMSO; 1991:41.

27. Cai QY, Chen XS, Zhu LZ et al. Biochemical and morphological changes in the lenses of selenium and/or vitamin E deficient rats. Biomed Environ Sci 1994; 7:109–115.

28. Bunker VW. Free radicals, antioxidants and ageing. Med Lab Sci 1992; 49:299–312.

29. Csallany AS, Zaspel BJ, Ayaz KL. Selenium and ageing. In: Spallholz JE, Martin JL, Ganther HE, eds. Selenium in biology and medicine. Westport, CT: Avi; 1981:118–131.

30. Hafeman DG, Hoekstrta WG. Lipid peroxidation in vivo during vitamin E and selenium deficiency in rat as monitored by ethane evolution. J Nutr 1977; 107:666–672.

Chapter **2.6**

Carotenoids

John Nolan and Kumari Neelam

INTRODUCTION

The term 'carotenoid' refers to a class of fat-soluble coloured pigments, found primarily in plants, where they play a critical role in the photosynthetic process. They are also found in non-photosynthetic microorganisms (bacteria, yeast and moulds), where they are known to protect against the detrimental effect of excess light and oxygen. A similar action of carotenoids has been proposed to exist at the macula in the human eye.

BIOCHEMICAL STRUCTURE

The majority of carotenoids are derived from a 40-carbon polyene chain ($C_{40}H_{56}$), which forms the molecular backbone. The chain is terminated by cyclic end-groups (rings), and may be complemented with oxygen-containing functional groups. Changes in geometrical configuration about the double bonds located in the backbone result in the formation of *cis* and *trans* isomers. Carotenoids can be subdivided into carotenes, and their derivatives xanthophylls.

Carotenes

The hydrocarbon carotenoids are known as carotenes and include β-carotene, α-carotene and lycopene. β-Carotene, the principal carotenoid found in carrots, is a major source of vitamin A for the human body.

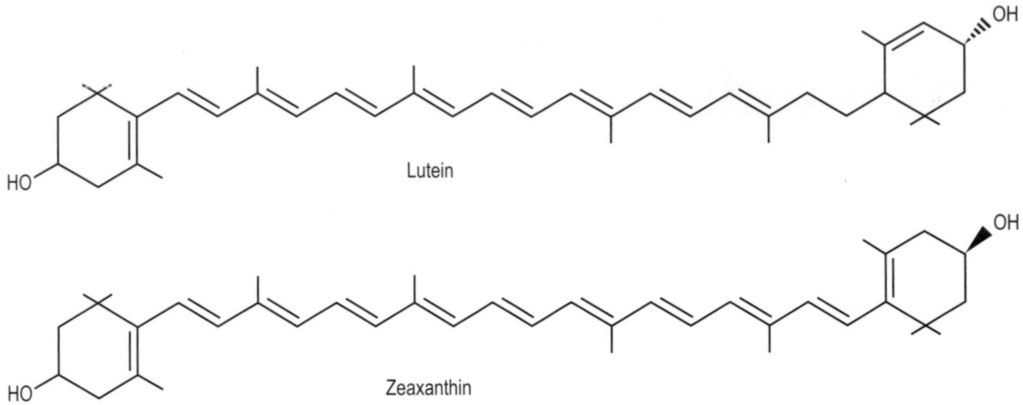

Figure 2.6.1 Chemical structures of lutein and zeaxanthin.

Table 2.6.1 Differences between lutein and zeaxanthin

Property	Lutein	Zeaxanthin
Maximum absorption spectrum	Below 500 nm	Above 500 nm
Orientation in lipid bilayer membrane	Two types of orientation: perpendicular (similar to zeaxanthin) or parallel to membrane	Perpendicular to the membrane
Scavenging action	As effective as β-carotene in quenching singlet oxygen	As effective as β-carotene in preventing auto-oxidation of lipids

Xanthophylls

The xanthophylls are oxygenated derivatives of carotenes. Two xanthophylls, lutein (L) and zeaxanthin (Z) accumulate at the macula where they make up macular pigment (MP). In the human eye, the MP optical density (MPOD) is not uniformly distributed across the retina.[1] It reaches its peak concentration in the central 1–2° of the fovea, and declines in an exponential fashion to optically negligible levels by 5–10° radial eccentricity.[2]

Structurally, L is an isomer of Z (Figure 2.6.1), which differs in the position of the double bond in the 6-carbon ring located on the right side of the carbon chain. Other differences between these two carotenoids are listed in Table 2.6.1. Of note, all three stereoisomers of Z are found in the macula, namely RRZ ({3R,3′R}-β,β-carotene-3,3′diol) meso-Z ({3R,3′S}-β,β-carotene-3,3′diol), and SSZ ({3S,3′S}-β,β-carotene-3,3′diol). The predominance of Z in the macula may be explained by the fact that L can be metabolised to Z.[3]

SPATIAL DISTRIBUTION OF MACULAR CAROTENOIDS

The MP is the most conspicuous accumulation of carotenoids in the human body. The concentration in the most central part of the macula has been estimated to be around 1 mmol/l, threefold higher than the typical carotenoid concentration in any other human tissue.

However, other adjacent ocular tissues such as the RPE/choroid and the ciliary body contain a much wider spectrum of carotenoids, including lycopene, β-carotene and β-cryptoxanthin (Figure 2.6.2).

According to Bone et al., an average mass of carotenoids per unit retinal area is 1.33 ng/mm² at

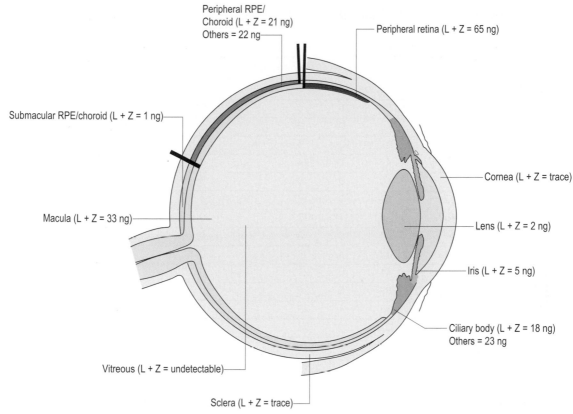

Peripheral RPE/
Choroid (L + Z = 21 ng)
Others = 22 ng

Peripheral retina (L + Z = 65 ng)

Submacular RPE/choroid (L + Z = 1 ng)

Cornea (L + Z = trace)

Macula (L + Z = 33 ng)

Lens (L + Z = 2 ng)

Iris (L + Z = 5 ng)

Ciliary body (L + Z = 18 ng)
Others = 23 ng

Vitreous (L + Z = undetectable)

Sclera (L + Z = trace)

Figure 2.6.2   Levels of lutein (L) and zeaxanthin (Z) in the human eye. RPE, retinal pigment epithelium. Modified from Bernstein PS. New insights into the rate of the macular carotenoids in age-related macular degeneration. Resonance Raman Studies. Pure Appl Chem 2002;74(8):1419–1425.

the centre of the fovea, and 0.81 ng/mm^2 at 1.6–2.5 mm eccentricity. Thus, there is a decrease in the total mass of pigment per unit area from central to the peripheral retina by a factor of almost 300.[4] L and Z do exist, albeit at insignificant levels, throughout the peripheral retina. Within the layer structure of the retina, the maximum concentration of carotenoids is found in the Henle fibre layer, the axons of the photoreceptors and the inner plexiform layer.

Sources

Carotenoids are not synthesised de novo by animals and therefore are entirely of dietary origin. Furthermore, carotenes cannot be converted to xanthophylls, and vice versa. Over 600 carotenoids have been identified from natural sources,[5] with up to 20 of these found in a typical western diet.[6] The highest amounts of L and Z,

combined, are found in egg yolk (54 mol% of L and 35 mol% of Z). However, maize and orange pepper have been shown to contain the highest amounts of L (60 mol%) and Z (37 mol%), respectively. Other rich sources of carotenoids include dark-green leafy vegetables and coloured fruits (Table 2.6.2).[7] However, the colour of the carotenoids is not evident in green leafy vegetables due to the masking effect of chlorophyll. Green leafy vegetables are good sources of xanthophylls, whereas yellow and orange vegetables contain predominantly carotenes. Gou qi zi, *Lycium barabarum*, deserves special mention. This small red berry, which is commonly used in home cooking in China, is a well-accepted herbal medicine to preserve good vision based on centuries of traditional experience in China.[8] It is tempting to hypothesise that the putative beneficial effect is attributable to its high content of Z (up to 5 mg/100 g).[9]

Table 2.6.2   Dietary sources of carotenoids (mol%)

	Xanthophylls			Carotenes			
	L and Z	L	Z	Cryptoxanthin	Lycopene	α-carotene	β-carotene
Egg yolk	89	54	35	4	0	0	0
Maize (corn)	86	60	25	5	0	0	0
Kiwi	54	54	0	0	0	0	8
Red grapes	53	43	10	4	5	3	16
Zucchini squash	52	47	5	24	0	0	5
Pumpkin	49	0	0	0	0	0	21
Spinach	47	47	0	19	4	0	16
Orange pepper	45	8	37	22	0	8	21
Yellow squash	44	44	0	0	0	28	9
Cucumber	42	38	4	38	0	0	4
Pea	41	41	0	21	0	0	5
Green pepper	39	36	3	20	0	0	12
Red grape	37	33	4	29	0	1	6
Butternut squash	37	37	0	34	0	5	0
Orange juice	35	15	20	25	0	3	8
Honeydew	35	17	18	0	0	0	48
Celery (stalks, leaves)	34	32	2	40	1	13	0
Green grapes	31	25	7	52	0	0	7
Brussels sprouts	29	27	2	39	0	0	11
Spring onions	29	27	3	35	4	0	0
Green beans	25	22	3	42	0	1	5
Orange	22	7	15	12	11	8	11
Broccoli	22	22	0	49	0	0	27
Apple (red delicious)	20	19	1	23	13	5	17
Mango	18	2	16	4	6	0	20
Green lettuce	15	15	0	36	0	16	0
Tomato juice	13	11	2	2	57	12	16
Peach	13	5	8	8	0	10	50
Yellow pepper	12	12	0	1	0	1	0
Nectarine	11	6	6	23	0	0	48
Red pepper	7	7	0	2	8	24	3
Tomato (fruit)	6	6	0	0	82	0	12
Carrots	2	2	0	0	0	43	55
Cantaloupe	1	1	0	0	3	0	87
Dried apricots	1	1	0	9	0	0	87
Green kidney beans	0	0	0	28	0	0	0

L, lutein; Z, zeaxanthin.

Digestion, absorption and transport

The digestion, absorption and transport processes of carotenoids are quite complex, and not well understood. Naturally occurring carotenoids are found in the form of protein matrices called carotenoproteins, which are the most important factor limiting carotenoid absorption in the gastrointestinal tract.[10]

Heating of food influences the availability of the carotenoids by denaturing the carotenoproteins, thus improving its accessibility. However, excess heating reduces their availability by isomerisation of all-*trans* double bonds to *cis* configurations. Thus, 60% of the xanthophylls, and 15% of the carotenes, present in foods are destroyed during the cooking process. Of the xanthophylls, L appears to be most heat-stable. Other dietary and non-dietary variables that affect carotenoid concentration in the human body are listed in Table 2.6.3.

Absorption of carotenoids takes place in the duodenum, involving formation of micelles, and is dependent on the action of existing bile juice and pancreatic lipases. This is followed by passive transfer of carotenoids into the mucosal cells. Hereafter, they enter the blood circulation by lymphatic duct, are taken up by the liver and are re-secreted on plasma lipoproteins.

Table 2.6.3 Factors affecting the bioavailability of carotenoids

Dietary factors
Size of food particle
Digestibility of food matrix
Fibre content
Fat level
Other carotenoids

Non-dietary factors
Intestinal malabsorption
Intestinal parasites
Drug interactions
Ethanol
P450 inducers

Liver disease

Kidney disease

In plasma, only six carotenoids have been identified: (1) lycopene; (2) β-carotene; (3) α-carotene; (4) β-cryptoxanthin; (5) L; and (6) Z. The carotenoids are exclusively transported in the non-polar core of lipoproteins, with the distribution largely determined by the physical properties of the carotenoids. L and Z are found predominantly in high-density lipoproteins (HDL: 53%), with lower proportions in LDL and very-low-density lipoproteins (VLDL) – 31% and 16%, respectively.

Accumulation of carotenoids in cells and tissues is largely determined by their polarity. The non-polar carotenoids, L and Z, are known to accumulate in the eye, liver and spleen,[11] with highest concentrations in adipose tissue (>80%).[11,12] Further, there is evidence of an inverse relationship between body fat and optical density of MP in the human eye.[13–15] In plasma, only a single isomer of L and Z is found, and this contrasts with the macula, where all three possible stereoisomers of Z are present.

The uptake and stabilisation of L and Z at the macula are unique, and they are evenly distributed between the cytosolic and membrane fractions. The cytosolic fraction, which is water-soluble, is passively deposited by tubulin in a non-specific manner.[16] The abundance of tubulin in the retina may explain, at least in part, the accumulation of L and Z at the macula to the exclusion of other carotenoids found in serum. However, specific xanthophyll-binding proteins are responsible for the accumulation of the membrane-associated fraction of carotenoids.

A typical western diet contains more L than Z, represented by an estimated ratio of 7 : 1.[17] Also, a similar finding has been reported in serum, with levels close to 5 : 1.[15–18] However, in the macula the ratio is reversed, with Z predominating over L (2 : 1). The latter finding may be explained by the observation that L can be isomerised to meso-zeaxanthin by a based-catalysed reaction involving shifting of a double bond.

Functions

In humans, carotenoids can serve several important functions. The most widely studied and well-known function of carotenoids is their provitamin

A activity. Vitamin A can be produced within the body from certain carotenoids, notably β-carotene, α-carotene and cryptoxanthin (for details, see Chapter 2.5). To date, the exact role of macular carotenoids remains elusive. However, the two main putative functions of the macular carotenoids, which are particularly attractive in terms of maintaining macular health, include blue light filtration and antioxidant activity.

Optical filter

The absorbance spectrum of MP peaks at 460 nm (blue light), thereby protecting the macula from photo-oxidative damage.[19] The fundamental means of blue light-induced damage is the photodynamic generation of free radicals (see page 102) from a toxic blend of light and oxygen.[20] It has been estimated that MP reduces the amount of blue light incident on the fovea by approximately 40%.[19] The relationship between wavelength of blue light and its potential to induce damage in the retina, expressed as the blue light hazard function, is maximised around 450 nm, the wavelength at which macular carotenoids absorb light.[21,22]

The filtering function of MP is particularly important in young individuals (30–40 years), when the lens is virtually transparent to blue light. This means that young individuals are at higher risk of macular exposure to blue light, and this may represent a risk for AMD. In newborns and infants, the retinal carotenoids are derived from human breast milk.[23]

In addition, the absorption of short-wavelength blue light by MP reduces chromatic aberration, as blue light has been primarily implicated in the image degradation at the fovea.[24,25]

Antioxidant properties

Kirschfeld apparently was the first to formulate the concept that carotenoids protect the macula via their antioxidant property.[26] However, the firm evidence that macular carotenoids act as antioxidants was provided by Khachik and co-workers in 1997,[27] by demonstrating the presence of direct oxidation products of macular carotenoids in the human retina.

Apoptosis (programmed cell death) plays a fundamental role in homeostasis, by maintaining a balance between cell division and elimination. Recent studies have observed that oxidative stress activates apoptosis. Carotenoids, by virtue of their antioxidant activity, may protect against this phenomenon.

FUNDAMENTAL CHEMISTRY

Singlet–oxygen quenching

The carotenoids quench singlet oxygen primarily by a physical mechanism, in which the excess energy of singlet oxygen is transferred to the electron-rich structure of the carotenoid. This added energy results in excitation of the carotenoid molecules into the triplet state ($^3Car^*$), and then the carotenoid relaxes to its ground state (^1Car) by losing the extra energy as heat. Because this is a physical mechanism (as opposed to a chemical reaction), the structure of the carotenoids remains unchanged. This activity is most significant to the retina, where there is abundance of polyunsaturated membranes located in the outer segments of the photoreceptors (for details, see Chapter 2.7).

$$^1O_2{}^* + {}^1Car \rightarrow {}^3O_2 + {}^3Car^*$$

$$^3Car^* \rightarrow {}^1Car + heat$$

The relative singlet-oxygen quenching ability of a given carotenoid is based on the number of its conjugated double bonds, and is given in Table 2.6.4. Hence, Z containing 11 double bonds is a more effective quencher of singlet oxygen, when compared with L.

The quenching activity of carotenoids in vivo is dependent on various parameters, such as concentration and solubility in the biological tissues, oxygen partial pressure, ionic strength, viscosity, cell structural complexity and presence of other redox-capable molecules or ions.

Radical scavenging

Carotenoids can scavenge free radicals in two ways. Firstly, the free radical obtains its 'missing' electron by taking one from the electron-rich

Table 2.6.4   Quenching capacity of different carotenoids

Carotenoid	Number of conjugated carbon–carbon double bonds	Terminal rings	Relative rates
Lycopene	11	0	103
Astaxanthin	11 (2)	2	80
Canthaxanthin	11 (2)	2	70
α-Carotene	10	2	63
β-Carotene	11	2	47
Zeaxanthin	11	2	33
Lutein	10	2	27
Cryptoxanthin	11	2	20

carotenoid. Secondly, the free radical adds itself to a carotenoid in its attempt to pair its single electron, thus forming a covalent bond. In either case, the electron-rich structure of the carotenoids makes them attractive to radicals, thus sparing other cell components (lipids, proteins, DNA) from oxidative damage.

CAROTENOIDS AND VISION

Carotenoids may play a vital role in maintaining ocular health, as many age-related eye diseases are thought to represent the end-stage of cumulative oxidative injury.

Cataract

Age-related cataract is the most common cause of visual impairment in elderly people worldwide.[28] Initially, the single-layered epithelium of the lens is damaged, followed by aggregation and cross-linkage of lens proteins, leading to cataract formation. It has been proposed that reactive oxygen species are generated through photo-oxidation and metabolic processes in the lens, leading to the afore-mentioned changes and thus contributing to the genesis of cataract. See Chapter 4.5 for more details on cataract.

Age-related macular degeneration

AMD is the commonest cause of visual impairment in the western world,[28] and oxidative stress represents an increasingly plausible aetiological mechanism for this condition. The retina is an ideal environment for generation of reactive oxygen intermediates due to its high content of polyunsaturated fatty acids, its exposure to high levels of visible light and oxygen, its wealth of chromophores and the continual process of phagocytosis by the retinal pigment epithelium. The function of macular carotenoids remains uncertain; however, they may protect against AMD through its filtering property, alone or in combination with its antioxidant activity. See Chapter 4.6 for more details on AMD.

Retinitis pigmentosa (RP)

RP is a genetically and clinically heterogeneous group of incurable retinal degenerative diseases. Aleman and co-investigators investigated MP in retinitis pigmentosa patients, and observed no significant difference between patients and controls. In addition, when supplemented with L, augmentation of MP density is observed in retinitis pigmentosa patients but is unaccompanied by an improvement in central visual acuity.[29] See Chapter 3.4 for more details on RP.

Choroideraemia

Choroideraemia is an X-linked progressive retinal degeneration affecting photoreceptors, retinal pigment epithelium cells and the choroid. Duncan and co-workers have studied the role of the L supplementation in a subset of patients having this disease, but no short-term change in central vision was seen in spite of MP augmentation.[30]

Stargardt's disease

Stargardt's disease is a dystrophy of the macula, and recent studies have reported that MP levels correlate well with the visual acuity in these patients.[31]

Diabetic retinopathy

Diabetic retinopathy is a complication of diabetes mellitus and is a leading cause of blindness.

Currently, studies are investigating the role of MP in diabetic patients.

CONCLUSION

There is a biologically plausible rationale which suggests that MP will protect the central retina from cumulative blue-light and/or oxidative damage, and any disease which is the result of at least one of these processes. However, a well-designed and large-scale, randomised, placebo-controlled trial of carotenoid supplements in the prevention and/or delay and/or modification of AMD has not yet been undertaken, and is required.

References

1. Bone RA, Landrum JT, Tarsis SL. Preliminary identification of human macular pigment. Vision Res 1985; 25:1531–1535.
2. Bone RA, Landrum JT, Dixon Z et al. Lutein and zeaxanthin in the eyes, serum and diet of human subjects. Exp Eye Res 2000; 71:239–245.
3. Khachik F, Englert G, Daitch CE. Isolation and structural elucidation of the geometrical isomers of lutein and zeaxanthin in extracts from human plasma. J Chromatogr 1992; 582:153–166.
4. Bone RA, Landrum JT, Ferandez L, Tarsis SL. Analysis of the macular pigment by HPLC: retinal distribution and age study. Invest Ophthalmol Vis Sci 1988; 29:843–849.
5. Ong ASH, Tee ES. Natural sources of carotenoids from plants and oils. Methods Enzymol 1992; 213:142–167.
6. Khachik F, Beecher G, Smith C. Lutein, lycopene, and their oxidative metabolites in chemoprevention of cancer. J Cell Biochem 1995; 22:236–246.
7. Sommerburg O, Keunen JEE, Bird AC, van Kuijk FJGM. Fruits and vegetables that are sources for lutein and zeaxanthin: the macular pigment in human eyes. Br J Ophthalmol 1998; 82:907–910.
8. Chai SS, Lee SF, Ng GP et al. Gou qi zi and its chemical composition. Chin Pharmacol Bull 1986; 11:31–43.
9. Lei Z, Leung I, Tso MOM, Lam KW. The identification of diapalmityl zeaxanthin as the major carotenoid in gou qi zi by high pressure liquid chromatography and mass spectrometry. J Ocul Pharm Ther 1999; 15:557–560.
10. Bryant JT, McCord JD, Unlu LK, Erdman JW. The isolation and partial characterization of α and β-carotene carotenoprotein(s) from carrot root chromoplasts. Food Chem 1988; 40:545–549.
11. Thomson LR, Toyoda Y, Langner A et al. Elevated retinal zeaxanthin and prevention of light-induced photoreceptor cell death in quail. Invest Ophthalmol Vis Sci 2002; 43:3538–3549.
12. Olson JA. Serum levels of vitamin A and carotenoids as reflectors of nutritional status. J Natl Cancer Inst 1984; 73:1439–1444.
13. Hammond BR, Ciulla TA, Snodderly DM. Macular pigment density is reduced in obese subjects. Invest Ophthalmol Vis Sci 2002; 43:47–50.
14. Johnson EJ, Hammond BR, Yeum KJ et al. Relation among serum and tissue concentrations of lutein and zeaxanthin and macular pigment. Am J Clin Nutr 2000; 71:1555–1562.
15. Nolan J, O'Donovan O, Kavanagh H et al. Macular pigment and percentage body fat. Invest Ophthalmol Vis Sci 2004; 45:3940–3950.
16. Bernstein PS, Balashov NA, Tsong ED, Rando RR. Retinal tubulin binds macular carotenoids. Invest Ophthalmol Vis Sci 1997; 38:167–175.
17. Nutrient Data Laboratory. US Department of Agriculture, Agriculture Research Service. 1998. Available online at: www.nal.usda.gov/fnic/foodcomp/
18. Bone RA, Landrum JT, Hime GW et al. Stereochemistry of the human macular carotenoids. Invest Ophthalmol Vis Sci 1993; 34:2033–2040.
19. Snodderly DM, Auran JD, Delori FC. The macular pigment II. Spatial distribution in primate retinas. Invest Ophthalmol Vis Sci 1984; 25:674–685.
20. Ruffolo JJJ, Ham WT, Mueller HA. Photochemical lesions in the primate retina under conditions of elevated blood oxygen. Invest Ophthalmol Vis Sci 1984; 25:893–898.
21. Ham WT, Mueller HA, Sliney DH. Retinal sensitivity to radiation damage from short wavelength light. Nature 1976; 260:153–158.
22. Hammond BR, Wooten BR, Snodderly DM. Protection of the retina by macular pigment. Invest Ophthalmol Vis Sci 1996; 37:3062.

23. Khachik F, Spangler CJ, Smith JC et al. Identification, quantification and relative concentrations of carotenoids and their metabolites in human milk and serum. Anal Chem 1997; 69:1873–1881.

24. Pease PL, Adams AJ, Nuccio E. Optical density of human macular pigment. Vision Res 1987; 27:705–710.

25. Reading VM, Weale RA. Macular pigment and chromatic aberration. J Am Optom Assoc 1974; 64:231–234.

26. Kirschfeld K. Carotenoids pigments: their possible role in protecting against photooxidation in eyes and photoreceptor cells. Proc R Soc Lond 1982; 216:71–85.

27. Khachik F, Bernstein PS, Garland DL. Identification of lutein and zeaxanthin oxidation products in human and monkey retinas. Invest Ophthalmol Vis Sci 1997; 38:1802–1811.

28. Stark WJ, Sommer A, Smith RE. Changing trends in intraocular lens implantation. Arch Ophthalmol 1989; 107:1441–1444.

29. Aleman TS, Duncan JL, Bieber ML et al. Macular pigment and lutein supplementation in retinitis pigmentosa and Usher syndrome. Invest Ophthalmol Vis Sci 2001; 42:1873–1881.

30. Duncan JL, Aleman TS, Gardner LM et al. Macular pigment and lutein supplementation in choroideremia. Exp Eye Res 2002; 74:371–381.

31. Zhang XY, Hargitai J, Tammur J et al. Macular pigment and visual acuity in Stargardt macular dystrophy. Graefes Arch Clin Exp Ophthalmol 2002; 240:10.

Chapter **2.7**

Oxidative stress and the eye

John Nolan, Kumari Neelam and Stephen Beatty

INTRODUCTION

The process of oxidation is essential if a cell is to provide energy for vital functions. During this process, 95–98% of the oxygen consumed is reduced to water, but the remaining fraction is converted to unstable and damaging ROI. At physiologic levels, ROI function as signalling and regulatory molecules, whereas at pathologic levels they are highly deleterious and act as cytotoxic oxidants. Even at low concentrations, prolonged exposure to ROI results in DNA mutation, tissue injury and disease.[1]

However, the body has an inherent defence system, consisting of antioxidants and antioxidant enzymes, which act synergistically in scavenging the ROI and thus protecting the underlying tissues. Oxidative stress occurs when the level of oxidants in a system exceeds the detoxifying capacity of its antioxidants, thus leading to oxidative damage to macromolecules with consequential injury to cells/tissues.

In this chapter, an overview of oxidative stress as it relates to different components of the eye, such as the retina, the lens and the trabecular meshwork, is discussed, as are its implications for age-related ocular diseases that affect these tissues, such as AMD, cataract and glaucoma, respectively.

OXIDATIVE PROCESSES

Chemical reactions which involve oxidation and reduction of molecules occur in every cell.

Chemically, oxidation refers to the removal of electrons, and reduction refers to the gain of electrons. The TCA cycle is responsible for most of the oxidation of dietary carbohydrates, proteins and lipids to CO_2 and H_2O. The energy yielded is conserved in the form of the reduced electron-accepting coenzymes, nicotinamide adenine dinucleotide (NADH) and flavin adenine dinucleotide ($FADH_2$). The electrons of these coenzymes can be used to reduce O_2 to H_2O via the electron transport chain, and this reaction releases energy for the conversion of adenosine diphosphate and inorganic phosphate to ATP in a process known as phosphorylation. Oxidative phosphorylation occurs in the mitochondrion and is catalysed by ATP synthase. The electron transport chain accounts for approximately 90% of our total O_2 consumption, the remainder being utilised by reactions involving oxidases or oxygenases. The majority of ROI are formed during energy generation from mitochondria, or during the detoxifying reactions involving the liver cytochrome P450 enzyme system.

Table 2.7.1 Reactive oxygen intermediates in living organisms

Radicals		Non-radicals	
Hydroxyl	$OH^•$	Peroxynitrite	$ONOO^-$
Superoxide	$O_2^{•-}$	Hypochloric acid	HOCL
Nitric oxide	$NO^•$	Hydrogen peroxide	H_2O_2
Thyl	$RS^•$	Singlet oxygen	$^{-1}O_2$
Peroxyl	$RO_2^•$	Ozone	O_3
Lipid peroxyl	$LOO^•$	Lipid peroxide	LOOH

$$Fe^{2+} + H_2O_2 \rightarrow FE^{3+} + OH^• + OH^-$$
$$Fe^{3+} + H_2O_2 \rightarrow FE^{2+} + OOH^• + OH^+$$

Figure 2.7.1 Fenton reaction. The hydroxyl radical is generated from hydrogen peroxide by the transfer of single electrons. $OH^•$, hydroxyl radical; H_2O_2, hydrogen peroxide.

REACTIVE OXYGEN INTERMEDIATES

Most ROI are the inevitable byproducts of normal and essential metabolic reactions, such as energy generation from mitochondria. However, pollution, asbestos, fungal or viral infections, cigarette smoking, excess consumption of alcohol, irradiation (mainly blue wavelength light), inflammation and ageing are all known to be associated with increased production of ROI.

ROI can be classified according to their reactivity towards biological targets, their site of production, their chemical nature, or their free radical or non-radical subgroups. In this section we describe ROI in terms of their free radical and non-radical subgroups (Table 2.7.1).

Free radicals are molecules that contain one or more unpaired electrons in their outer orbits.[2] In order to achieve a stable state, free radicals extract electrons from other molecules, which are themselves rendered unstable by this interaction, and a cytotoxic oxidative chain reaction results. Non-radical ROI contain their full complement of electrons, but in an unstable state. The most important among them is hydrogen peroxide and singlet oxygen. Hydrogen peroxide can generate free radicals through the Fenton reaction (Figure 2.7.1) and singlet oxygen can damage molecules as it converts back to normal oxygen.

ROI and cellular damage

Every component of the eye is vulnerable to damage from ROI; however, the retina is particularly susceptible. There are several reasons for the vulnerability of the retina, including: high concentrations of polyunsaturated fatty acid (PUFA); constant exposure to visible light; high consumption of oxygen; an abundance of photosensitisers in the neurosensory retina and the RPE; and the process of phagocytosis by the RPE, which is known to generate hydrogen peroxide.

The high concentrations of PUFA (50%) are found in the lipid bilayer of the outer segment of the rod photoreceptors, and docosahexaenoic acid, the most highly PUFA occurring in nature, accounts for approximately 50% of the vertebrate rod photoreceptor phospholipids.

The susceptibility of an unsaturated fatty acid to oxidation correlates directly with the number of its double bonds. Hence, PUFAs are particularly susceptible to free radical damage because their conjugated double bonds are convenient sources of hydrogen atoms, which contain one electron. The lipid radical thus formed then combines with oxygen to form lipid peroxyl radicals and lipid peroxides, which can only be stabilised by acquiring a quenching electron, probably from an adjacent PUFA. Thus, a cascade of reactions that consumes valuable PUFAs ensues.

A series of special conditions imposed upon photoreceptors puts them in what can only be termed a high-risk, pro-oxidant environment. Rod photoreceptor outer segments contain a high proportion of PUFAs which are readily oxidised, while the inner segments contain a considerable number of mitochondria, which leak a small but significant fraction of newly formed ROI. Also, it has been shown that the partial pressure in this environment is higher than found elsewhere in the body.[3]

Under normal conditions, the production of ROI is met by an ample supply of the detoxifying enzyme, SOD, whereas catalase and glutathione reductase are readily available to cope with hydrogen peroxide. These enzymes, in concert with antioxidant proteins and small molecular reductants, form an effective antioxidant defence within the photoreceptor. When overwhelmed, lipid peroxidation within the outer segment results.

Proteins make up the remaining 50% of the lipid bilayer of the rod outer segment. Fragmentation, cross-linking and aggregation of proteins, as well as enhanced vulnerability to proteolysis, can result from oxidation of their amino acids. The oxidised bases of DNA, arising from interactions with ROI, are believed to contribute significantly to ageing and age-related disorders involving many organ systems, including the eye.[4]

Assessments of ROI activity

There are various methods for assessing ROI activity; however, a consensus with respect to which is the most valid and reliable technique is still lacking. The three most commonly used techniques are: (1) determination of endogenous antioxidant levels; (2) measurement of the products of oxidised macromolecules; and (3) direct detection of ROI.

Antioxidant levels

The concentration of antioxidants in plasma and cells, and the cellular activities of antioxidant enzymes, can be used as a reflection of ROI activity.

Products of oxidised macromolecules

ROI damage may be identified, indirectly, by the presence of degradation products of lipids, such as malondialdehyde, in blood and/or urine. For assessing ROI-induced protein oxidation, protein nitrotyrosine has been widely used as a convenient and stable marker. Finally, urinary excretion of 8-hydroxydeoxyguanosine represents a useful means of assessing DNA base oxidation in humans.

Direct detection of ROI

Direct detection of ROI can be assessed using electron spin resonance and spin-trapping techniques. The electron spin resonance technique is suitable for detecting ROI in vitro, but it has limited application in vivo. The spin-trapping technique involves the conversion of ROI to relatively inert radicals, which are then detected by electron spin resonance analysis.

DEFENCE MECHANISMS AGAINST OXIDATIVE STRESS

Various defence mechanisms exist, which protect tissues against oxidative damage. These include quenching and/or removal of ROI by the antioxidant defence system, which comprises enzymatic and exogenous components, cellular compartmentalisation and repair. The most important is the antioxidant defence system (Figure 2.7.2).

An antioxidant is a substance that significantly delays or prevents oxidation of a substrate.

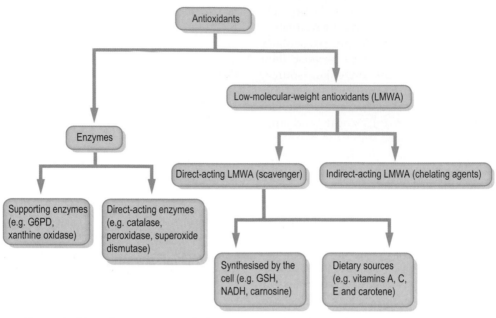

Figure 2.7.2   The antioxidant defence system. G6PD, glucose-6-phosphate dehydrogenase; GSH, reduced glutathione; NADH, nicotinamide adenine dinucleotide.

Sources of antioxidants may be classed as endogenous or exogenous. The endogenous antioxidants include glutathione, SOD and catalase, and they function by catalysing the decomposition of oxidants and free radicals.

The exogenous antioxidants include vitamins A, C and E, the carotenoids, bioflavonoids, selenium and zinc. These substances alleviate the oxidant load by directly quenching ROI before they damage vital cellular components.

ENDOGENOUS ANTIOXIDANTS

Glutathione

Glutathione is a universal antioxidant, and is abundant in cytoplasm, nuclei and mitochondria of cells, and is dependent on selenium as a cofactor. The concentration of cellular glutathione has a major effect on its antioxidant capacity, and it varies considerably as a result of nutrient limitation, exercise and oxidative stress (Figure 2.7.3). Glutathione exists in the following forms: the

antioxidant reduced glutathione, known as GSH and the oxidised form, known as glutathione disulphide (GSSG). The GSSG/GSH ratio in a living cell is believed to reflect oxidative stress.

Superoxide dismutases

SODs are metalloproteins, some of which contain manganese, whereas others contain copper or zinc. SOD catalyses the quenching of the superoxide anion to produce hydrogen peroxide and oxygen (see Chapter 2.5).

Catalase

Catalase is an iron-dependent enzyme that scavenges H_2O_2, either catalytically or peroxidatively. It has been demonstrated in human retina and RPE, where its activity has been shown to decline with increasing age. Also, a reduction in retinal catalase activity has been demonstrated in eyes with AMD.

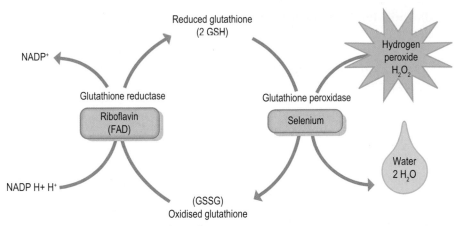

Figure 2.7.3 Glutathione oxidation reduction (redox) cycle. One molecule of hydrogen peroxide is reduced to two molecules of water, while two molecules of glutathione (GSH) are oxidised in a reaction catalysed by the selenoenzyme, glutathione peroxidase. Oxidised glutathione (GSSG) may be reduced by the flavin adenine dinucleotide (FAD)-dependent enzyme, glutathione reductase. NADP, nicotinamide adenine dinucleotide phosphate; NADPH, reduced NADP.

EXOGENOUS ANTIOXIDANTS

Vitamin A

It is believed that vitamin A may protect photoreceptor membranes against oxidative damage by breaking the chain reaction during lipid peroxidation. In addition, vitamin A is also involved in the repair of cells that have been injured by oxidation.

Vitamin C

Vitamin C is a major water-soluble antioxidant. It is an ideal scavenger because of its water solubility, stability and mobility, and because it can be transported, reabsorbed and recycled. Compared to plasma, all ocular tissues have very high concentrations of vitamin C.

Vitamin E

Vitamin E acts synergistically with carotenoids in scavenging free radicals. In the presence of vitamin E deficiency, various changes indicative of oxidative damage are seen in the rod outer segments and RPE, suggesting that this vitamin protects the retina against such injury.

Carotenoids

Carotenoids act as antioxidants by virtue of their free radical scavenging and singlet-oxygen-quenching capacity. The macular carotenoids are increasingly believed to protect the macula against oxidative damage by at least one of the following two mechanisms: filtering blue light at a prereceptorial level, thus limiting photochemical reactions; quenching free radicals. Consequently, carotenoids may protect against eye diseases putatively linked to oxidative stress, most notably age-related macular degeneration (for details, see Chapter 2.6).

Bioflavonoids

Bioflavonoids are large polyphenolic molecules, which are derived from the peel and coverings of teas, berries, grapes and bark. They exhibit a myriad of properties, such as anti-inflammatory, antibacterial and antioxidant activity. Of the sources of bioflavonoids, such as red wine, green tea and English blueberry, green tea produces the most potent antioxidants known to humans. Numerous studies have shown their unique role in protecting vitamin C from oxidation in the body, thereby allowing the body to reap more benefits from vitamin C.

OXIDATIVE STRESS AND AGE-RELATED MACULAR DEGENERATION

AMD is the late stage of age-related maculopathy (ARM), and is the leading cause of blind registration in the western world.[5] AMD results in loss of central vision due to choroidal neovascularisation with consequential subretinal fibrosis, or by atrophic changes of the RPE and overlying neurosensory retina.

The exact cause of AMD still remains elusive; however, oxidative stress has been increasingly linked to its aetiopathogenesis. As AMD is, by definition, an age-related disorder, the free radical and the evolutionary theories of ageing are of particular relevance to this discussion.

The free radical theory of ageing proposes that ageing and age-related disorders are the result of cumulative damage resulting from reactions involving ROI. If this theory applies to the eye, an altered antioxidant/oxidant balance should be evident for age-related eye disease such as AMD. The evolutionary theory of ageing proposes that there is a decline in the force of natural selection with increasing age, and that we may have evolved with genes which promote senescence once we have passed our period of procreation. In other words, we do not eliminate genes that have a detrimental effect in later life if they have a beneficial effect, or no effect, in early life.

Evidence of oxidative stress can be seen in the RPE and in the neurosensory retina with increasing age, and this damage is most prominent in the region of the retina where early AMD changes are seen. It has been shown that the concentration of lipofuscin, an age pigment, in the RPE increases with increasing age.[6] Lipofuscin consists of lipid/protein byproducts resulting from, at least in part, oxidatively damaged photoreceptor outer segments.[7] Further, it has been shown that lipofuscin compromises RPE cellular function.[8] But also, and of equal interest, lipofuscin generates ROI in response to irradiation with blue light, and therefore contributes further to oxidative stress in the local environment.[2] Various investigators have proposed that the age-related changes within the

RPE, the role of which is metabolically to maintain and support the photoreceptors, represent the earliest changes which ultimately lead to AMD. In brief, therefore, it appears that RPE dysfunction contributes to the pathogenesis of ARM/AMD, and that this dysfunction is related to lipofuscin accumulation, which, in turn, is related to oxidative injury. See Chapter 4.6 for more details on ARM/AMD.

MACULAR PIGMENT AND AMD

Macular pigment (MP) was first described as a yellow spot in the centre of the human eye, and was later found to be composed of two hydroxycarotenoids, lutein and zeaxanthin. MP is entirely of dietary origin, and is found in high concentrations in green leafy vegetables, fruits and egg yolk, and dietary modification can augment the optical density of MP.

The function of macular pigment remains uncertain, but it is likely that MP protects the retina from photochemical (oxidative) damage directly, by acting as a free radical scavenger, and indirectly, by filtering damaging blue light at a prereceptorial level. In addition, MP is known to reduce chromatic aberration.

Although the aetiopathogenesis of AMD remains a matter of debate, there is a growing body of evidence that cumulative oxidative damage, attributable, at least in part, to long-term blue light retinal injury, plays a role. Consequently, it has been postulated that the optical and antioxidant properties of MP confer protection against AMD, and that the augmentation of MP through dietary modification could delay, or even avert, the onset of AMD.[9]

The evidence in support of the view that MP protects against AMD can be classed as observational or epidemiological. Observational studies suggest that a lack of MP is associated with several known risk factors for AMD, including female gender, smoking, light iris colour, increasing age and disease in the fellow eye. However, these studies are often limited by small numbers of subjects, and are inconsistent.

Some epidemiological studies have shown a reduced risk of ARM/AMD in subjects with a higher intake of lutein and zeaxanthin, or higher plasma concentrations of these compounds,[10] while other epidemiological studies have failed to show such an association.[11]

ANTIOXIDANT AND AMD

The exact role antioxidants play in the protection against AMD remains unclear. Several large studies have examined the role of antioxidant supplementation in ARM/AMD, the largest of which was the AREDS. AREDS was a multicentre, prospective study of 4757 individuals aged 55–80 years, designed to assess the effect of dietary antioxidant supplements (vitamin E, vitamin C, β-carotene and zinc) on the clinical course of AMD. AREDS reported a beneficial effect of supplementation with this formulation, with reduced risk for disease progression by 25% and vision loss by 19%.[12]

OXIDATIVE STRESS AND CATARACT

ROI can be generated in the lens as a result of exogenous (UV light) or endogenous factors (enzymes). UV light represents an important factor, since the exposure of the lens to these wavelengths renders it vulnerable to ROI production, with consequential protein modification, lipid peroxidation and DNA fragmentation, all of which are believed to contribute to the genesis of cataract. Of these, the most important insult is protein modification, which includes protein disulphide cross-links and high-molecular-weight aggregation.

With increasing age, the protection and repair mechanism against oxidation in the lens, the key component of which is GSH, slowly deteriorates and becomes ineffective. As the lens ages, de novo synthesis and the recycling system of GSH become less efficient, resulting in a net decline in its concentration. Protein sulfhydryl groups can undergo oxidation, thus contributing to cataract formation. See Chapter 4.5 for more details on cataract.

OXIDATIVE STRESS AND GLAUCOMA

Glaucoma is a progressive and potentially blinding condition that affects approximately 70 million people around the world,[13] and open-angle glaucoma is the commonest variety seen in clinical practice. It is believed that raised intraocular pressure in primary open-angle glaucoma is attributable to malfunction of the trabecular meshwork (TM) – Schlemm's canal outflow system. The TM is believed to be exposed to chronic oxidative stress because of the presence of ROI in the aqueous humour,[14] and because of the generation of ROI by mechanical stress[15] and intracellular metabolism.[16]

Like other tissues, the TM possesses several protective mechanisms to deal with oxidative stress. One of these is proteasome, which protects the TM from oxidative injury by eliminating the altered proteins damaged by ROI. However, it has been suggested that the function of proteasome can be impaired by excessive exposure to oxidative stress by at least one of the following two mechanisms: (1) saturation of the proteasome by the presence of an excessive number of altered proteins; and/or (2) direct oxidation of proteasome components.[17] This impaired function of proteasome, and the consequential reduced capacity of the TM to protect itself from oxidative damage, has been proposed to underlie the pathophysiology of glaucoma. See Chapter 4.4 for more details on glaucoma.

OXIDATIVE STRESS AND RETINITIS PIGMENTOSA (RP)

RP is a progressive degeneration of the retina, and is best described as a phenotypic description of several related, yet distinct, dystrophies of the photoreceptors and the pigment epithelium. Apoptosis represents the final common pathway of cell death in RP, and it has been demonstrated that ROI act as mediators of retinal cell apoptosis in this condition. See Chapter 3.4.

OXIDATIVE STRESS AND RETINOPATHY OF PREMATURITY (ROP)

In paediatric medicine, oxidative stress has been implicated in the pathogenesis of numerous conditions. ROP deserves special mention; there is a general consensus that ischaemia–reperfusion injury, with consequential generation of ROI during the metabolism of ATP, results in ROP. ATP is degraded intracellularly via adenosine monophosphate to adenosine, which is further degraded to inosine and hypoxanthine outside the cell. Under normal conditions, hypoxanthine is metabolised to uric acid by the enzyme xanthine dehydrogenase (XDH), but under conditions of ischaemia or anoxia XDH is converted to xanthine oxidase (XO). Metabolism of hypoxanthine by XO results in release of superoxide anions, and consequential oxidative injury.

References

1. Mccord JM. The evolution of free radicals and oxidative stress. Am J Med 2000; 108:652–659.
2. Beatty S, Koh HH, Henson D, Boulton M. The role of oxidative stress in the pathogenesis of age-related macular degeneration. Surv Ophthalmol 2000; 45:115–134.
3. Alder VA, Cringle SJ, Constable IJ. The retinal oxygen profile in cats. Invest Ophthalmol Vis Sci 1983; 24:30–36.
4. Yannuzzi LA, Sorenson JA, Sobel RS et al. Risk factors for neovascular age-related macular degeneration. Arch Ophthalmol 1992; 110:1701–1708.
5. Bird AC, Bressler NM, Bressler SB et al. An international classification and grading system for age-related maculopathy and age-related macular degeneration. The International ARM Epidemiological Study Group. Surv Ophthalmol 1995; 39:367–374.
6. Wing GL, Blanchard GC, Weiter JJ. Topography and age relationship of lipofuscin concentration in retinal-pigment epithelium. Invest Ophthalmol Vis Sci 1978; 17:601–607.
7. Boulton M, Dontsov A, Jarvisevans J et al. Lipofuscin is a photoinducible free-radical generator. J Photochem Photobiol B-Biol 1993; 19:201–204.
8. Dorey CK, Wu G, Ebenstein D et al. Cell loss in the aging retina – relationship to lipofuscin accumulation and macular degeneration. Invest Ophthalmol Vis Sci 1989; 30:1691–1699.
9. Snodderly DM. Evidence for protection against age-related macular degeneration by carotenoids and antioxidant vitamins. Am J Clin Nutr 1995; 62:S1448–S1461.
10. Broekmans WMR, Berendschot TTJM, Klopping-Ketelaars IAA et al. Macular pigment density in relation to serum and adipose tissue concentrations of lutein and serum concentrations of zeaxanthin. Am J Clin Nutr 2002; 76:595–603.
11. Mares-Perlman JA, Brady WE, Klein R et al. Serum antioxidants and age-related macular degeneration in a population based case control study. Arch Ophthalmol 1995; 113:1518–1523.
12. Age-Related Eye Disease Study Research Group. Risk factors associated with age-related macular degeneration: a case-control study in the Age-Related Eye Disease Study: Age-Related Eye Disease Study report number 3. Ophthalmology 2004; 107: 2224–2232.
13. Quigley HA. Number of people with glaucoma worldwide. Br J Ophthalmol 1996; 80:389–393.
14. Spector A, Ma WC, Wang RR. The aqueous humor is capable of generating and degrading H_2O_2. Invest Ophthalmol Vis Sci 1998; 39:1188–1197.
15. Gonzalez P, Epstein DL, Borras T. Genes upregulated in the human trabecular meshwork in response to elevated intraocular pressure. Invest Ophthalmol Vis Sci 2000; 41:352–361.
16. Shringarpure R, Grune T, Davies KJA. Protein oxidation and 20S proteasome-dependent proteolysis in mammalian cells. Cell Mol Life Sci 2001; 58: 1442–1450.
17. Carrard G, Bulteau AL, Petropoulos I, Friguet B. Impairment of proteasome structure and function in aging. Int J Biochem Cell Biol 2002; 34:1461–1474.

SECTION 3

Nutrition deficiency and ocular disease

Chapter **3.1**

Vitamin A deficiency

Hannah Bartlett

INTRODUCTION

The term 'nutritional deficiency' has varying connotations, depending upon which part of the world is under discussion. In the extreme case, we can talk about starvation, commonly associated with the Third World. The various types of malnutrition that can occur have been summarised as follows:[1]

Total inanition: absence or insufficiency of all nutriment
Complete total inanition: an entire absence of food. The subject subsists on water alone
Incomplete total inanition: a diet that is insufficient in quantity in all respects
Aqueous-deficiency inanition: no nutriment of any kind (food or water) is ingested.

However, secondary deficiency may occur in the presence of an adequate diet. This can result from failure of metabolism of nutrients within the body and may be caused by disorders of digestion, absorption, transport or cellular metabolism.[2]

VITAMIN A DEFICIENCY

Vitamin A deficiency (VAD) is usually caused by prolonged dietary deprivation, and is endemic in areas where foods lacking in carotene are staple. An example is southern and east Asia, where rice is the main dietary component. Secondary VAD may be caused by inadequate conversion of carotene to vitamin A, or to interference with absorption, storage or transport of vitamin A.

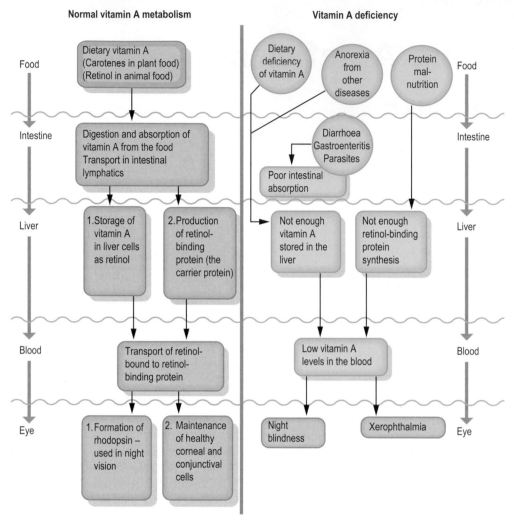

Figure 3.1.1   Normal vitamin A metabolism compared with the main causes of vitamin A deficiency. (Reproduced from Sandford-Smith J. Eye diseases in hot climates. Oxford: Butterworth-Heinemann; 1997:151, with permission.[3])

This may occur with conditions such as coeliac disease, cystic fibrosis and pancreatic disease. VAD is also common in protein–energy malnutrition (PEM), which retards growth and development and weakens the child's resistance to infection. Transport of vitamin A from the liver to the tissues relies upon production of retinol-binding protein (RBP). In protein deficiency there is insufficient RBP synthesised by the liver, which means that less retinol enters the blood stream and less vitamin A reaches the tissues[3] (Figure 3.1.1).

Function of vitamin A

Vitamin A is an essential nutrient for humans because it cannot be synthesised within the body. It is obtained from two sources: (1) preformed vitamin A from animal products; and (2) provitamin A (carotene), from plant products. Animal sources include milk, meat, fish and liver; plant sources include green leafy vegetables, yellow fruit and red palm oil.[4] Vitamin A is essential for maintenance of the integrity of epithelial tissues, and normal growth and differentiation of epithelial cells. It is also involved with reproduction, and the growth of developing bony structures.[4,5] The role of vitamin A in vision, specifically dark adaptation, was first shown by Wald.[6] In studies of sheep, pigs and frogs, he found vitamin A in the retinal pigment epithelium (RPE) and choroid.[7]

Histological effect of vitamin A deficiency

In the absence of vitamin A, keratinisation of epithelial tissue occurs, a process that can result in death.[8] In mucous membranes, secretory function is destroyed. Atrophy of the normal epithelial layer is followed by proliferation of basal cells, which in the epithelia of the cornea and conjunctiva tends to produce a continuous, keratinised layer. This replacement epithelium begins as one or two layers of flat cells, but epidermis-like tissue is soon formed and the original epithelium shed. The basal cells retain their ability to produce the appropriate epithelium however, and do so following administration of vitamin A.[9]

Primary vitamin A deficiency (xerophthalmia)

VAD is a public health problem in 118 countries, especially in Africa and South-East Asia.[10] Those at greatest risk of VAD are malnourished children born to vitamin A-deficient mothers. The World Health Organization (WHO) approximates that 228 million children worldwide are affected by VAD, making it the leading cause of childhood blindness.[11] VAD results in blindness in 350 000 children every year, and increases the chance of dying in childhood by 20%.[12] These high levels of mortality occur because affected children are susceptible to respiratory and intestinal infections.[13,14] VAD also increases susceptibility to potentially fatal childhood illnesses such as diarrhoeal disease and measles.[10]

Children become vitamin A-deficient for two main reasons: (1) their mothers are deficient and produce breast milk low in vitamin A; and (2) they are weaned on to diets that contain too little vitamin A. Another contributing factor is that they spend much of their childhood being ill, when anorexia and malabsorption further deteriorate

Table 3.1.1 World Health Organization classification of the clinical signs of xerophthalmia

Classification	Signs
XN	Night blindness
X1A	Conjunctival xerosis
X1B	Bitot's spots
X2	Corneal xerosis
X3A	Corneal ulceration–keratomalacia involving one-third or less of the cornea
X3B	Corneal ulceration–keratomalacia involving one-half or more of the cornea
XS	Corneal scars
XF	Xerophthalmic fundus

their vitamin A status.[15] In addition to having a dietary deficiency of vitamin A, women in developing countries spend a large proportion of their lives breast-feeding, which increases their requirement for the vitamin. In developed countries women have an average of 1.6 children[16] and breast-feed for an average of 5 months.[17] This means that they spend 8 months out of their 30 reproductive years breast-feeding. In underdeveloped countries, women have an average of five children and breast-feed each for 2 years.[16,17] This means that they spend one-third of their reproductive years breast-feeding, with a diet that provides less than one-third of the recommended daily allowance for vitamin A.

The use of the term 'xerophthalmia' has been adopted by the WHO to describe primary VAD[18] and will be used to indicate the clinical syndrome as a whole. The clinical signs of xerophthalmia were reclassified by the WHO in 1980[19] (Table 3.1.1).

Night blindness

Vitamin A is associated with specific proteins (opsins) in the form of visual pigments within the rods and cones. These opsins are different for each type of photoreceptor; the rods are especially sensitive to low-intensity light and the cones are sensitive to high-intensity light and colour. The retinal form of vitamin A is an active component of the photosensitive pigment in rods and cones. In the rods, retinal is found associated with opsin in the form of the visual pigment, rhodopsin. In cones, retinal is combined with other forms of opsin; the type of opsin determines the wavelength of light that can be absorbed by the retinal. When exposed to light, the rhodopsin is broken down into retinal and opsin, a process known as bleaching (see page 50 for details on the bleaching pathway). The reformation of rhodopsin requires a fresh supply of vitamin A. Incomplete reformation of rhodopsin, found in those who are vitamin A-deficient, results in poor dark adaptation. This is also known as night blindness.

Night blindness is the earliest and most common manifestation of VAD. Its presence can be confirmed by electroretinography even during subclinical VAD.[20] In early stages of VAD night blindness is reversible with systemic administration of vitamin A, and responds within 24–48 hours.

Conjunctival xerosis

The term 'xerosis' refers to drying of the conjunctiva and results from damage to the secretory function of mucous membranes and proliferation of basal cells. It typically affects the temporal, interpalpebral, bulbar conjunctiva and stains well with rose Bengal,[21] although it has been suggested that this staining is not specific enough to be diagnostic.[22] Signs include thickening, wrinkling and loss of pigmentation and transparency[2] (Figure 3.1.2).

Bitot's spots

Bitot's spots occur on the bulbar conjunctiva, most commonly temporally and usually confined to the interpalpebral fissure. They are classically triangular, although in practice many shapes are found.[2] They consist of keratinised epithelial debris which most often gives rise to a punctate granular appearance[23] (Figure 3.1.3).

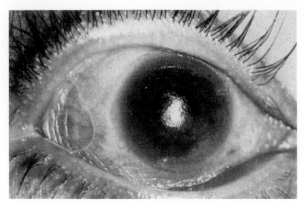

Figure 3.1.2 Conjunctival and corneal xerosis. The conjunctiva is dry, thickened and slightly pigmented. The light reflection from the corneal surface is altered and stringy mucus can also be seen. (Reproduced from Sandford-Smith J. Eye diseases in hot climates. Oxford: Butterworth-Heinemann; 1997:159, with permission.[3])

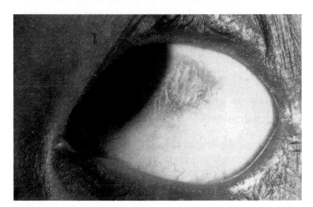

Figure 3.1.3 The Bitot's spot is characteristic in its triangular shape. It is also pigmented with foamy deposits on the surface. (Reproduced from Sandford-Smith J. Eye diseases in hot climates. Oxford: Butterworth-Heinemann; 1997:157, with permission.[3])

Corneal xerosis

Early stages of corneal involvement may present as haziness and dryness of the cornea, with small erosions or punctate superficial infiltrations.[5] The disorder is usually preceded by night blindness and Bitot's spots. Without intervention, the keratopathy progresses to epithelial defects, stromal oedema and keratinisation in the interpalpebral fissure.[24] Further progression results in ulceration of partial or full thickness, with potential for bacterial infection[21] (Figure 3.1.4).

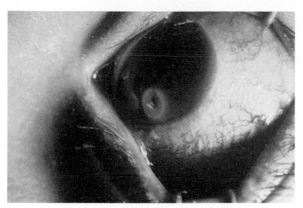

Figure 3.1.4   Corneal xerosis with ulceration, which is stained with fluorescein. (Reproduced from Sandford-Smith J. Eye diseases in hot climates. Oxford: Butterworth-Heinemann; 1997:159, with permission.[3])

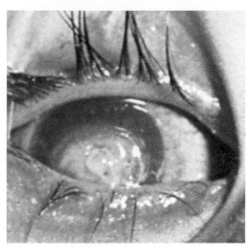

Figure 3.1.5   Keratomalacia. (Reproduced from McLaren D. Clinical manifestations of human vitamin and mineral disorders: a resume. In: Ross A, ed. Modern nutrition in health and disease. Baltimore, MD: Williams & Wilkins; 1999, with permission.[45])

Keratomalacia

This consists of liquefactive necrosis of the cornea, occurring rapidly and resulting in melting of the corneal structure into a gelatinous mass. In severe cases loss of the anterior chamber and extrusion of the lens may occur.[2] Vitamin A supplementation speeds healing, although other systemic diseases such as measles, diarrhoea or respiratory infection may be implicated in the development of keratomalacia. This more advanced stage of xerophthalmia may also be related to PEM[25] (Figure 3.1.5).

Xerophthalmic fundus

This condition was first described as a collection of small white spots on the fundus, similar in appearance to retinitis punctata albicans.[26] It usually occurs with night blindness and Bitot's spots and resolves with systemic administration of vitamin A within 1–4 months.[27] The spots have been classified as focal pigment epithelium defects by fluoroscein angiography.[28]

Treatment of xerophthalmia

Table 3.1.2 shows the WHO recommendations for vitamin A dosage. Most vitamin A preparations

are combined with small doses of vitamin E, which appears to aid vitamin A absorption and utilisation. Vitamin E supplementation has been demonstrated to prevent changes to the cornea and conjunctiva due to vitamin A deficiency.[29] Vitamin A accelerates the development of the epithelium, prevents keratinisation of the epithelium and provides fatty acids that combine with vitamin A.[30–32] Vitamin E is involved with membrane stabilisation and maintaining epithelial structures.[33] The preventive effect of vitamin E against vitamin A deficiency-induced corneal and conjunctival damage may be explained by the strong antioxidant effect of vitamin E, although the mechanism is not clear.

Studies show that this is an effective prevention programme.[34,35] Intermittent doses of vitamin A are sufficient as retinol is stored effectively by the liver and adequate serum levels can be maintained for up to 6 months.[3] Much lower doses are recommended for pregnant women to prevent teratogenic effects on the fetus. However, the need for supplementation during pregnancy was demonstrated by a group who found that the risk of mortality in the first 6 months of life was 63% higher among infants of night-blind than

Table 3.1.2 World Health Organization recommendations for vitamin A dosage

Emergency treatment of children with xerophthalmia or corneal ulcers

	Dose by mouth		
	mg	IU	
Day 1	110	200 000	
Day 2	110	200 000	
Two weeks later	110	200 000	
For children less than 1 year old these doses should be halved			

Preventive treatment within the community

	mg	IU	
Children under 1 year old	55	100 000	Repeat every 4–6 months
Children over 1 year old	110	200 000	
Children at birth	27.5	50 000	
Mothers just after giving birth	165	300 000	
Pregnant and lactating mothers	5.5	10 000	Daily for 2 weeks

non-night-blind women.[36] Active corneal xerophthalmia is uncommon in older children and adults, except in severe famines. However, most people with this condition go blind within 24–48 hours unless treated with vitamin A.[25] It is generally thought that the low-dose regimes set out for women of child-bearing age are not sufficient to prevent blindness in these cases. In the main, clinicians and women accept that the need to save the woman's sight outweighs the risk of damage to an unborn fetus, even if she is aware that she is pregnant.[37]

Secondary vitamin A deficiency

Disorders of digestion, absorption, transport, storage, cellular metabolism, elimination or basic requirements may be responsible for secondary vitamin A deficiency.[2] In the case of vitamin A, there are accounts of night blindness and xerosis of the conjunctiva associated with chronic liver disease,[38] and xerosis of the conjunctiva in chronic alcoholism.[32] Vitamin A deficiency has also been implicated in various intestinal diseases[39] and cirrhosis.[40]

Chapter **3.2**

Vitamin C deficiency and ocular disease

Hannah Bartlett

CHAPTER CONTENTS

Clinical vitamin C deficiency is known as 'scurvy' and was once widespread amongst sailors and explorers who depended upon preserved meat in a diet devoid of fruit and vegetables. Today, scurvy is far less common but may be found in infants who have been fed an exclusive cow's milk–formula diet with no supplements. Another susceptible group is ulcer patients who consume diets made up principally of milk, cream, eggs and cereals. The incidence of scurvy may reach epidemic proportions within groups of otherwise healthy individuals who undergo long periods of eating easily stored, non-perishable foods. An example is the soldiers of South Korea, during and immediately after the Korean war.[5] In practice, the group most likely to be affected by vitamin C deficiency are poor, elderly men,[41] especially those who are institutionalised, housebound or chronically sick.[42]

Vitamin C is used in the formation of intercellular ground matrix. It is essential in the production of collagen,[43] required for wound-healing; chondroid and osteoid, required for normal skeletal development;[44] and intercellular cement, required for cohesion of endothelial capillary cells. Impaired cohesion of endothelial capillary cells results in increased capillary fragility and consequently an increased risk of haemorrhage.[5]

SCURVY IN INFANTS (BARLOW'S DISEASE)

Scurvy usually develops between the age of 5 and 14 months, and symptoms include failure to gain

Table 3.2.1   Clinical manifestations of vitamin C deficiency

Systemic
Perifollicular haemorrhages
Coiled hairs
Inflamed and bleeding gums
Hyperkeratosis – thickening of the skin
Difficulty breathing
Build-up of fluid within the joints
Pain within the joints
Impaired wound-healing
Weakness
Fatigue

Psychological and neurological
Lethargy
Depression
Hysteria
Hypochondriasis

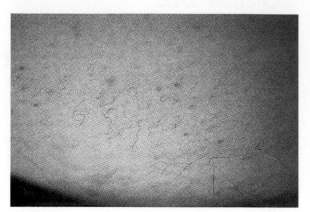

Figure 3.2.1   'Swan-neck' or corkscrew deformities of the hairs, characteristic of early adult scurvy. (Reproduced from McLaren D. Clinical manifestations of human vitamin and mineral disorders: a resume. In: Ross A, ed. Modern nutrition in health and disease. Baltimore, MD: Williams & Wilkins; 1999, with permission.[45])

weight, irritability, excessive crying and reduced appetite.[5] Pseudoparalysis (failure to move the limbs) most often involves the legs, and haemorrhages may occur, most commonly around erupting teeth. Painful haemorrhages may occur deep within the joints. A dose of 200 mg vitamin C orally every day for a week or 10 days provides rapid improvement.[2]

SCURVY IN ADULTS

The condition is most likely to affect those who are unable to cater for themselves adequately, and rely on long-life or preserved foods. However, scurvy is likely to take longer to develop than in infants as growth and skeletal development are not involved, and the body will have some stores of ascorbic acid. Table 3.2.1 gives an overview of the clinical manifestations of vitamin C deficiency.

Painful haemorrhages occur within the joints, accompanied by weight loss, loss of appetite, weakness and irritability.[5,45] As the condition advances, there are characteristic changes in the skin.[46] The first stage of skin involvement consists of acne, similar to that experienced by adolescents.

This is followed by hair deformity, consisting of broken, coiled hairs and a 'swan-neck' deformity, which refers to the hairs being flat instead of round in cross-section. The more noticeable symptoms of adult scurvy are perifollicular haemorrhages and perifollicular hyperkeratosis, usually affecting the thorax, forearms, thighs, legs and anterior abdominal wall. In extreme deficiency there is bleeding from the gums, which are spongy and swollen. Old wounds break down and new wounds are slow to heal.[45] In advanced stages there may be emotional changes such as hypochondriasis, depression or hysteria.[5] Convulsions and shock may result from bleeding into the brain or viscera and ultimately the patient may die[45] (Figure 3.2.1).

Treatment for adult scurvy is usually 100 mg vitamin C three to five times daily until 4 g has been administered, then 100 mg twice daily. Severe weakness and spontaneous bleeding should cease within 24 hours, pain and fever resolve within 48 hours, and gums and skin heal within 10–12 days.[2]

OCULAR MANIFESTATIONS OF VITAMIN C DEFICIENCY

The concentration of vitamin C (ascorbic acid) varies in different parts of the body, but is generally higher in the cells than in extracellular fluids. The aqueous and vitreous humours are the exception to this and have high concentrations of the vitamin, along with the lens.[2]

Animal studies have shown little effect of vitamin C deficiency on the lens.[8] The cornea, however, may be more prone to vascularisation following small standard heat injuries in scorbutic (affected by scurvy) than normal guinea pigs.[47]

Haemorrhages of the bulbar conjunctiva and retina[48] may be seen, as well as drying of the tear and salivary glands (Sjögren's syndrome).[5] Minute haemorrhages, or petechiae, have been reported on the lids, and intraorbital haemorrhage is common in infantile scurvy.[8] Subconjunctival haemorrhage was reported in a human vitamin C deprivation study, as well as conjunctival vessel dilation after 74 days and xerosis on day 91.[49]

Chapter **3.3**

Vitamin E deficiency

Hannah Bartlett

Vitamin E is a chain-breaking antioxidant that prevents propagation of free radical damage in cell membranes.[33,50,51] Free radical damage resulting from vitamin E deficiency may cause anaemia[52] and peripheral neuropathy due to nerve damage.[53] Deficiency is rare in humans as vitamin E is widely available in oils and fats; however, it may occur in genetic abnormalities, fat malabsorption syndromes, cystic fibrosis and chronic steatorrhoea (excessive discharge of fat in the faeces).[54]

Genetic defects occurring in the α-tocopherol transfer protein (α-TTP) are associated with the ataxia with vitamin E (AVED) syndrome, which causes neurological abnormalities. Symptoms are characterised by progressive peripheral neuropathy, resulting in ataxia.[55] Further deterioration of neurological function is normally preventable by oral administration of 800–1200 mg vitamin E.

Retinitis pigmentosa (RP) has been described in patients with AVED,[56] and the same defect in the α-TTP gene has been described in three such patients.[57] It is not known, however, whether this defect in the α-TTP gene causes RP, or whether vitamin E deficiency is responsible. Vitamin E supplementation slows the progression of RP caused by vitamin E deficiency.[59] It has been shown, however, that in RP not related to vitamin E deficiency, supplementation with vitamin E may have an adverse effect.[58]

Vitamin E deficiency is also related to genetic defects in lipoprotein synthesis. Specific lipoproteins are required for the effective transport and absorption of vitamin E. Clinical features include steatorrhoea, retarded growth, acanthocytosis (presence of abnormal red blood cells) and a chronic progressive neurological disorder with ataxia.[54]

Chapter **3.4**

Retinitis pigmentosa

Hannah Bartlett

RP is the commonest cause of registrable blindness in children and young adults in the USA, and has a prevalence of 1 in 4000.[59–61] The name refers to a group of heredofamilial diseases characterised by progressive visual field loss, night blindness and abnormal electroretinogram (ERG). ERG testing is used to detect RP early in life, and involves fitting a contact lens electrode on to a topically anaesthetised cornea. Responses to flashes of light are amplified and displayed on an oscilloscope. Patients with early stages of RP have ERGs that are reduced in amplitude and delayed in their temporal aspects.[62] Blindness can occur between the ages of 30 and 60 years, with a central visual field diameter of less than 20º. A characteristic ring of pigment can be seen with an ophthalmoscope, as well as attenuation of the peripheral vessels and, sometimes, a waxy pallor to the optic discs.[63] Pigment changes occur mainly in the periphery and often present around the vessels due to the pigment within the vessel walls. Bone corpuscular-like patterns are common, as are irregular clumps and spots. Histological studies suggest that the pigment originates from the RPE rather than the choroid[66] (Figure 3.4.1).

Diseases encompassed by the term RP may be primary (with ocular involvement only) or secondary (with systemic involvement).[64] Primary forms of RP include rod-cone degenerations, where the patient has a markedly reduced scotopic (rod) ERG but a relatively normal photopic (cone) ERG, and cone-rod degenerations, where the reverse is true. Within these groups, there are three different inheritance types of RP: (1) auto-

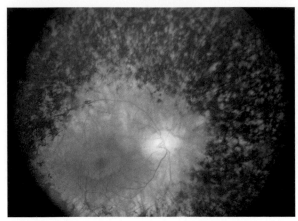

Figure 3.4.1   Advanced retinitis pigmentosa.
(Reproduced from Kanski JJ. Clinical ophthalmology, 5th
edn. Oxford: Butterworth-Heinemann; 2003:438, with
permission.[83])

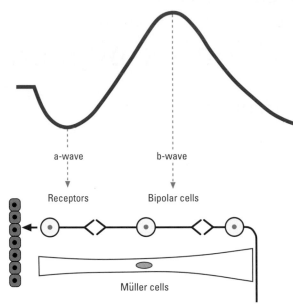

Figure 3.4.2   Origins of the electroretinogram.
(Reproduced from Kanski JJ. Clinical ophthalmology, 5th
edn. Oxford: Butterworth-Heinemann; 2003:438, with
permission.[83])

somal dominant; (2) autosomal recessive; and (3)
X-linked recessive. Primary RP may also be
congenital in onset (Table 3.4.1).[64]

INHERITANCE TYPES

Autosomal dominant

In autosomal dominant inheritance the trait is
transmitted by the affected person to 50% of the
offspring; the trait appears in every generation.
Unaffected persons do not transmit the trait and
both sexes are equally affected.

Autosomal recessive

When both parents carry the gene, there is a 25%
chance of each child inheriting the trait, so it does
not typically appear in every generation. Sexes are
equally affected.

X-linked recessive inheritance

The affected male gives the gene to all daughters,
who pass the trait on to half their sons. Only males
are severely affected and there is no history of
male-to-male transmission.

THE ELECTRORETINOGRAM

The ERG is a response evoked from the retina to
a flash of light. It is usually recorded from the
corneal surface by means of a contact lens or gold-
foil electrode. The ERG response is comprised of
an initial negative downward peak called an a-
wave, followed by a positive upward peak, called
the b-wave (Figure 3.4.2). The a-wave represents
repolarisation of the photoreceptors; it can be differentiated to a1, derived from the cones, and a2,
derived from the rods. The b-wave is derived from
the bipolar or Müller cells. Under certain circumstances a late positive c-wave can be recorded 2–3
seconds after the initial flash. This is an indicator
of the integrity of the RPE.

In order to obtain a photopic or cone-mediated
ERG (Figure 3.4.3), the background conditions
must be light such that the rods are bleached and
will not respond. Conversely, to obtain a rod-
mediated ERG, the patient must be dark-adapted
for at least 30 minutes and a dim blue or white
flash below cone threshold is used (Figure 3.4.4).

Table 3.4.1   Classification of retinitis pigmentosa (RP)

Primary form of RP	Cone-rod degeneration	Congenital onset
Rod-cone degenerations	Autosomal dominant	Leber's amaurosis congenital, typical form
Autosomal dominant	Autosomal recessive	Congenital RP with macular colobomata
Autosomal recessive	X-linked recessive	Juvenile Leber's amaurosis
X-linked recessive	Simplex/multiplex forms	Autosomal dominant form (rare)
Retinitis punctata albicans		
Preserved para-arteriolar retinal pigment epithelium (PPRPE)		
Choroideraemia		
Simplex/multiplex forms		

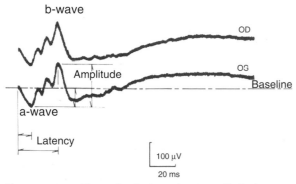

Figure 3.4.3 Photopic electroretinogram. Typical waveform of the cone system in which the first negative wave is called the a-wave, and the positive peak is called the b-wave. Oscillatory potentials can be seen on the ascending b-wave. OD, oculus dexter (right eye); OS, oculus sinister (left eye). (Reproduced from Heckenlively J. The diagnosis and classification of retinitis pigmentosa. In: Heckenlively J, ed. Retinitis pigmentosa. Philadelphia: JB Lippincott; 1988:7, with permission.[67])

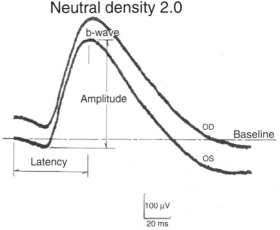

Figure 3.4.4 Scotopic electroretinogram. Typical waveform of the rod system. Neutral-density filters reduce the stimulus flash intensity below cone threshold. Rod-mediated electroretinogram waveforms have almost no a-wave. OD, oculus dexter (right eye); OS, oculus sinister (left eye). (Reproduced from Heckenlively J. The diagnosis and classification of retinitis pigmentosa. In: Heckenlively J, ed. Retinitis pigmentosa. Philadelphia: JB Lippincott; 1988:7, with permission.[67])

Use of ERG in classification of RP

In typical RP, the rods are more affected than the cones, and this preferential loss can be demonstrated by ERG testing. The rod-mediated ERG is more affected than the cone-mediated ERG, and this is termed the rod-cone degenerative pattern.[65] In some patients the cone-mediated ERG is more severely affected than the rod-mediated ERG; they often present with progressive field loss but no or late-onset night blindness. This is known as a cone-rod response.[66] Rod-cone degeneration patients generally exhibit diffuse rod loss, whereas cone-rod patients show areas of preservation of rod and cone function.[67]

Cone and rod b-wave amplitudes are evaluated to determine whether the patient has rod-cone or cone-rod degeneration. If the scotopic b-wave is of greater amplitude than the photopic b-wave and both are abnormal, then the patient has cone-rod degeneration. If the photopic b-wave is of greater amplitude than the scotopic b-wave, the patient has rod-cone degeneration. Where it is difficult to detect a difference between scotopic and photopic b-waves, a dark adaptation test may be employed; cone-rod patients are not markedly night blind until the visual field is less than 10°.[67] Patients are usually legally blind when their cone ERG amplitudes fall below 0.05 µV (normal values are 50–100 µV).[68]

Use of vitamin A and vitamin E supplementation in RP

A randomised controlled trial (RCT) to investigate the effect of vitamin A and vitamin E supplementation on the course of RP was instigated following 2-year observation of RP patients who were self-treating with these vitamins. The percentage of patients with a decline in ERG amplitude from baseline was lower among those taking vitamin A (11%) or vitamin E (21%) than among those taking only a multivitamin supplement (34%) or no supplement (41%).[60] In the RCT, patients were randomised into one of four treatment groups receiving 15 000 IU/day vitamin A, 15 000 IU/day vitamin A plus 400 IU/day vitamin E, trace amounts of both vitamins, or 400 IU/day vitamin E. The two groups taking 15 000 IU/day vitamin A had a lower average rate of decline of retinal function than the two groups not taking vitamin A ($P = 0.1$). Among 354 patients who had higher initial amplitudes, the two groups receiving 15 000 IU vitamin A were 32% less likely to have a decline in ERG amplitude of 50% or more from baseline in a given year than those not receiving vitamin A ($P = 0.1$). The two groups receiving 400 IU/day vitamin E were 42% more likely to have a decline in amplitude of 50% or more than those not receiving vitamin E ($P = 0.3$). The results suggest a beneficial effect of 15 000 IU/day vitamin A and suggest a possible adverse ef-

fect of 400 IU/day vitamin E on the course of RP.[58]

The mechanism by which vitamin A may be protective against progression of RP has yet to be established. Patients with the condition may have a diminished capacity to retain vitamin A in the retina due to impaired photoreceptors, or the fact that they have abnormal carrier proteins.[69,70] Daily vitamin A supplementation may protect against transient decreases in serum retinol concentration that may adversely affect photoreceptor function. Investigators suggest that the adverse affect of vitamin E on progression of RP may be explained by an inhibitory effect of vitamin E on vitamin A. They observed that patients receiving 400 IU/day vitamin E had a small but significant decrease in serum retinol levels compared with those not receiving 400 IU/day vitamin E ($P = 0.03$). Interestingly, vitamin E has been found to prevent changes in the cornea and conjunctiva, such as keratinisation, caused by vitamin A deficiency.[29] An investigation into the safety of vitamin A supplementation in RP patients found that prolonged daily consumption of < 25 000 IU/day can be considered safe in those aged between 18 and 54 years.[71]

Use of lutein supplementation in retinitis pigmentosa

A small amount of data has been published in which lutein slowed vision loss associated with RP in one[72] but not another[73] study.

BASSEN–KORNZWEIG SYNDROME

This condition is characterised by a malabsorption syndrome, generalised retinal degeneration, a diffuse neuromuscular disease and acanthocytosis. Patients can assimilate fat into the intestinal mucosa, but there is difficulty in its removal from this site because of the lack of chylomicra. Mutations in a gene encoding a microsomal triglyceride-transfer protein have been found in patients with this condition.[74] The liver and retina become devoid of vitamin A.

Patients with the condition are treated with a low-fat diet and supplements of the fat-soluble vitamins A, E and K. Elevated dark adaptation thresholds and reduced ERG responses have been restored to normal with vitamin A supplementation in patients with early stages of the condition. In some cases, supplementation of vitamin E and vitamin A has been advocated to stabilise retinal function.[75,76]

REFSUM DISEASE

This disease results from impairment of peroxisomes within the body. Peroxisomes are responsible for the breakdown of a branched-chain fatty acid called phytanic acid, which is obtained from the diet in foods like beef, lamb, milk, butter, cheese and green vegetables.[77] The symptoms of Refsum disease include RP, peripheral polyneuropathy, deafness, cerebellar ataxia, anosmia (loss of sense of smell), pupillary abnormalities, nystagmus, icthyosis (inflammatory scaliness of the skin) and epiphyseal dysplasia (abnormal function of the growth area at the end of bone, resulting in shortness of limbs).

The relationship between elevated serum phytanic acid and the symptoms of Refsum disease remains unclear. It may be that phytanic acid replaces phospholipids and triglycerides with consequent malfunction, or that its accumulation in the myelin lipid bilayer disrupts the packing of myelin.[68] Patients are advised to restrict milk products, animal fats and green leafy products containing phytol. Successful treatment depends upon the patient receiving enough calories; if not, body weight is reduced and phytanic acid is released from tissue stores. Subsequent increased serum levels of phytanic acid can exacerbate symptoms.

SORSBY FUNDUS DYSTROPHY

This is a rare autosomal dominant retinal degeneration. Patients experience night blindness in young adulthood and then progressive loss of central vision associated with subretinal neovascularisation and haemorrhage. In later stages, peripheral vision is lost as well.[78–80] The exact patheogenesis of the condition is not yet known, but it is thought that mutations in the *TIMP3* gene on chromosome 22[81] lead to an abnormal lipid-containing deposit interposed between the photoreceptors and their choroidal blood supply. Diffusion of nutrients to the photoreceptors is restricted. The disturbance in the extracellular matrix caused by this mutation may also impair storage of vitamin A in the RPE and/or its transport to the photoreceptors.

Sorsby fundus dystrophy patients have been treated with a dose of 50 000 IU/day oral vitamin A, which resulted in reversal of night blindness within 1 week in early stages of the disease. Macular rod sensitivity recovered after peripheral rod sensitivity and could not be maintained by a dose of 5000 IU/day vitamin A. Cone function in the central macula remained normal throughout the trial period, whereas rod function varied.[82] Further research is required to determine whether long-term safe doses of vitamin A (25 000 IU/day) could be administered to try and modify the course of the disease.[68]

References to Section 3

1. Jackson C. The effects of inanition and malnutrition upon growth and structure. Philadelphia: Blakiston; 1925.
2. McLaren D. Nutrition and its disorders, 2nd edn. Edinburgh: Churchill Livingstone; 1976.
3. Sandford-Smith J. Eye diseases in hot climates. Oxford: Butterworth-Heinemann; 1997.
4. Combs G. The vitamins: fundamental aspects in nutrition and health, 2nd edn. San Diego: Academic Press; 1998.
5. Burton B, Foster W. Human nutrition, 4th edn. New York: McGraw-Hill; 1988.
6. Wald G. Pigments of the bull frog retina. Nature 1935; 136:832–833.
7. Wald G. Vitamin A in eye tissues. J Gen Physiol 1935; 18:905–915.
8. McLaren DS. Nutritional ophthalmology. London: Academic Press; 1980.
9. Bessey O, Wolbach S. Vitamin A: physiology and pathology. J Am Med Soc 1938; 110:2072–2080.
10. World Health Organization. Micronutrient deficiencies. Combating vitamin A deficiency. Available online at: www.who.int/nut/vad.htm 28/01/04; 2003.
11. World Health Organization. Prevention of childhood blindness. Geneva: World Health Organization; 1994.
12. World Health Organization. Blindness and visual disability. Part III of VII: other leading causes worldwide. Fact sheet N 144 28/01/04. Geneva: World Health Organization; 1997.
13. Sommer A, Tarwotjo I, Djunaedi E et al. Impact of vitamin A supplementation on childhood mortality. A randomized controlled community trial. Lancet 1986; 1:1169.
14. Sommer A, Katz J, Tarwotjo I. Increased risk of respiratory disease and diarrhoea in children with preexisting vitamin A deficiency. Am J Clin Nutr 1984; 40:1090–1095.
15. Miller M, Hunphrey J, Johnson E et al. Why do children become vitamin A deficient? J Nutr 2002, 132:2867S–2880S.
16. UNICEF. State of the world's children. Available online at: www.unicef.org/sowc00 UNICEF; 2000.
17. World Health Organization. Complementary feeding of young children in developing countries: a review of current scientific knowledge. WS 130 98 CO. Geneva: World Health Organization; 1998.
18. World Health Organization. Vitamin A deficiency and xerophthalmia. Technical reporting service of the World Health Organization. Jakarta, Indonesia: World Health Organization; 1976:590.
19. World Health Organization. Control of vitamin A deficiency. Report of a joint WHO/UNICEF/USAAID/HKI/IVACG meeting. Geneva: World Health Organization; 1980.
20. Russell R, Multack R, Smith V et al. Dark-adaptation testing for diagnosis of subclinical vitamin A deficiency and evaluation of therapy. Lancet 1973; 302:1161–1164.
21. Harris EW, Loewenstein JI, Azar D. Vitamin A deficiency and its effects on the eye. Int Ophthalmol Clin 1998; 38:155–161.
22. Kusin J, Soewando W, Parlindungan Dinaga H. Rose Bengal and lissamine green vital stains: useful diagnostic aids for early stages of xerophthalmia? Am J Clin Nutr 1979, 32:1559–1561.
23. Bitot C. Sur une lésion conjonctivale non encore décrite, coincidant avec l'hémeralopie. Gas Hebd Med Chir 1863; 10:284.
24. Smith J, Steinemann TL. Vitamin A deficiency and the eye. Int Ophthalmol Clin 2000; 40:83–91.
25. Sommer A. Nutritional blindness: xerophthalmia and keratomalacia. New York: Oxford University Press; 1982.
26. Elliott R. Tropical ophthalmology. London: Frowde; 1920.
27. Sommer A. Vitamin A deficiency. In: Duane T, ed. Clinical ophthalmology (CD ROM). Philadelphia: Lippincott-Raven; 1998.
28. Carr R, Margolis S, Siegel I. Fluorescein angiography and vitamin A and oxalate levels in fundus albipunctatus. Am J Ophthalmol 1976; 82:549.

29. Fujikawa A, Gong HQ, Amemiya T. Vitamin E prevents changes in the cornea and conjunctiva due to vitamin A deficiency. Graefes Arch Clin Exp Ophthalmol 2003; 241:287–297.

30. Anderson JA, Richard NR, Rock ME, Binder PS. Requirement for vitamin-A in long-term culture of human cornea. Invest Ophthalmol Vis Sci 1993; 34:3442–3449.

31. Hatchell DL, Ubels JL, Stekiel T, Hatchell MC. Corneal epithelial wound-healing in normal and diabetic rabbits treated with tretinoin. Arch Ophthalmol 1985; 103:98–100.

32. Sullivan W, McCully J, Dohlman C. Return of goblet cells after vitamin A therapy in xerosis of the conjunctiva. Am J Ophthalmol 1973; 75:720–725.

33. Burton GW, Joyce A, Ingold KU. Is vitamin-E the only lipid-soluble, chain-breaking antioxidant in human-blood plasma and erythrocyte-membranes? Arch Biochem Biophys 1983, 221:281–290.

34. Vijayaraghavan G, Naidu A, Rao N, Sritkantia S. A simple method to evaluate the massive dose vitamin A prophylaxis programme in preschool children. Am J Clin Nutr 1975; 28:1189–1193.

35. Tarwotjo I, Gunawan S, Reedy S et al. An evaluation of the vitamin A prevention pilot project in Indonesia 1973–1975. New York: American Foundation for Overseas Blind; 1975.

36. Christian P, West K, Khatry S et al. Maternal night blindness increases risk of mortality in the first 6 months of life among infants in Nepal. J Nutr 2001; 131:1510–1512.

37. Ross D. Recommendations for vitamin A supplementation. J Nutr 2002; 131:2902S–2906S.

38. Moore T. Vitamin A. Amsterdam: Elsevier; 1957.

39. Vahlqquist A, Sjolund K, Norden A et al. Plasma vitamin A transport and visual dark adaptation in diseases of the intestine and liver. Scand J Clin Lab Invest 1978; 38:301–308.

40. Bronte-Stewart J, Foulds W. Acquired dyschromatopsia in vitamin A deficiency. Modern Probl Ophthalmol 1972; 11:168–173.

41. Life Sciences Research Office. Nutrition monitoring in the United States – an update report on nutrition monitoring. Prepared for the US Department of Agriculture and the US Department of Health and Human Services. DHHS publication no. (PHS) 89-1255. Federation of American Societies for Experimental Biology. Washington DC: Government Printing Office; 1989.

42. Monget AL, Galan P, Preziosi P et al. Micronutrient status in elderly people. Int J Vit Nutr Res 1996; 66:71–76.

43. Englard S, Seifter S. The biochemical functions of ascorbic acid. Annu Rev Nutr 1986; 6:365–406.

44. Ronchetti I, Quaglino DJ, Bergamini G. Ascorbic acid and connective tissue. In: Harris JR, ed. Subcellular biochemistry, vol. 25. Ascorbic acid: biochemistry and biomedical cell biology. New York: Plenum Press; 1996:249–264.

45. McLaren D. Clinical manifestations of human vitamin and mineral disorders: a resume. In: Ross A, ed. Modern nutrition in health and disease. Baltimore, MD: Williams & Wilkins; 1999:485–504.

46. Hodges R, Hood J, Canham J. Clinical manifestations of ascorbic acid deficiency in man. Am J Clin Nutr 1971; 24:432–443.

47. Campbell F, Ferguson I. The role of ascorbic acid in corneal vascularization. Br J Ophthalmol 1950; 34:329–334.

48. Kitamura S. Ein Beitrag zur Kerntrus der Netzhautver-anderungen beim Skorbut. Dtsche Med Wochenschr 1910; 36:403.

49. Hood J, Hodges R. Ocular lesions in scurvy. Am J Clin Nutr 1969; 22:559–567.

50. Burton GW, Ingold KU. Vitamin E – application of the principles of physical organic chemistry to the exploration of its structure and function. Accounts Chem Res 1986; 19:194–201.

51. Ingold KU, Webb AC, Witter D et al. Vitamin E remains the major lipid-soluble, chain-breaking antioxidant in human plasma even in individuals suffering severe vitamin-E-deficiency. Arch Biochem Biophys 1987; 259:224–225.

52. Kayden H, Silber R. The role of vitamin E deficiency in the abnormal autohemolysis of acanthocytosis. Trans Assoc Am Phys 1965; 78:334–341.

53. Traber MG, Sokol RJ, Ringel SP et al. Lack of tocopherol in peripheral nerves of vitamin-E-deficient patients with peripheral neuropathy. N Engl J Med 1987; 317:262–265.

54. Traber MG. Vitamin E. In: Ross A, ed. Modern nutrition in health and disease. Baltimore, MD: Williams & Wilkins; 1999:347–362.

55. Sokol RJ, Kayden HJ, Bettis DB et al. Isolated vitamin-E-deficiency in the absence of fat malabsorption – familial and sporadic cases – characterization and investigation of causes. J Lab Clin Med 1988, 111:548–559.

56. Matsuya M, Matsumoto H, Chiba S et al. [A sporadic case of essential vitamin E deficiency manifested by sensory-dominant polyneuropathy and retinitis pigmentosa.] Brain Nerve (Tokyo) 1994; 46:989–994.

57. Yokota T, Shiojiri T, Gotoda T, Arai H. Retinitis pigmentosa and ataxia caused by a mutation in the gene for the alpha-tocopherol transfer protein. N Engl J Med 1996; 335:1770–1771.

58. Berson E, Rosner B, Sandberg M et al. A randomized trial of vitamin A and vitamin E supplementation for retinitis pigmentosa. Arch Ophthalmol 1993; 111:761–772.

59. Ammann F, Klein D, Franceschetti A. Genetic and epidemiological investigation of pigmentary degeneration of the retina and allied disorders in Switzerland. J Neurol Sci 1965; 2:183–196.

60. Boughman J, Conneally P, Nance W. Population genetic studies of retinitis pigmentosa. Am J Hum Genet 1980; 32:223–235.

61. Bunker C, Berson E, Bromley W et al. Prevalence of retinitis pigmentosa in Maine. Am J Ophthalmol 1984; 97:357–365.

62. Berson EL. Nutrition and retinal degenerations. Int Ophthalmol Clin 2000; 40:93–111.

63. Berson EL. Retinitis pigmentosa – the Friedenwald lecture. Invest Ophthalmol Vis Sci 1993; 34:1659–1676.

64. Heckenlively JR. Retinitis pigmentosa. In: Heckenlively JR, ed. Retinitis pigmentosa. Philadelphia: Lippincott; 1988:1–5.

65. Krill A. Rod-cone dystrophies. In: Krill A, Archer D, eds. Krill's hereditary retinal and choroidal diseases. Hagerstown: Harper and Row; 1977:227–276.

66. Berson E, Gouras P, Gunkel R. Progressive cone-rod degeneration. Arch Ophthalmol 1968; 80:68–76.

67. Heckenlively J. The diagnosis and classification of retinitis pigmentosa. In: Heckenlively J, ed. Retinitis pigmentosa. Philadelphia: JB Lippincott; 1988:6–24.

68. Berson E. Nutrition and retinal degenerations. Int Ophthalmol Clin 2000; 40:93–111.

69. Goodman D. Vitamin A and retinoids in health and disease. N Engl J Med 1984; 310:1023–1031.

70. Blomhoff R, Green M, Berg T, Norum K. Transport and storage of vitamin A. Science 1990; 250:399–404.

71. Sibulesky L, Hayes KC, Pronczuk A et al. Safety of < 7500RE (< 25 000IU) vitamin A daily in adults with retinitis pigmentosa. Am J Clin Nutr 1999; 69:656–663.

72. Dagnelie G, Zorge I, McDonald T. Lutein improves visual function in some patients with retinal degeneration: a pilot study via the internet. Optometry 2000; 71:147–164.

73. Aleman TS, Duncan JL, Bieber ML et al. Macular pigment and lutein supplementation in retinitis pigmentosa and Usher syndrome. Invest Ophthalmol Vis Sci 2001; 42:1873–1881.

74. Narcisi T, Shoulders C, Chester S et al. Mutations of the microsomal triglyceride-transfer-protein gene in abetalipoproteinemia. Am J Hum Genet 1995; 57:1298–1310.

75. Runge P, Muller D, McAllister J et al. Oral vitamin E supplements can prevent the retinopathy of abetalipoproteinemia. Br J Ophthalmol 1986; 70:166–173.

76. Rader D, Brewer H. Abetalipoproteinemia: new insights into lipoprotein assembly and vitamin E metabolism from a rare genetic disease. JAMA 1993; 270:865–869.

77. Masters-Thomas A, Bailes J, Bilimoria J et al. Heredopathia atactica polyneuritiformis (Refsum's disease): 2. Estimation of phytanic acid in foods. J Hum Nutr 1980; 34:251–254.

78. Fraser H, Wallace D. Sorsby's familial pseudo-inflammatory macular dystrophy. Am J Ophthalmol 1971; 72:1216–1220.

79. Carr R, Noble K, Nasaduke I. Hereditary hemorrhagic macular dystrophy. Am J Ophthalmol 1978; 85:318–328.

80. Sorsby A, Joll Maseon M. A Fundus dystrophy with unusual features. Br J Ophthalmol 1949; 33:67–97.

81. Weber B, Vogt G, Pruett R et al. Mutations in the tissue inhibitor of metalloproteinases-3 (TIMP3) in patients with Sorsbys fundus dystrophy. Nature Genet 1994; 8:352–366.

82. Jacobson S, Cideciyan A, Regunath G et al. Night blindness in Sorsbys-fundus dystrophy reversed by vitamin A. Nature Genet 1995; 11:127–132.

83. Kanski JJ. Clinical ophthalmology, 5th edn. Oxford: Butterworth-Heinemann; 2003:438.

SECTION 4

Nutrition and ocular senescence

SECTION CONTENTS

Chapter **4.1**

Nutrition and malnutrition in older people

Jayne V Woodside and Ian S Young

CHAPTER CONTENTS

INTRODUCTION

The World Health Organization defines elderly persons as being of 60 years of age and older. Based on this definition, the proportion of elderly people in Europe is currently around 20%, with a predicted increase to 25% by 2020.[1]

Within this elderly group, the most dramatic demographic change is amongst those in the oldest age group (80 years and over). In Europe it is estimated that the number of people aged over 80 years will grow from 21.4 million in 2000 to 35 million in 2025.[1] This increase in the proportion of older adults in the population arises both from an increasing average life expectancy as well as from a declining birth rate.

Ageing is a complex biological phenomenon, with evidence supporting at least five common characteristics of ageing in mammals (Box 4.1.1). Ageing is often accompanied by socioeconomic changes that can have a great impact on the nutritional needs and status of elderly individuals. The incidence of disability increases with ageing, with over a third of the elderly population limited by chronic conditions and unable to carry on normal daily living activity.[2] Arthritis, hypertension, cardiovascular disease, hearing impairment, orthopaedic impairment, cataracts, age-related macular degeneration and diabetes are the main health problems in the elderly that affect normal daily activity.[2] Therefore, as the elderly population increases, so will both the incidence of these diseases and the prevalence of the population with disability. Strategies that will reduce the

---

Box 4.1.1   Characteristics of ageing

1. Increased mortality with increasing age after maturation
2. Change in the biochemical composition of tissues with increasing age
3. Progressive decrease in physiological capacity with increasing age
4. Reduced ability to respond adaptively to environmental stimuli with increasing age
5. Increased susceptibility to disease with increasing age

Box 4.1.2   Common theories of ageing

Immunological breakdown
Reduction in cellular proliferation
Reduction in basal metabolic rate
Reduction in telomere length
Reduction in DNA repair activity
Free radical damage
Reduction in rate of protein synthesis and catabolism

---

age-related decline in mobility and reduce chronic disease prevalence will be important for healthy ageing, and for maintaining elderly independence and the ability to carry out normal daily living activities.[2]

THE AGEING PROCESS

Ageing is a gradual process that takes place over many decades. Most theories of ageing relate to impaired DNA replication and loss of cell viability and hence the viability of the body's organs.[3] The most common theories of ageing are shown in Box 4.1.2.

NUTRITION AND THE AGEING PROCESS

Some major biological changes seen amongst elderly people occur primarily as an irreversible result of the ageing process. However, many of the health problems and physiological changes experienced by older people, commonly attributed to the ageing process, are now recognised to be linked to lifestyle or environmental factors.[4] Good nutrition and other lifestyle factors, such as being physically active and not smoking, are essential to ensure that people have long, healthy and active lives, continuing to live independently for as long as possible.[4] The strongest evidence that nutrition can affect longevity and the ageing process comes from animal studies.

Dietary restriction experiments with animal models

Experimental studies in a variety of species, including rats, mice and fish, indicate that moderate energy restriction markedly extends the life span of experimental animals, compared with control animals.[5] It is also known that dietary restriction decreases the incidence of several chronic diseases such as glomerulonephritis, atherosclerosis and cancer.[6] The eventual response to the dietary restriction appears to depend on the severity, age of initiation and duration of dietary perturbation, as well as the species and strain of laboratory animals.[5,6]

Dietary restriction by selective removal of individual macronutrients such as fat, carbohydrate and protein has also been carried out.[6] However, without an overall decrease in energy intake, little alteration in life span has been demonstrated. Dietary excess of protein or fat has been shown to increase tumour incidence and decrease the time to appearance of certain physical, biochemical and immunological indices of early maturational development and ageing.[6]

The mechanism or mechanisms through which this prolongation of life occurs are unclear. Caloric restriction reduces metabolic rate and oxidative stress, improves insulin sensitivity, and alters neuroendocrine and sympathetic nervous system function in animals.[5]

Whether prolonged caloric restriction increases life span or improves biomarkers of ageing in humans is unknown. A number of studies have subjected humans to periods of non-volitional partial starvation, but the diets in these cases have generally been of poor quality.[5] Studies of good-quality, calorie-restricted diets are unlikely to occur due to ethical and methodological issues.[5]

MALNUTRITION PREVALENCE IN OLDER PEOPLE

Relatively little is known regarding actual malnutrition prevalence among older people.[7] At present, there are not even generally accepted criteria for the diagnosis of malnutrition.[8] Morley and Silver[9] highlighted that malnutrition is common among nursing-home residents, and that protein–energy undernutrition prevalence ranges from 17 to 65% in this setting. Neel[10] suggested that approximately 50% of residents in care homes in the USA are undernourished, whilst Crogan et al.[11] found the rate in some homes to be as high as 85%.

In the UK, there has been a marked lack of research examining malnutrition prevalence in the elderly in long-term care.[7] However, the UK National Diet and Nutrition Survey of people aged 65 years and older examined 453 older people from 155 care homes, and found that 15% of women and 16% of men were malnourished, compared to figures of 6 and 3% respectively of those living in the community independently.[12] A report by the Malnutrition Advisory Group[7] has highlighted that, in developed countries, suboptimal nutrition is common among hospital patients and older people resident in care homes, and it is frequently unrecognised and untreated. In the Survey in Europe on Nutrition and the Elderly: A Concerted Action (SENECA) study, which sampled a cohort of community-dwelling subjects born between 1913 and 1918 in 12 European countries, a relatively high risk of malnutrition was found (47% for vitamin D, 23.3% for vitamin B_6, 2.7% for vitamin B_{12} and 1.1% for vitamin E).[13,14]

FACTORS AFFECTING NUTRITIONAL STATUS

Older people are a special type of population when compared to other age groups in that they are a particularly heterogeneous group in terms of capabilities and levels of functioning. Elderly persons are more likely to be in marginal nutritional health and thus to be at higher risk of frank nutritional deficiency in times of stress or health care problems.[6] Physical, social and emotional problems may interfere with appetite or affect the ability to purchase, prepare or consume an adequate diet.[15] These factors include whether or not a person lives alone, how many daily meals are eaten, who does the cooking and shopping and any physical impediments such as problems in chewing and denture use, adequate income to purchase appropriate foods, and alcohol and medication use.[6]

THE PHYSICAL EFFECTS OF AGEING

Throughout life, the body goes through changes in composition, physical strength and physiological functioning. There is a great deal of inter-individual variation in the degree to which cells, systems and the whole body age and suffer from a progressive loss of adaptability.[4]

Body composition

In general, older people tend to lose bone and muscle and gain body fat.[16] Loss of muscle, known as sarcopenia, can be significant in later years and its consequences may be dramatic.[17] Loss of muscle mass reduces energy requirements and may also reduce mobility.[4] As people lose their ability to move and maintain balance, falls become more likely.[18] The limitations that accompany the loss of muscle and its strength would appear to play a key role in the diminishing health that often accompanies ageing. Optimal nutrition and regular physical activity can help maintain muscle mass and strength and minimise the changes in body composition associated with ageing.[18]

Energy expenditure and physical activity

Energy expenditure tends to decrease as people age. The basal metabolic rate (BMR) of 70-year-olds is approximately 9–12% lower than that of adults aged 18–30 years, mainly because of a reduction in lean body mass.[4]

As people grow older, physical activity may decrease as they become increasingly sedentary. However, activity levels in the elderly do vary widely, ranging from the physically active recently retired to the frail and chair-bound. Even in the eighth decade of life, activity levels of some people can equate to those of younger and middle-aged people.[19] Reduced activity levels lead to accelerated loss of muscle (although sarcopenia does occur regardless of activity levels), with the resultant declines in muscle strength and mass leading to a reduced BMR.[4] The degree of loss may be ameliorated by resistance training exercise, which can increase muscle mass and strength even in individuals suffering from chronic disease.[20]

Bone loss

Bone density is reduced with increasing age, and this process is more predominant in women. Up until about the age of 30, the rate of new bone formation exceeds that of bone degradation. Once peak bone mass is achieved at about this age this process is reversed, and minerals and collagen matrix are removed from bone faster than new bone tissue is added.[4] There are many factors that influence the rate of age-related bone loss, such as immobility, thinness, cigarette smoking, alcohol intake, physical activity, obesity and hormone replacement therapy use.[21]

Taste changes

Studies of sensitivity in taste amongst older people show a gradual decline with age,[22] and this is likely to have an impact on food selection. The loss of taste and/or smell is highly variable, and certain medical conditions and some drugs may affect taste, smell and appetite, thus affecting food intake.[20,23]

In addition to altered taste perception, a person's enjoyment of eating may be impaired by reduced salivary flow and a resulting dry mouth. These do not usually arise as an inevitable consequence of ageing, but rather as a side-effect of medication, or the presence or treatment of disease (e.g. with radiotherapy).[4]

Decreased thirst sensation may exacerbate the problem of a dry mouth, and can contribute towards dehydration. A stroke can affect a person's swallow reflex, making eating and drinking difficult. Older adults are at risk of dehydration due to reduced fluid intake and increased fluid losses.[4]

Neurological and cognitive function

Mental impairment and dementia, as a result of chronic degenerative brain disease, can have a severe impact on a person's autonomy and independence.[4] Cognitive impairment is thought to be sensitive to vitamin and mineral status, and this will be discussed in a later section.

Immune function

Considerable evidence indicates that ageing is associated with altered regulation of the immune system, and this contributes to the increased incidence of infections seen in older people, and to their prolonged recovery period post-illness.[1] Studies have shown that undernutrition contributes to the decline of the immune response with ageing.[24] However, it is not yet clear whether this effect is due to protein–energy undernutrition,[25] micronutrient deficiency or deficiency of some other dietary component.

Dentition

Poor dentition can have a major impact on the foods, and therefore nutrients, that can be consumed. The National Diet and Nutrition Survey of people aged 65 years and over in the UK found that those who had their own teeth had better vitamin and mineral intakes and better nutritional status than those who had lost most or all of their teeth.[26] Those with no or few natural teeth ate a more restricted range of foods, because of their perceived inability to chew.

Digestive function

It is thought that the digestive and absorptive efficiency of the gastrointestinal (GI) tract declines with age.[20] The intestinal wall loses strength and elasticity with age, and GI hormone secretions change.[27] All of these actions slow motility, and as a result constipation is much more common in the elderly than in the young.

The most significant change in GI function with ageing is the reduction in gastric acid output in older people who have atrophic gastritis. Atrophy of the stomach mucosa becomes more common in old age and is estimated to affect about 30% of those over 60 years.[20] Gastric acid, intrinsic factor and pepsin secretion are reduced, which impairs the digestion and absorption of nutrients, most notably vitamin B_{12}, but also biotin, folate, calcium, iron and zinc.[28] Pancreatic enzyme secretion also appears to decline with age, impairing the digestion of fat and protein when consumed in large amounts. Sensitivity of the gallbladder to cholecystokinin (a hormone that influences the release of bile from the gallbladder) may be reduced in older people and this may also have adverse effects on fat digestion.[27,29]

Eyesight

Deteriorating eyesight can make buying food more difficult, in terms of getting to the supermarket (an inability to drive, for example), reading food labels and counting money. Failing eyesight can also affect a person's ability to prepare food.

NUTRITIONAL NEEDS OF OLDER ADULTS

The physiological changes that occur with ageing may affect requirements for several nutrients, and the higher prevalence of disease and drug administration in older people may also affect nutritional requirements and nutritional status.[4,30] UK recommendations for macro- and micronutrients for the elderly will be considered in the following sections, and a comparison between UK and US recommendations (for the elderly, or the closest age group to elderly if no specific recommendation has been made) is presented in Table 4.1.1.

Energy and macronutrients

Older adults often have reduced energy needs because of their reduced energy expenditure.[31] If energy intakes are lower, it becomes crucially important that the foods that are consumed are micronutrient-dense so that other nutritional needs are still met. Foods with high nutrient density that are low in fat, such as lean meat, fish,

eggs, low-fat milk and vegetables and fruits, are helpful in that they provide the protein, vitamins and minerals the elderly need with relatively few calories.

The report of the UK Panel on Dietary Reference Values states that data on energy requirements of the elderly in the UK are limited.[32] The Panel do calculate estimated average requirements, but recognise that these are likely to vary considerably depending on whether elderly people are free-living, institutionalised or bed-ridden.[32]

Data on protein requirements of the elderly are limited, but the currently available evidence suggests that, in healthy elderly people, a mean intake of 0.75–0.8 g protein/kg body weight per day results in nitrogen balance.[32,33]

Recommendations for carbohydrate and fat are similar for healthy elderly people and for healthy younger adults, but for elderly people with small appetites, fat may be substituted for starchy carbohydrates to make up energy needs.[30,32,33]

Micronutrients

Ageing affects requirements for certain micronutrients, but it is difficult to distinguish changes in nutrient needs resulting from the ageing process alone from those resulting from disorders prevalent in older people.[30] Low-to-inadequate dietary intake may account for much of the poor vitamin status observed in the elderly.[34]

Vitamins

There is accumulating evidence that older people may have greater needs for vitamins B_{12}, B_6 and folate owing to the prevalence of disorders that reduce absorption (e.g. atrophic gastritis).[32]

Elderly people may also have increased requirements for vitamin D, which is necessary for the absorption of calcium and important for bone health. Deficiency of vitamin D in older people is a significant risk factor for hip fractures, and therefore represents a major public health problem. For most adults in Europe, the main source of vitamin D is from the action of sunlight on skin, but for older people, particularly for those in residential or nursing homes, exposure to the sun may be limited. Older skin also has a reduced ability to

Table 4.1.1 Comparison of macronutrient, vitamin and mineral UK estimated average requirements (EAR) and US recommended daily intakes (RDAs) for the elderly

Macronutrient	UK EAR	US RDA
Energy	51–59 years 2550 kcal (males) 1900 kcal (females) 75+ years 2100 kcal (males) 1810 kcal (females)	>51 years 2300 kcal (males) 1900 kcal (females)
Protein	>50 years – reference nutrient intake 53.3 g/day (males) 46.5 g/day (females)	>51 years 0.8 g/kg per day
Fat	All ages – population average Total fatty acid intake 30%: 10% SFA 12% MFA 6% PUFA	All ages Total fatty acid intake 30%: <10% SFA 10–15% MFA <10% PUFA
Fibre	All ages 18 g/day	All ages 25 g/day
Vitamin	UK RNI (>50 years)	US RDA (>51 years)
A	600–700 µg/day	800–1000 µg/day
B₆	1.2–1.4 mg/day	1.6–2.0 mg/day
B₁₂	1.5 µg/day	2.0 µg/day
Folate	200 µg/day	180–200 µg
C	40 mg/day	60 mg/day
D	>65 years 10 µg/day	5 µg/day
Thiamin	0.8–0.9 mg/day	1–1.2 mg/day
Riboflavin	1.1–1.3 mg/day	1.2–1.4 mg/day
Niacin	12–16 mg/day	13–15 mg/day
Mineral	UK RNI (>50 years)	US RDA (>51 years)
Calcium	700 mg/day	800 mg/day
Iron	9 mg/day	10 mg/day
Zinc	7.1–9.4 mg/day	12–15 mg/day
Copper	1.2 mg/day	1.5–3 mg/day
Selenium	63–71 µg/day	55–70 µg/day
Magnesium	262–295 mg/day	280–350 mg/day

RNI, reference nutrient intake; SFA, saturated fatty acids; MFA, monounsaturated fatty acids; PUFA, polyunsaturated fatty acids.
Reproduced from Department of Health. Dietary reference values for food energy and nutrients for the United Kingdom. Report of the panel on dietary reference values of the Committee on Medical Aspects of Food Policy. London: HMSO; 1991.[32] and Food and Nutrition Board, National Research Council. Recommended dietary allowances, 10th edn. Washington, DC: National Academy Press, 1989.[50]

synthesise the previtamin D_3, and declining kidney function may result in impaired synthesis of active metabolites of vitamin D.[30] A UK study of people aged 65 years and over found low vitamin D status amongst those living in institutions.[12] To maintain winter 25-hydroxyvitamin D at or above 8 ng/ml would require summer values to reach 16 ng/ml, which is 2–3 times higher than the elderly, particularly those over 75 years, reach in practice.[32] Diet is a secondary source of vitamin D, as only a few foods such as oily fish, meat and fortified margarines contain substantial amounts of vitamin D. Thus intake is frequently well below the recommended level. The UK Dietary Reference Value Panel recommends that the population over 65 years of age should consume 10 µg of vitamin D daily, through diet and/or supplements, to achieve plasma 25-hydroxyvitamin D values at the lower end of the normal range found in younger adults.[32]

Oxidative stress is believed to be an important factor in ageing and many age-associated degenerative diseases. Dietary antioxidants are regarded as being important in modulating oxidative stress. In the UK, many elderly people have low blood vitamin C levels, low body stores, and occasionally even clinical deficiency.[32] However, there are no special dietary reference values for vitamin C or vitamin E in the elderly.[32]

Minerals

The body's requirements for iron are lowest in old age, as iron is not required for growth and there is no menstrual blood loss. However, factors associated with old age may increase the risk of iron-deficiency anaemia, and the consequences of this can be life-threatening.[35] Factors that may increase the risk of iron deficiency include chronic blood loss from ulcers or other disease conditions, poor iron absorption due to reduced stomach acid secretion or medicines like aspirin that can cause blood loss from the GI tract.[20] Older people should be encouraged to consume foods containing bioavailable haem iron, such as red meat, liver and meat products.[30]

Osteoporosis and associated bone fractures are one of the major causes of disability and are a major and increasing public health problem in Europe. The World Health Organization has defined osteoporosis as the second leading health care problem after cardiovascular disease. Calcium absorption is reported to decline with age.[1] Adequate dietary calcium is essential throughout life, especially for women after the menopause to protect against osteoporosis. Therefore the elderly should continue to include calcium-rich foods such as milk and dairy products in their diets. The Committee on Medical Aspects of Food Policy (COMA) Dietary Reference Value Panel does not however recommend any increase in calcium intakes in the elderly, and dietary reference values are the same as for those >50 years old.[32]

Based on the nutritional requirements outlined above, the International Dietary Energy Consultative Group Working Group has produced recommendations on diet and lifestyle for healthy ageing (Box 4.1.3).[4,36]

NUTRITIONAL REQUIREMENTS WITH AGEING – POTENTIAL PREVENTION OF DISEASE?

Nutrition may play a greater role than has been realised in preventing many changes that were once thought to be inevitable consequences of growing older. Nutrition may provide at least some protection against some of the conditions associated with ageing, and several of these are considered below.

Cataracts and age–related macular degeneration

Cataracts are age-related thickenings in the lenses of eyes that impair vision. If not surgically removed, they ultimately lead to blindness. Being overweight appears to be associated with cataract, although the mechanism has not been identified. Factors that accompany overweight, such as physical inactivity, diabetes or hypertension, do not explain the association.[37] Oxidative stress appears to play a significant role in the development of cataracts, and the antioxidant micronutrients may protect against their development.

Like cataracts, risk factors for age-related macular degeneration include oxidative stress, e.g. from sunlight. Antioxidant vitamins and

Box 4.1.3 International Dietary Energy Consultative Group recommendations on diet and lifestyle for healthy ageing

1. Aerobic and resistance exercise promotes health and contributes to better quality of life in the elderly
2. Increased vitamin D and dietary calcium intake may help to slow the development of osteoporosis
3. Maintain a healthy weight – overweight and obesity predispose to comorbidities, including hypertension, cardiovascular disease, diabetes, osteoarthritis and some cancers
4. Cessation of smoking improves health at any age
5. A diet with a relatively high variety of fruits and vegetables is highly beneficial
6. Diets relatively low in saturated fatty acids can reduce the risk of cardiovascular disease
7. Consumption of alcohol in moderation is compatible with good health; however it is better to abstain than to consume alcohol in excess
8. Salt intake should be moderate
9. For elderly people in nursing homes, physical and social activities and a varied diet are important, and assistance, for example with eating, should be provided where necessary
10. A major contributor to morbidity in the elderly is falls associated with poor balance and coordination that can be improved by activities which promote balance

carotenoids have therefore been proposed to be protective against the disease.[38] Dietary fat may also be a risk factor for macular degeneration,[39] whilst the omega-3 fatty acids of fish oils may be protective.[39] This will be dealt with in detail later in the book.

Arthritis

Over 40 million people in the USA have some form of arthritis, and, as the population ages, the preva-lence is expected to increase.[18] In the UK it is esti-mated that more than 7 million adults (15% of the population) have long-term health problems due to arthritis and related conditions.[40]

Osteoarthritis is the commonest type of arthri-tis that disables older people. One known con-nection between osteoarthritis and nutrition is overweight.[18] Weight loss may relieve some of the symptoms, as the joints affected are often the weight-bearing joints. Aerobic activity and strength-training produce modest improvements in physical performance and pain relief.[41]

Rheumatoid arthritis has a possible link to diet through the immune system. The integrity of the immune system depends on adequate nutri-tion, and a poor diet may worsen rheumatoid arthritis. The essential omega-3 fatty acids eicosa-pentaenoic acid and docosahexaenoic acid appear to have an anti-inflammatory effect on rheumatoid arthritis.[42]

Alzheimer's disease

Much attention has focused on the abnormal de-terioration of the brain caused by Alzheimer's disease (AD), which affects 10% of US adults by age 65 and 30% of those over 85 years old.[43] An estimated 15 million people worldwide suffer from AD.[44] AD is a neurodegenerative disorder characterised by loss of memory and progressive decline of cognitive abilities.[45]

Oxidative stress may be central to the neurode-generative process. Brain tissue is highly suscep-tible to free radical damage because of its low levels of endogenous antioxidants, and antioxi-dants may have a potential therapeutic role in AD.[46,47] Homocysteine, an amino acid which is ele-vated in those with inadequate B-vitamin status, also seems to play a role in the pathophysiology of dementia in older people.[48,49] As yet, it is still unknown whether supplementation with antioxi-dants or B-group vitamins would reduce the risk of AD.

CONCLUSION

The potential impact of dietary manipulation on the maintenance of physical and cognitive function throughout old age has profound consequences for the optimisation of health, independence and well-being in the elderly, which is particularly important in this era of an ageing population. Encouraging better nutrition and taking exercise is a cost-effective way of decreasing the incidence and progression of age-related disease.

References

1. WHO (World Health Organization). Keeping fit for life: meeting the nutritional needs of older persons. Geneva: WHO; 2002.
2. Meydani M. Nutrition interventions in aging and age-associated disease. Proc Nutr Soc 2002; 61:165–171.
3. Harman D. Aging: overview. Ann NY Acad Sci 2001; 928:1–21.
4. Phillips F. Nutrition for healthy ageing. Nutr Bull 2003; 28:253–263.
5. Heilbronn LK, Ravussin E. Caloric restriction and aging: review of the literature and implications for studies in humans. Am J Clin Nutr 2003; 78:361–369.
6. Ausman LM, Russell RM. Nutrition in the elderly. In: Shils ME, Olson JA, Shike M, Ross AC, eds. Modern nutrition in health and disease, 9th edn. Baltimore, MD: Lippincott, Williams & Wilkins; 1999:869–881.
7. Malnutrition Advisory Group (MAG) and British Association for Parenteral and Enteral Nutrition (BAPEN). Guidelines for detection and management of malnutrition. BAPEN; 2000.
8. Seiler WO. Clinical pictures of malnutrition in ill elderly subjects. Nutrition 2001; 17:496–498.
9. Morley JE, Silver AJ. Nutritional issues in nursing home care. Ann Intern Med 1995; 123:850–859.
10. Neel AB. Malnutrition in the elderly: interactions with drug therapy. Ann Long Term Care 2001; 9:24–30.
11. Crogan NL, Shiltz JA, Adams CE, Massey LK. Barriers to nutrition care for nursing home residents. J Geront Nursing 2001; 12:25–31.
12. Finch S, Doyle W, Lowe C et al. National diet and nutrition survey: people aged 65 years and older, vol. 1. Report of the diet and nutrition survey. London: HMSO; 1998.
13. De Groot CP, van Staveren WA, on behalf of the SENECA group. Undernutrition in the European SENECA studies. Clin Geriatr Med 2002; 18:699–708.
14. Haller J. The vitamin status and its adequacy in the elderly: an international overview. Int J Vitam Nutr Res 1999; 69:160–168.
15. Russell RM, Sahyoun NR. The elderly. In: Paige EM, ed. Clinical nutrition, 2nd edn. Washington, DC: CV Mosby; 1988:110–116.
16. Young VT. Macronutrient needs in the elderly. Nutr Rev 1992; 50:454–462.
17. Rosenberg IH. Sarcopenia: origins and clinical relevance. J Nutr 1997; 127:990S–991S.
18. Whitney EN, Cataldo CB, Rolfes SR. Understanding normal and clinical nutrition, 6th edn. Wadsworth, CA: West; 2002.
19. Black AE, Coward WA, Cole TJ, Prentice AM. Human energy expenditure in affluent societies: an analysis of 574 doubly-labelled water measurements. Eur J Clin Nutr 1996; 50:72–92.
20. Howarth C. Nutrition and ageing. In: Mann J, Truswell AS, eds. Essentials of human nutrition, Oxford: Oxford University Press; 2002:551–565.
21. Branca F. Physical activity, diet and skeletal health. Public Health Nutr 1999; 2:391–396.
22. Schiffman S. Changes in taste and smell: drug interactions and food preferences. Nutr Rev 1994; 52:S11–S14.
23. Hetherington MM. Taste and appetite regulation in the elderly. Proc Nutr Soc 1998; 57:625–631.
24. Lesourd B, Mazari L. Nutrition and immunity in the elderly. Proc Nutr Soc 1999; 58:685–695.
25. Morley JE. Protein-energy malnutrition in older subjects. Proc Nutr Soc 1998; 57:587–592.
26. Steele JG, Sheiham A, Marcenes W et al. National diet and nutrition survey: people aged 65 years and older, vol. 2: report of the oral health survey. London: HMSO; 1998.
27. MacIntosh CG, Andrews JM, Jones KL et al. Effects of age on concentrations of plasma cholecystokinin, glucagons like peptide 1 and peptide YY and their relation to appetite and pyloric motility. Am J Clin Nutr 1999; 69:999–1006.
28. Russell RM. Factors in aging that effect the bioavailability of nutrients. J Nutr 2001; 131:1359–1361.
29. Russell RM. Changes in gastrointestinal function attributed to ageing. Am J Clin Nutr 1992; 55:1203–1207S.
30. BNF (British Nutrition Foundation). Nutrition in older people. London: British Nutrition Foundation; 1996.
31. Beaufrere B, Castaneda C, de Groot L et al. Report of the IDECG working group on body weight and body composition of the elderly. Eur J Clin Nutr 2000; 54:S162–S163.
32. Department of Health. Dietary reference values for food energy and nutrients for the United Kingdom. Report of the panel on dietary reference values of the Committee on Medical Aspects of Food Policy. London: HMSO; 1991.
33. Garrow JS, James WPT. Human nutrition and dietetics, 9th edn. Edinburgh: Churchill Livingstone; 1993.
34. Suter PM, Russell RM. Vitamin requirements of the elderly. Am J Clin Nutr 1987; 45:501–512.
35. Izaks GJ, Westendorp RG, Knook DL. The definition of anaemia in older persons. JAMA 1999; 281: 1714–1717.

36. Roubenoff R, Scrimshaw N, Shetty P et al. Report of the IDECG working group on the role of lifestyle including nutrition for the health of the elderly. Eur J Clin Nutr 2000; 54:S164–S165.

37. Schaumberg DA, Glynn RJ, Christen WG et al. Relations of body fat distribution and height with cataract in men. Am J Clin Nutr 2000; 72:1495–1502.

38. Chopdar A, Chakravarthy U, Verma D. Age related macular degeneration. Br Med J 2003; 326:485–488.

39. Seddon JM, Cote J, Rosner B. Progression of age-related macular degeneration: association with dietary fat, transunsaturated fat, nuts, and fish intake. Arch Ophthalmol 2003; 121:1728–1737.

40. Arthritis Research Campaign. Available online at: http://www.arc.org.uk/about_arth/astats.htm, accessed 21 April 2004.

41. Ettinger WH Jr, Burns R, Messier SP et al. A randomised trial comparing aerobic exercise and resistance exercise with a health education program in older adults with knee osteoarthritis: the Fitness Arthritis and Seniors Trial (FAST). JAMA 1997; 277:25–31.

42. Kremer JM. N-3 fatty acid supplements in rheumatoid arthritis. Am J Clin Nutr 2000; 71:349S–351S.

43. Cullum CM, Rosenberg RN. Memory loss – when is it Alzheimer's disease? JAMA 1998; 279:1689–1690.

44. Ohno M, Sametsky EA, Younkin LH et al. BACE1 deficiency rescues memory deficits and cholinergic dysfunction in a mouse model of Alzheimer's disease. Neuron 2004; 41:27–33.

45. Gonzalez-Gross M, Marcos A, Pietrzik K. Nutrition and cognitive impairment in the elderly. Br J Nutr 2001; 86:313–321.

46. Lethem R, Orrell M. Antioxidants and dementia. Lancet 1997; 349:1189–1190.

47. Riviere S, Birlouey-Aragon I et al. Low plasma vitamin C in Alzheimer patients despite an adequate diet. Int J Geriatric Psych 1998; 13:749–754.

48. Clarke R, Smith AD, Jobst KA et al. Folic acid, vitamin B_{12}, and serum homocysteine levels in confirmed Alzheimer's disease. Arch Neurol 1998; 55:1449–1455.

49. Snowdon DA, Tully CL, Smith CD et al. Serum folate and the severity of atrophy of the neocortex in Alzheimer disease: findings from the Nun Study. Am J Clin Nutr 2000; 71:993–998.

50. Food and Nutrition Board, National Research Council. Recommended dietary allowances, 10th edn. Washington, DC: National Academy Press, 1989.

Chapter **4.2**

The ageing eye

Ruth Hogg

CHAPTER CONTENTS

Ageing seems to be the only available way to live a long life[1] and is a universal and inescapable phenomenon which, when considered, raises many interesting questions. How do we define it? How do we distinguish between normal ageing and pathological ageing? What causes it? And can we delay or prevent it? How does ageing affect the eye, and what are the functional consequences of these changes? All of these questions will be addressed in this chapter.

DEFINITIONS OF AGEING

Ageing could be defined as 'an innate process caused by chemical reactions that arise in the course of normal metabolism which, collectively, produce diverse deleterious changes that occur with the passage of time that increase the chance of death and disease'.[2] Life expectancy, in contrast, is 'the age at which 50% of a given population survive'.[3]

Despite ageing being the major risk factor for disease and death in developing countries after age 28,[2] it is worth noting that death remains the ultimate consequence of ageing, and that there is no clear relationship between ageing and death.

The past hundred years have seen a dramatic rise in life expectancy in the USA, from 57 years in 1900 to 80 years in the 1980s. This marked rise has been attributed to better diet, health care and reduced infant mortality. The inevitable consequence of reducing mortality in infancy, childhood and young adulthood has been the clustering of

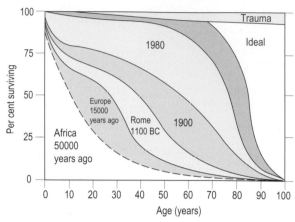

Figure 4.2.1   Survival curves for humans at different times in history, and their relationships with varying environments, nutrition and medical care. (Reproduced from Troen BR. The biology of ageing. Mount Sinai J Med NY 2003; 70:3–22.[3])

morbidity to the latter part of life, and this is clearly illustrated in Figure 4.2.1.

The upper limit of a life span is determined by the production in individuals of ageing changes associated with environment and disease, along with those indeterminate and innate changes associated with ageing. Therefore, the dramatic increase in life expectancy is now considered to be reaching a plateau. However, improved outcomes of medical care of cancer and cardiovascular disease have the potential to further increase life expectancy at birth by 3 and 6 years, respectively.[4] But future dramatic increases in average life expectancy in developed countries will only be achieved by slowing the rate of changes attributable to ageing.

THEORIES OF AGEING

Although various theories have been proposed, it is generally recognised that ageing is both complex and multifactorial. Researchers are faced with a process in which precisely defined and easily measurable biomarkers are absent, and one which produces changes ranging from a molecular to organism level, where environmental factors may affect experimental observations and where secondary effects complicate the elucidation of primary mechanisms.[3]

Various reviews have been published summarising the proposed theories which can be categorised in different ways. Weinert and Timiras produced an interesting classification, which reflects the universal impact of ageing from a molecular to organism level.[5]

Evolutionary theories

These theories basically argue that ageing results from a decline in the force of natural selection. Evolutionary pressures select for a minimum successful life, which includes the ability to reach reproductive age, procreate and care for offspring until they are weaned.

Mutation accumulation

Detrimental, late-acting mutations that affect older age are not selected against, and therefore may accumulate within a population and ultimately lead to pathology and senescence.

Disposable soma

The somatic organism is effectively maintained only for reproductive success, after which it is disposable; longevity has a cost and therefore the balance of resources invested in longevity versus reproductive fitness determines the life span.

Antagonistic pleiotropy

Genes that are beneficial at a younger age become deleterious at an older age. An example is the *p53* tumour suppressor gene which appears to require a fine equilibrium in order for the organism to achieve a long life span. Too little *p53* results in death from cancer whereas too much *p53* leads to death by accelerated ageing.[3]

Molecular theories

Gene regulation

Ageing is caused by changes in the expression of genes regulating development and ageing.

Codon restriction

Fidelity/accuracy of mRNA translation is impaired due to the inability to decode codons in mRNA.

Error catastrophe

This theory proposes that random errors in synthesis eventually occur in proteins that synthesise DNA or other 'template' molecules, leading to rapid accumulation of error-containing molecules that would be incompatible with normal function and life.

Somatic mutation

Random damage to vital molecules accumulates to a sufficient level to result in the physiological decline associated with ageing.

Dysdifferentiation

Gradual accumulation of random molecular damage impairs regulation of gene expression.

Cellular theories

Cellular senescence – telomere theory[3,5,6]

Phenotypes of ageing are considered to be caused by an increase in the frequency of senescent cells. Senescence may result from cellular stress (cellular senescence) or telomere shortening (replicative senescence). Telomeres are specialised structures composed of repeating DNA sequence, and are located at the ends of each chromosome. Cell division results in ever-shorter telomeres, altered telomere structure, and, ultimately, replicative senescence. In this context, environmental influences such as exposure to high levels of oxidative stress, and thus damage, have been shown to accelerate telomere shortening.

Free-radical theory[2,3,4,5,7–9]

This theory postulates that the ageing process is the consequence of free-radical reactions. Free radicals are responsible for the progressive deterioration of biological systems over time because of their unstable state.

Wear and tear

This involves accumulation of normal injury.

Apoptosis

Apoptosis is programmed cell death from genetic events or genome crisis.

System-based theories

Neuroendocrine

Functional decrements in neurons and their associated hormones that control homeostasis may result in age-related physiological changes.

Immunological

Decline of immune function (decreased T-cell response) with ageing results in decreased incidence of infectious diseases but increased incidence of autoimmunity (e.g. increased serum antibodies).

Rate of living

The rate of living assumes a fixed amount of metabolic potential for every living organism (live fast, die young).

At present, the exact cause of ageing remains unclear. Overall, it seems likely that the integration of selected models and theories which take into account the interactions among intrinsic (genetic), extrinsic (environmental) and stochastic (random damage to vital molecules) factors will yield a plausible model that explains the ageing process.

ANATOMICAL AND PHYSIOLOGICAL AGE-RELATED CHANGES IN THE EYE

The eye, like all organs, is not isolated from the universal process of ageing. Therefore, distinguishing between physiological and pathological age-related ocular change is difficult.

Cornea

The changes which occur in the cornea can be divided into three main categories: (1) changes in shape and optical properties; (2) corneal degeneration; and (3) physical and biological changes.[10]

Changes in shape and optical properties

Steepening of keratometry occurs, with a shift from with-the-rule to against-the-rule astigmatism.[11,12] This change is thought to be due to decreasing pressure from the lids as they become more lax with age. A recent report has suggested that ageing influences changes in patterns of astigmatism differently in men and women, with the corneas of older men flatter than those of older women. Men also have a significantly higher potential for against-the-rule astigmatism than women.[13] Transparency is unaffected in the central cornea by physiological ageing.[14]

The average corneal radius decreases with age, and the cornea becomes more spherical, resulting in significantly more spherical aberration in middle-aged and older corneas.[15] Image quality, as quantified by the modulation transfer function, is therefore degraded with age as a consequence of increased wave aberrations.[16] Indeed, monochromatic aberrations and age have been shown to fit a quadratic model.[17]

Ultrastructurally, intramolecular and interfibrillar spacing in collagen increases with age, possibly via increased protein glycation.[18,19] Also, the number of corneal endothelial cells decreases as they do not regenerate, and neighbouring cells expand to fill the space, resulting in a departure from the classical uniform six-sided endothelial cell appearance (polymorphism).[20]

Corneal degenerations

The development of age-related corneal degenerations is thought to be influenced by genetic factors and environmental exposure.

Cornea farinata (Figure 4.2.2)   This innocuous condition is characterised by the presence of minute, usually flour-like deposits in the deep corneal stroma that are most prominent centrally.

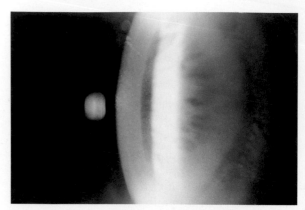

Figure 4.2.2   Cornea farinata.

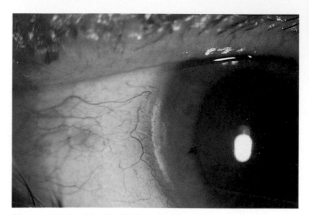

Figure 4.2.3   Vogt's limbal girdle.

Vogt's limbal girdle (Figure 4.2.3)   This common, innocuous, bilateral, asymptomatic, age-related finding is characterised by narrow, crescenteric, white opacities of the peripheral cornea in the interpalpebral zone along the nasal and temporal limbus. It is seen in all patients over the age of 80, and in 50% of normal eyes of people between the ages of 40 and 60.[21]

Deep crocodile shagreen (Figure 4.2.4)   This is usually asymptomatic, and appears as bilateral, polygonal, greyish-white opacities which can occur either in the anterior two-thirds of the stroma (anterior crocodile shagreen) or more posteriorly (posterior crocodile shagreen). These are thought to be due to changes in the collagen lamellae accompanied by widely spaced collagen fibres.

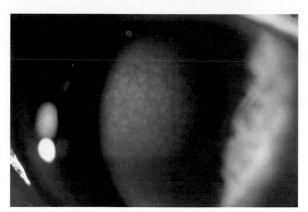

Figure 4.2.4 Deep crocodile shagreen.

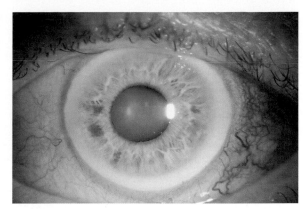

Figure 4.2.6 Arcus senilis.

Figure 4.2.5 Hassall–Henle bodies.

Hassall–Henle bodies (Figure 4.2.5) These are defined as small hyaline excrescences on the posterior surface of Descemet's membrane at the periphery of the cornea.

Arcus senilis (Figure 4.2.6) This is the most common peripheral corneal opacity. It appears as bilateral grey, white or yellowish circumferential deposits in the peripheral cornea. The sharp peripheral edge is usually separated from the limbus by a lucid area, and this clear zone may occasionally undergo thinning. Its presence is due to increased permeability of local blood vessels to lipids, and is related to serum cholesterol level.

Physical and biological changes

Resistance to corneal infection is reduced with increasing age,[22] as is the number of phagocytically active cells following infection.[23] Other age-related features include: failure to upregulate intercellular adhesion molecule-1 (ICAM-1) and reduced inflammatory cell infiltration;[24] a decline in high energy metabolism;[25] increased tear contact time;[26] increased epithelial permeability to fluorescein;[22] and reduced corneal sensitivity.[27]

Iris

A large number of elderly people with normal eyes display increased bowing of the iris, even in the absence of optic nerve atrophy or elevation of intraocular pressure at the time of examination.[28] A study investigating ultrastructural changes in the iris found that age-related changes of the iris included: duplication of the basal lamina of the posterior iris pigment epithelial cells; formations of atrophic invaginations in the posterior cell membranes containing interlacing basal lamina; and formation (or deposition) of microfibrils and electron-dense material.[29]

Vitreous

The vitreous gel is attached at the vitreous base, which is a 3–4-mm-wide zone straddling the ora serrata; it is also attached at the optic disc and the macula. In general, the ageing of the human vitreous is characterised by a thickening of the basal lamina of the retina, an increase in the liquid vitreous volume, the collapse of the gel and the aggregation of collagen fibrils into large fibres.[30,31] By about 80–90 years, more than half the total vitreous volume is liquid, and the vitreous volume begins to decrease. Another common ageing change is detachment of the posterior vitreous, where the cortical vitreous gel separates from the basal lamina, and this represents the end-point of the normal ageing of the vitreous. Posterior vitreous detachment may cause serious visual disturbances by at least one of two mechanisms: (1) by causing traction on the retina, which, in turn, results in functional and structural changes in this tissue; or (2) by creating optical heterogeneity in the vitreous, thus interfering with clear image formation. These image disturbances can include photopsia (caused by traction on the nerve fibre layer), metamorphopsia (through retinal oedema) and floaters (shadows cast on the central visual area by the collapsed structures of the gel). Detachment of the posterior vitreous may occasionally act as a precipitating factor for retinal tears and detachments. Other age-related features include Cloquet's canal becoming less distinguishable, an increase in degradative enzymes[32] and age-related changes in the basal retinovitreous adhesion.[33]

Recent evidence has shown a significant correlation between increased vitreous liquefaction and increased risk of nuclear cataracts, suggesting that preservation or replacement of the vitreous gel may protect patients from nuclear cataract.[34] The total reactive antioxidant potential of the vitreous has also been shown to decrease with age, and this phenomenon was shown to correlate directly with decreases in photoreceptor density, and to correlate inversely with increases in the autofluorescent intensity of the retina and the thickness of Bruch's membrane, providing possible new insights into the oxidative stress hypothesis of age-related macular degeneration (AMD).[35] Several investigators have also reported that AMD patients are less likely to have a posterior vitreous detachment,[36,37] thus suggesting that vitreoretinal adherence may have a role in the pathogenesis and/or progression of this disease.

Aqueous formation

The rate of aqueous formation diminishes with age, such that from the age of 10 it declines by 3.2% per decade.[21] Investigation of aqueous humour dynamics in older eyes compared to younger eyes has revealed several significant differences, including a smaller anterior chamber volume, a reduced aqueous flow and reduced uveoscleral outflow in the aged eyes.[38]

Lens

The lens presents as an interesting case as regard to ageing because, despite growth throughout life, none of the cells are cast off and, therefore, time is represented spatially across the lens profile. Although growth occurs throughout life, it is maximal in fetal life.[39] Growth up to the age of about 30 is concentrated in the equatorial plane of the lens, after which it is approximately zero, whereas continued lens growth in the adult eye is primarily in the sagittal direction. These changes cause an increase in the dioptric power of the lens, which is attenuated by a compensatory decrease in refractive index of the lens with time. A recent study using magnetic resonance imaging has shown that age-related lens growth is confined to the anterior portion.[40]

Increased absorption and scatter of optical radiation with age cause the lens to become yellow and fluorescent, contrasting sharply with the young human lens, which has an almost 100% transmission. The increased scatter is attributed to the accumulation of high-molecular-weight crystalline aggregates. Recent data suggest that the increased fluorescence is thought to be due to an age-related increase in the tryptophan-derived fluorophore: reduced glutathione (GSH)-3-hydroxylkynurenine. The absorption of optical radiation by the lens rises exponentially with age, with absorption greatest for shorter wavelengths in the blue end of the spectrum,[41,42] due to the postnatal accumulation of yellow chromophores. This optical factor of lenticular senescence is the main contributor to the age-related changes observed in colour vision.[43] The functional consequence of ultraviolet light excitation fluorescence within the crystalline lens, which results in intraocular stray light, is a decrease in low-contrast acuity and this loss increases linearly with age.[44]

Optic nerve

Ageing is associated with an increase in mean diameter of the optic nerve due to an increase in the optic nerve/meningeal membrane ratio, and an increase in the mean number of astrocytes. The mean number of nerve fibres of large diameter decreases with increasing age.[45] The cup and disc areas, and the cup-to-disc ratios, increase with age, whereas the retinal nerve fibre layer thickness decreases during the course of normal senescence.[46]

Capillary blood flow in the retina, neuroretinal rim and lamina cribrosa decreases with advancing age.[47] The resilience of the lamina cribrosa also decreases with age, suggesting an increased susceptibility to plastic flow and permanent deformation.[48] From a histological point of view, alterations in the composition of the lamina cribrosa with age include: increased elastin and decreased fibronectin; a decreased lipid content; and decreased total sulphinated glycosaminoglycans. There is no change, however, in cellularity or water content.[49]

Pupil size

Pupillary diameter decreases with increasing age, resulting in decreased retinal illuminance. Pupil size is independent of gender, refractive error or iris colour.[50–52]

Sclera

The sclera is an envelope of dense collagenous tissue of thickness 0.4–0.6 mm at the equator of the globe, 0.8 mm at the limbus and 1.0–1.35 mm at the posterior pole. The literature is inconsistent with regard to age-related changes in scleral thickness.[21] An increase in yellowing is often noted in the ageing sclera, which can be attributed to an increase in lipid composition in common with other connective tissues. Focal hyalinisation of the sclera results in what is known as Cogan's scleral

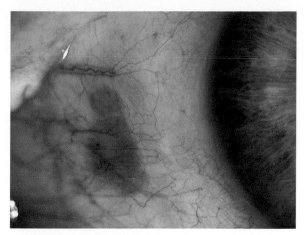

Figure 4.2.7   Scleral plaque. (Courtesy of Department of Ophthalmology, Edward S. Harkness Eye Institute, Columbia University, New York, USA.)

plaque, a common bilateral, asymptomatic, sharply demarcated zone of increased scleral translucency which is commonly situated just in front of the medial and lateral recti (Figure 4.2.7).

The number of elastic fibres also increases with age, as does scleral rigidity. Interestingly, increased scleral rigidity has been proposed as a risk factor for the development of AMD.[53] An age-related loss of glycosaminoglycans is accompanied by a loss of scleral tissue hydration.[54] However, scleral permeability to hydrophilic compounds is unaffected by age.[55] The transport capability of the sclera has important implications for drug delivery, and a recent report suggests that delivery is more readily achieved across the posterior sclera compared with the anterior sclera, and that the ease of delivery decreases with time.[56]

Choroid

The choroid is divided into three layers: (1) the vessel layer; (2) capillary layer; and (3) Bruch's membrane, and it assumes several important roles. Firstly, because of its rich vasculature it supplies nutrition to the overlying retinal pigment epithelium (RPE) and the outer third of the neurosensory retina as far as the outer plexiform layer, and secondly, the choroid acts to exchange heat and waste material produced by retinal metabolism.

Morphological analysis of age-related changes in the choroid has revealed thickening of Bruch's membrane, decreased density and diameter of the choriocapillaris and thinning of the entire choroid.[57,58] Interestingly, the age-related thickening of Bruch's membrane has been shown to correlate directly with age-related RPE autofluorescence.[59]

The transport capability of the choroid is also reduced with age, due to reduced choroidal blood flow and increased lipid/cholesterol content of Bruch's membrane.[60–63] Bruch's membrane, in particular, is considered to assume importance in the physiology of the eye due to its strategic location between the metabolically active photoreceptors and the choriocapillaris. As well as providing support and an attachment for the RPE, it forms a semipermeable filtration barrier through which major metabolic exchange takes place, thus allowing nutrients to reach the photoreceptors and RPE from the choriocapillaris and waste products of cellular reactions to travel in the opposite direction.[64] Age-related changes in Bruch's membrane have been consistently shown to be greater in the posterior pole than in the periphery.[58,65,66] Altered nutrition as a consequence of these changes in the extracellular matrix and Bruch's membrane results in dysfunction of the RPE and photoreceptors, and has been postulated as a major influence on the development of disease and its subsequent outcome. Also, calcification of Bruch's membrane may occur, thus rendering the tissue brittle.[67] Examination of donor eyes has revealed progressive accumulation of lipids in Bruch's membrane, with an exponential increase over 50 years of age. It is thought that the material is cellular in origin, and is not derived from plasma.[64] A recent study, however, found a massive accumulation of esterified cholesterol leading to the conclusion that Bruch's membrane is altered in the same way as the arterial intima in cardiovascular disease.[68]

The diffuse accumulation of extraneous material characteristic of ageing Bruch's membrane is believed to be derived from the pigment epithelium as a result of a failure of debris to traverse Bruch's membrane into the choriocapillaris. Though there is no consensus regarding the actual mechanism involved in drusen formation, it is generally considered they form as a consequence of RPE metabolic activity rather than being directly derived from outer-segment material. Recently, an inflammatory process has been proposed, suggesting that a chronic local inflammatory component is initially associated with the formation of drusen, and that the debris derived from altered RPE cells may act as a chronic inflammatory stimulus for drusen formation.[69]

Retina

The neural retina consists of three basic classes of neuron: (1) photoreceptors, which absorb quanta of light and transform them into chemical signals in the form of glutamic acid (glutamate); (2) bipolar cells, which connect the photoreceptors to the ganglion cells; and (3) ganglion cells, which collect the information generated in the retina and transmit it to the brain (Figure 4.2.8). These three classes of cell are commonly referred to as the vertical retinal pathway; in addition, there are laterally integrating interneurons which can be divided into two major classes, according to the layer within the retina where they make their synaptic connections: (1) horizontal cells, which have their terminals in the outer synaptic (plexiform) layer; and (2) amacrine cells, which connect exclusively in the inner plexiform layer. The retinal photoreceptors and ganglion cells are part of the central nervous system, and therefore do not replicate in life. Therefore, they are subject to cumulative changes with age.

A recent study using optical coherence tomography (OCT) has shown that both total retinal thickness and nerve fibre layer thickness significantly decrease with increasing age,[70] particularly in the superior quadrant. Indeed, the evoked potentials from the neurons comprising this layer showed attenuation by a near-equivalent amount.[71] Actual density of ganglion cells subserving the central 11° of vision is reduced by one-fourth in old eyes when compared with young eyes.[72]

Studies investigating photoreceptor topography have revealed a dichotomy between the influence of age on the cell types, with rods being more vulnerable to loss by ageing than cones.[73,74] Peak density of cones varied considerably but appeared remarkably stable throughout life, whereas the

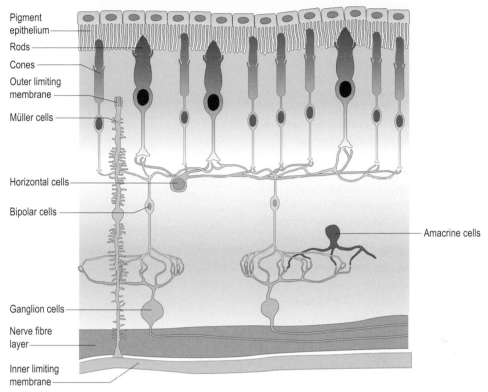

Pigment epithelium
Rods
Cones
Outer limiting membrane
Müller cells
Horizontal cells
Bipolar cells
Amacrine cells
Ganglion cells
Nerve fibre layer
Inner limiting membrane

Figure 4.2.8 Retina. (Courtesy of Helga Kolb.)

number of rods in the macular retina of the same eyes decreased by 30%, and this loss was maximal in the parafovea (4–6 mm, 3.5–10° from fixation). The kinetics of rod loss is not sigmoidal, which indicates that cell death is not related to cumulative damage.[75,76] Even in eyes with disrupted retinal architecture due to large drusen and thick basal deposits, the appearance and density of the foveal cone mosaic is normal when compared with other age-matched controls without these characteristics.[77] By contrast, however, the few rods that remained in the parafovea appeared large and misshapen. In late age-related macular degeneration, virtually all surviving photoreceptors were cones. Another study confirmed this finding in that there was a preferential loss of rods over cones found in three-quarters of early and late ARM eyes examined.[78]

Structurally, the net increase in the number of disc membranes with age is not accompanied by an increase in axial length of the rod outer segment, and therefore most individuals over the age of 45 display convolutions in their outer segments.[79]

Vascular changes with age include endothelial loss from retinal capillaries and thickening of the basal membranes of these capillaries, which can induce ischaemia. There is also a reduction in the number of astrocytes with age, which display higher levels of glial fibrillary acidic protein and more cytoplasmic organelles. This reactive astrocyte population may protect neurons from free radicals by upregulating enzymatic and non-enzymatic antioxidant defences.[80] Mitochondrial DNA deletions and cytochrome c oxidase-deficient cones also accumulate in the ageing retina, particularly in the foveal region, and it has been hypothesised that these changes may contribute to the changes in macular function observed in ageing and age-related maculopathy.[81]

Retinal pigment epithelium

The RPE consists of a single layer of epithelial cells; it lies just behind the neural retina and is interposed between the photoreceptor cells and their supporting blood supply in the choroid (Figure 4.2.9). This continuous sheet of cells forms the equivalent of the blood–brain barrier between the choroidal capillaries and the photoreceptors.[82,83]

The RPE performs and controls many important processes within the retina, which are essential for maintaining normal photoreceptor cell function and survival. It regulates the delivery of nutrients and metabolites to the photoreceptors, directs retinoid and interphotoreceptor metabolism, controls neuroretinal adhesion, absorbs stray light through its melanosomes, constitutes the blood–eye barrier and is responsible for outer-segment phagocytosis.[75] Photoreceptor outer segments must undergo continuous turnover; however, unlike other phagocytes, RPE cells remain in situ for a lifetime, with the RPE residual body content increases with age. Loss of RPE cells results in increased metabolic demand on each cell.[64] Impairment of outer-segment phagocytosis by the RPE has been shown to result in photoreceptor cell degeneration.[84,85] The RPE also plays a role in the antioxidant defences within the retina as it is rich in vitamin E, superoxide dismutase, catalase, glutathione peroxidase and melanin.

Generally, increasing age is characterised by a loss of melanin and accumulations of lipofuscin. There is a net reduction in the number of RPE cells across the retina with age, and this results in the expansion of the remaining cells to cover the deficits.[86–88] This decrease is slower in whites than in blacks.[86] Melanin distribution also decreases from the equator to the posterior pole with increasing age, with a significant peak at the macula.[88,89] It decreases by about 25% in the macula between early and late decades, and is accompanied by an age-related change in the spectral properties of melanin with age.[90]

Lipofuscin is a generic name given to a heterogeneous group of complex, autofluorescent lipid and protein aggregates present in a wide variety of neuronal and non-neuronal tissues.[75] Lipofuscin shows an almost linear accumulation with age,

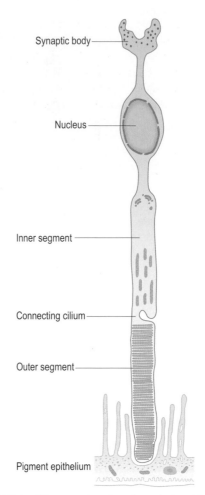

Figure 4.2.9   Diagram showing the relationship of a rod photoreceptor cell with the retinal pigment epithelium (RPE). Photoreceptors are long cylindrical cells organised into the distinct regions shown. The outer segment grows continually by addition of new material at its base adjacent to the connecting cilium. Periodically, the apical portion of the outer segment is shed from the cell and is taken up by the RPE via phagocytes. (Modified from Katz ML. Bernard Strehler – inspiration for basic research into the mechanisms of aging. Mechanisms Ageing Dev 2002; 123:831–840, with permission.[82])

correlates negatively with longevity and is widely assumed to play a role in the ageing process.[91] In the eye, lipofuscins notably accumulate in the vicinity of the RPE and Bruch's membrane.

Lipofuscins have three primary defining characteristics: (1) they consist of intracellular secondary lysosomes; (2) they have yellow autofluorescent emission when excited by near ultra-violet or blue light; and (3) they accumulate during normal senescence. The accumulation of lipofuscin appears to have several functional consequences. Near the end of the life span, in post-mitotic cells, such as those found in the retina, large quantities of lipofuscin can accumulate that cannot be removed, resulting in progressive cellular dysfunction. This interferes with important autophagic processes, preventing cellular removal, and resulting in accumulation of damaged cellular constituents.[92] It also appears to sensitise lysosomes and aged neurons to oxidative stress by binding to transition metals such as copper and iron, whose concentration increases in the central nervous system with time. Of particular concern is the fact that lipofuscin is a photoinducible generator of reactive oxygen species. In the RPE, which lies in a highly metabolically active environment where the generation of reactive oxygen species is high,[93] the presence of lipofuscin is likely to increase the damage induced by visible light, which may explain the increased risk of developing macular degenerative disease in aged individuals. Indeed, exposure of lipofuscin to blue light has been shown to generate superoxide ions, singlet oxygen, hydrogen peroxide and lipid peroxides.[94] The generation of superoxide ions on exposure of lipofuscin to light is wavelength-dependent, and is greatest when exposed to blue light (400–520 nm).[95] A2E, the fluorophore of lipofuscin, appears to mediate the blue-light-induced apoptosis of RPE cells by inhibiting the degradative capacity of lysosomes and by disrupting membrane integrity through phototoxicity.[96–98] Lipofuscin accumulation only occurs when visual cycle retinoids are present in the retina.[91] It is now generally accepted that oxidative stress is involved in promoting lipofuscin accumulation in the RPE.[82,99] In support of this view, a recent report showed significantly reduced formation of lipofuscin when the antioxidants lutein, zeaxanthin, lycopene or tocopherol were added to rabbit and bovine RPE cells exposed to normobaric hyperoxia and photoreceptor outer segments.[100]

While there is increasing indirect evidence that accumulation of lipofuscin is involved in the development of AMD,[93,100–102] the fundamental question on whether or how it results in impairment of cellular function remains.[83] This has proved difficult to determine as the same factors that influence lipofuscin accumulation may also have effects on cell function independent of their effects on the rate at which lipofuscin accumulates. Although a cause-and-effect relationship has not been established, it has been noted that:[83]

1. RPE accumulation is accompanied by progressive decreases in photoreceptor cell densities in both humans and rats.
2. RPE lipofuscin content has been shown to be higher in individuals with AMD.
3. RPE lipofuscin content has been shown to be greatly elevated in subjects with a form of inherited retinal degeneration.
4. The ability of RPE to mediate photoreceptor outer-segment turnover appears to be reduced during senescence.
5. Age-related accumulation of lipofuscin in the RPE is accompanied by significant changes in the morphological features of this cell line, as well as the morphology of its extracellular matrix. In particular, the accumulation of extracellular material on the basal side of the RPE has been associated with the development of AMD.
6. Experimental manipulations that cause an increase in RPE lipofuscin accumulation have also been shown to result in photoreceptor losses.

The study of fundoscopically visible autofluorescence due to lipofuscin has also attracted much attention. Lipofuscin fractions from all age groups exhibit a strong broadband fluorescence emission spectrum, with a peak at 600 nm, when excited at 364 nm.[90] The autofluorescence has been shown to follow closely the normal distribution of rods, i.e. low in the foveal centre and high at 2–4 mm eccentricity.[103] Changes in autofluoresence have also been shown to be associated with drusen and geographic atrophy.[104,105]

PHYSIOLOGICAL FUNCTIONAL CHANGES

A multitude of the structural age-related changes that occur in the eye will have functional consequences. However, it is worth noting that relating anatomic changes to specific functional changes may be difficult, as the location of such complex perceptions often remains unclear, and may well be multicentric.[106]

Visual acuity

Visual acuity represents the ability to discriminate small detail, and is a measure of the spatial-resolving ability of the visual system under conditions of very high contrast.[107] Although all studies agree that acuity declines with age, even when patients are wearing their best optical correction for the test distance, it is difficult to find a definitive rate of decline with age as different studies use different case-definitions of what constitutes good eye health.[108] A cross-sectional study of 78 subjects aged 21–68 years revealed that the expected loss of acuity over a lifetime is approximately 0.1–0.2 log units.[109]

Visual acuity, contrast sensitivity (CS), disability glare and visual field were measured in 3654 subjects in the epidemiological Blue Mountain Eye Study. All tests of visual function were observed to decrease with increasing age, and disability glare was the only test that was selectively impaired in patients with identifiable eye disease. A longitudinal study carried out in Sweden, in which the cohort was followed from the age of 70 to 88 years, found that at age 70 nearly 100% of the sample had an acuity of 6/7.5 or better; at age 82, however, this had dropped to 50%, and at age 88 this had further reduced to 25%.[110]

Vernier acuity, which measures the ability to discriminate displacement, samples a smaller part of the retina and does not seem to vary with age.[111,112] However, this finding may be restricted to static targets because a marked age-related effect is observed once oscillation is introduced.[113,114]

Macular function

Macular function declines significantly throughout adulthood.

Central visual pathways

Alterations in the physiological properties of neural elements in both the retina and visual cortex are associated with normal ageing.[115,116] It has, however, been suggested that ageing has only minor effects on the retina–geniculo-striate pathway, since rod losses are compensated for, ganglion cell loss is small compared to individual-to-individual variability and no massive cell loss occurs in lateral geniculate nucleus (LGN) or striate cortex.[117] Functional studies of LGN suggest their retinal inputs are not affected significantly by ageing, and pattern-evoked electroretinograms (PERG) suggest that electrical properties are likewise unaffected. Comparisons between PERG and cortical evoked potentials suggest that some neural change occurs, but its location is unknown.

Electrophysiology has been used to show that mechanisms sensitive to high spatial and low temporal frequencies are selectively degraded by ageing.[118] An alternative theory proposes that a shortage of γ-aminobutyric acid (GABA)-mediated inhibition in the visual cortex might underlie age-related visual deficits. GABA production is reduced in older animals and, if reduced inhibition underlies age-related functional defects in widespread cortical regions, the GABA system could represent an important target for the treatment of sensory, motor and cognitive age-related deficits.[119]

Visual fields

Visual field thresholds decline with age at a rate of about 0.5–1.0 dB per decade;[120–121] therefore, most automated perimeters incorporate an age-related correction into the analysis. The borders of the visual field are constricted in older adults compared to younger adults,[122,123] and there is a generalised loss in sensitivity throughout the central 30° of the field. There is possibly a slightly greater loss of sensitivity in the more peripheral field.[124–126] These alterations are thought to be primarily the results of neural changes.[126]

A study which investigated normal observers aged 20–83 years using conditions mediated by chromatic opponent mechanisms found that average visual field sensitivity decreases for opponent mechanisms by approximately 0.7 dB per decade. These are similar to data obtained on standard automated perimetry. By comparison, short-wavelength sensitive mechanisms exhibited age-related losses that were more than twice as large, even after lenticular transmission was accounted for.[127]

Colour vision

The elderly tend to show acquired colour vision deficiencies, typically the loss of colour discrimination, especially along the blue–yellow axis.[121,128] These changes are indicative of problems in the short-wavelength system, and the optical factor of lenticular senescence has been shown to be the main contributor to the age-related changes observed in colour vision.[43] Despite this diminished ability to discriminate subtle differences in hue, both young and old have similar colour-naming functions, loci of achromatic points and loci of unique hues for yellow and blue. Therefore, the visual system somehow continuously recalibrates the strength of colour signals, maintaining colour constancy throughout the life span.[129,130]

Accommodation and presbyopia

The most common problem encountered in vision with ageing is presbyopia, a loss of accommodative amplitude of the crystalline lens. This loss begins in early teens, but is not noticeable until the 40s, when patients note they are unable to read fine print up close. Some of the factors thought to contribute to presbyopia include changes in the shape, structure and position of the ciliary body, increases in the stiffness of the cortex of the lens, increased curvature of the anterior lens surface and altered zonular insertion.[39,120]

Contrast sensitivity

CS measures the ability to perceive differences between an object and its background. Clinical measures of CS are often considered to be more representative of a patient's functional vision than traditional measures of visual acuity. CS is the reciprocal of the contrast threshold, and is defined as the ratio of the difference in the luminance of the target and background to the lower or higher of these luminance values.[107]

Several studies have shown that CS decreases with age for medium and high spatial frequen-

cies.[131,132] Investigators have attempted to separate the relative optical and neural contributions to the decline in CS at medium and high spatial frequencies. In brief, optical changes included increased optical blur, pupillary miosis, increased light-scattering and lens-yellowing. Although both play a role, most consider the neural contributions to be more important, though some disagree.[117,133] They attribute the loss of CS in age to the increase in intraocular scattering of light with age, and the fact that there also appears to be an increment in ocular aberration that causes an additional reduction in the contrast of retinal images.[134] However, most agree that optical factors do not contribute significantly,[135–137] as it has been demonstrated that pupillary miosis is not responsible for the accentuated loss in CS at low luminance.[138]

To resolve these uncertainties, studies of age-related optical changes through simulation were undertaken to compare spatiotemporal CS in younger age groups with older people. The younger group were consistently better, suggesting that under normal viewing conditions it is primarily neural factors that underlie the deterioration in visual quality experienced by older observers.[139] Sampling efficiencies (how effectively the available stimulus information is utilised by the visual system) were also found to be significantly lower in the older group, while internal noise showed no significant change, thus suggesting that the neural system plays a major role in the loss of CS in ageing, but otherwise healthy, eyes.[140] Reduced retinal illuminance due to increased lens density, and reduced retinal contrast due to increased light scatter, would shift the function along the abscissa or ordinate, respectively, but would not lead to the observed increase in the slope, adding further weight to the argument rejecting optical factors.[141]

From a practical point of view, when tested at high spatial frequencies (16 cpd), older adults in their 70s require about three times more contrast to detect a target than do young adults in their 20s.[133] Statistically significant age-related declines in scotopic CS have been found for all spatial frequencies at or below 1.2 cpd. An age-related and statistically significant decrease in high-frequency cut-off with age has also been observed.[142] An explanation of these results in terms of optical factors was rejected, as the authors felt the results were consistent with age-related changes in the magnocellular pathway.

Binocular summation and stereopsis

Binocular summation refers to the enhancement in visual function resulting from neural interactions between signals originating in the two eyes, a processing task which occurs at the level of the visual cortex of the brain where the inputs from the two eyes are combined. It is the ratio of binocular sensitivity to sensitivity measured with the better-seeing eye. This has been shown to decline with age, implying that the visual centres become unaware that two eyes have been stimulated.[143,144] The increasing incidence of anisometropia with age, and decreased prism adaptation amplitude, is consistent with this.[120,145]

Stereopsis arises from the fact that objects at different depths are imaged on different parts of the two eyes (binocular disparity), and thus provides an important source of depth information. Ever-larger disparities are required with age in order to perceive depth from a particular cue,[130,146] and the decline appears to be attributable to alterations in the early stages of visual processing.[147] Defective stereopsis is very common in the elderly in the absence of ocular morbidity. A survey of over 700 elderly people with healthy eyes living in an inner city found that only 27% had full stereopsis, and 29% had no stereopsis.[113]

Scotopic sensitivity

Anatomically, it is evident that the rods are particularly vulnerable throughout the ageing process; therefore, it is not surprising that older healthy adults demonstrate an average of 0.1 log unit elevation in absolute threshold under dark-adapted conditions, even after correcting for lens density.[148] This age-related deficit does not vary by eccentricity or by meridian, and therefore does not correspond with the age-related loss of rods in the perifoveal region. By middle to later decades of life, scotopic impairment is typically more severe than photopic impairment, and it progresses at a greater rate than photopic sensitivity impairment

as a function of decade. It has been suggested that it is caused by alteration of RPE and Bruch's membrane that impedes the passage of vitamin A or other nutrients to the rod photoreceptors.[148]

Rod-mediated dark adaptation is also slowed with increasing age, by about 8 seconds per decade.[149] This is not correlated with scotopic sensitivity, however, indicating that the underlying mechanisms are not identical. Many consider the decreased rod sensitivity to be caused by neural factors,[150] and support for a postreceptoral basis for decreased scotopic sensitivity was fostered when it was found that no age-related difference was found in the amplitude of scotopic A-wave, yet a significant loss existed in the amplitude of the scotopic B-wave.[151–153] Significant losses were also reported in the amplitude of the rod pattern ERG, reflecting activity at the ganglion cell level.[115] The scotopic deficits reflect the subjective complaints of older adults who frequently cite difficulty driving at night and seeing in conditions of low illumination as primary visual problems.[154]

Photopic sensitivity

Photopic sensitivity shows a linear decrease with age, at a rate of 0.04 log units per decade.[148] Sensitivity for all three cone types, or at least one of their postreceptoral pathways, declines in older adults.[155] Various studies have demonstrated a decrease in short-wavelength sensitive pathways with age,[156–158] and some attribute this partly to preretinal absorption,[156,157] while others do not.[158] It has been suggested that the presence of high levels of macular pigment in older people may help maintain a high level of photopic sensitivity, as older subjects with low macular pigment levels had lower sensitivity than younger subjects, whereas the sensitivity of older subjects with high levels of macular pigment was not significantly different from that of young subjects.[159] A significant and positive correlation was also found between foveal macular pigment density and the short-, but not the middle- or long-, wavelength sensitive cones. This, however, was independent of age, and, therefore, was interpreted as being due to local gain changes resulting from differential filtering of incident light by the macular pigment between the fovea and the parafovea rather than because of the protection hypothesis.[160]

Critical flicker fusion

Critical flicker fusion (CFF) measures the temporal resolving capacity of the visual system. Older adults have reduced CFFs, as well as reduced temporal CS, particularly at intermediate and high spatial frequencies.[161,162] This loss is thought to be neurally based.[108]

Motion perception

The visual motion system performs numerous functions essential for survival in a dynamic visual world, including the ability to recover and represent the trajectories of objects in a form that facilitates behavioural responses to those movements.[163] Decreased sensitivity to moving targets has been demonstrated in association with increasing age, and cannot be explained by optical changes or cognitive factors, thus implicating age-related changes in the visual neural pathway.[164–166]

CONCLUSION

Real-life and practical consequences of age-related changes of the visual system and alteration in ocular structure tell only part of the story. Along with the other senses, vision makes a central contribution to a wide variety of cognitive abilities, including reasoning and memory.[130] The relationships between vision and ageing have real and important implications, for individuals in relation to quality of life, and for society in terms of public health.

References

1. Auber D, Esprit F. Age and ageing quotations. Available online at: www.quotationsbook.com/quotes/1389/view. Accessed 6 July 2005.
2. Harman D. The free radical theory of ageing. Antioxidants Redox Signal 2003; 5:557–561.
3. Troen BR. The biology of ageing. Mount Sinai J Med NY 2003; 70:3–22.
4. Harman D. The ageing process: major risk factor for disease and death. Proc Natl Acad Sci USA 1991; 88:5360–5363.
5. Weinert BT, Timiras PS. Invited review: theories of ageing. J Appl Physiol 2003; 95:1706–1716.
6. Jennings BJ, Ozanne SE, Hales CN. Nutrition, oxidative damage, telomere shortening, and cellular senescence: individual or connected agents of ageing? Mol Genet Metab 2000; 71:32–42.
7. Halliwell B. Antioxidant defence mechanisms: from the beginning to the end (of the beginning). Free Radical Res 1999; 31:261–272.
8. Wickens AP. Ageing and the free radical theory. Resp Physiol 2001; 128:379–391.
9. Harman D. Ageing and oxidative stress. J Int Fed Clin Chem/IFCC 1998; 10:24–27.
10. Faragher RG, Mulholland B, Tuft SJ et al. Ageing and the cornea. Br J Ophthalmol 1997; 81:814–817.
11. Hayashi K, Hayashi H, Hayashi F. Topographic analysis of the changes in corneal shape due to ageing. Cornea 1995; 14:527–532.
12. Hayashi K, Masumoto M, Fujino S et al. [Changes in corneal astigmatism with ageing.] Nippon Ganka Gakkai Zasshi 1993; 97:1193–1196.
13. Goto T, Klyce SD, Zheng X et al. Gender- and age-related differences in corneal topography. Cornea 2001; 20:270–276.
14. van den Berg TJ, Tan KE. Light transmittance of the human cornea from 320 to 700 nm for different ages. Vision Res 1994; 34:1453–1456.
15. Guirao A, Redondo M, Artal P. Optical aberrations of the human cornea as a function of age. J Opt Soc Am 2000; 17:1697–1702.
16. McLellan JS, Marcos S, Burns SA. Age-related changes in monochromatic wave aberrations of the human eye. Invest Ophthalmol Vis Sci 2001; 42:1390–1395.
17. Brunette I, Bueno JM, Parent M et al. Monochromatic aberrations as a function of age, from childhood to advanced age. Invest Ophthalmol Vis Sci 2003; 44:5438–5446.
18. Malik NS, Meek KM. Vitamins and analgesics in the prevention of collagen ageing. Age Ageing 1996; 25:279–284.
19. Malik NS, Moss SJ, Ahmed N et al. Ageing of the human corneal stroma: structural and biochemical changes. Biochem Biophys Acta 1992; 1138:222–228.
20. Hollingsworth J, Perez-Gomez I, Mutalib HA et al. A population study of the normal cornea using an in vivo, slit-scanning confocal microscope. Optom Vision Sci 2001; 78:706–711.
21. Buckley RJ. The ageing eye – changes in the anterior segment with age. Optom Today 2003; 44–49.
22. Chang SW, Hu FR. Changes in corneal autofluorescence and corneal epithelial barrier function with ageing. Cornea 1993; 12:493–499.

23. Hazlett LD, Kreindler FB, Berk RS et al. Ageing alters the phagocytic capability of inflammatory cells induced into cornea. Curr Eye Res 1990; 9:129–138.

24. Hobden JA, Masinick SA, Barrett RP et al. Aged mice fail to upregulate ICAM-1 after *Pseudomonas aeruginosa* corneal infection. Invest Ophthalmol Vis Sci 1995; 36:1107–1114.

25. Lass JH, Greiner JV, Merchant TE et al. The effects of age on phosphatic metabolites of the human cornea. Cornea 1995; 14:89–94.

26. Nzekwe EU, Maurice DM. The effect of age on the penetration of fluorescein into the human eye. J Ocular Pharmacol 1994; 10:521–523.

27. Millodot M. The influence of age on the sensitivity of the cornea. Invest Ophthalmol Vis Sci 1977; 16:240–242.

28. Ochiai H, Chihara E, Chuman H et al. Age and increased incidence of forward bowing of the iris in normal eyes. J Glaucoma 1998; 7:408–412.

29. Khalil AK, Kubota T, Tawara A et al. Ultrastructural age-related changes on the posterior iris surface. A possible relationship to the pathogenesis of exfoliation. Arch Ophthalmol 1996; 114:721–725.

30. Balazs EA, Delinger JL, Sekuler R, eds. Ageing changes in the vitreous. In: Ageing and human visual function. New York: Alan R. Liss; 1982:45–57.

31. Bishop PN, Holmes DF, Kadler KE et al. Age-related changes on the surface of vitreous collagen fibrils. Invest Ophthalmol Vis Sci 2004; 45:1041–1046.

32. Vaughan-Thomas A, Gilbert SJ, Duance VC. Elevated levels of proteolytic enzymes in the ageing human vitreous. Invest Ophthalmol Vis Sci 2000; 41:3299–3304.

33. Wang J, McLeod D, Henson DB et al. Age-dependent changes in the basal retinovitreous adhesion. Invest Ophthalmol Vis Sci 2003; 44:1793–1800.

34. Harocopos GJ, Shui YB, McKinnon M et al. Importance of vitreous liquefaction in age-related cataract. Invest Ophthalmol Vis Sci 2004; 45:77–85.

35. Berra A, Ferreira S, Stanga P et al. Age-related antioxidant capacity of the vitreous and its possible relationship with simultaneous changes in photoreceptors, retinal pigment epithelium and Bruchs' membrane in human donors' eyes. Arch Gerontol Geriatr 2002; 34:371–377.

36. Lambert HM, Capone A Jr, Aaberg TM et al. Surgical excision of subfoveal neovascular membranes in age-related macular degeneration. Am J Ophthalmol 1992; 113:257–262.

37. Ondes F, Yilmaz G, Acar MA et al. Role of the vitreous in age-related macular degeneration 1. Jpn J Ophthalmol 2000; 44:91–93.

38. Toris CB, Yablonski ME, Wang YL et al. Aqueous humor dynamics in the ageing human eye. Am J Ophthalmol 1999; 127:407–412.

39. Patel CK, Bron AJ. The ageing lens. Optom Today 2001; 27–30.

40. Strenk SA, Strenk LM, Semmlow JL et al. Magnetic resonance imaging study of the effects of age and accommodation on the human lens cross-sectional area. Invest Ophthalmol Vis Sci 2004; 45:539–545.

41. Boettner EA, Wolter JR. Transmission of the ocular media. Invest Ophthalmol Vis Sci 1962; 1:776–783.

42. Said FS, Weale RA. The variation with age of the spectral transmissivity of the human crystalline lens. Gerontology 1959; 3:213–231.

43. Nguyen-Tri D, Overbury O, Faubert J. The role of lenticular senescence in age-related color vision changes. Invest Ophthalmol Visual Sci 2003; 44:3698–3704.

44. Elliott DB, Yang KC, Dumbleton K et al. Ultraviolet-induced lenticular fluorescence: intraocular straylight affecting visual function. Vision Res 1993; 33:1827–1833.

45. Cavallotti C, Pacella E, Pescosolido N et al. Age-related changes in the human optic nerve. Can J Ophthalmol 2002; 37:389–394.

46. Kergoat H, Kergoat MJ, Justino L et al. Age-related topographical changes in the normal human optic nerve head measured by scanning laser tomography. Optom Vision Sci 2001; 78:431–435.

47. Embleton SJ, Hosking SL, Roff Hilton EJ et al. Effect of senescence on ocular blood flow in the retina, neuroretinal rim and lamina cribrosa, using scanning laser Doppler flowmetry. Eye 2002; 16:156–162.

48. Albon J, Purslow PP, Karwatowski WS et al. Age related compliance of the lamina cribrosa in human eyes. Br J Ophthalmol 2000; 84:318–323.

49. Albon J, Karwatowski WS, Easty DL et al. Age related changes in the non-collagenous components of the extracellular matrix of the human lamina cribrosa. Br J Ophthalmol 2000; 84:311–317.

50. Loewenfield IE, Thompson H, Daroff R et al., eds. Pupillary changes related to age. In: Topics in neuro-ophthalmology. Baltimore, MD: Williams & Wilkins; 1979:124–150.

51. Birren JE, Casperson RC, Botwinick J. Age changes in pupil size. J Gerontol 1950; 5:216–221.

52. Winn B, Whitaker D, Elliott DB et al. Factors affecting light-adapted pupil size in normal human subjects. Invest Ophthalmol Vis Sci 1994; 35:1132–1137.

53. Friedman E, Ivry M, Ebert E et al. Increased scleral rigidity and age-related macular degeneration. Ophthalmology 1989; 96:104–108.

54. Brown CT, Vural M, Johnson M et al. Age-related changes of scleral hydration and sulfated glycosaminoglycans. Mechanisms Ageing Dev 1994; 77:97–107.

55. Olsen TW, Edelhauser HF, Lim JI et al. Human scleral permeability. Effects of age, cryotherapy, transscleral diode laser, and surgical thinning. Invest Ophthalmol Vis Sci 1995; 36:1893–1903.

56. Boubriak OA, Urban JP, Bron AJ. Differential effects of ageing on transport properties of anterior and posterior human sclera. Exp Eye Res 2003; 76:701–713.

57. Rymgayllo-Jankowska B, Szczesny P, Zagorski Z. [Morphological analysis of age-related changes in the human choroids.] Klinika Oczna 2002; 104:327–331.

58. Ramrattan RS, van der Schaft TL, Mooy CM et al. Morphometric analysis of Bruch's membrane, the choriocapillaris, and the choroid in ageing. Invest Ophthalmol Vis Sci 1994; 35:2857–2864.

59. Okubo A, Rosa RH Jr, Bunce CV et al. The relationships of age changes in retinal pigment epithelium and Bruch's membrane. Invest Ophthalmol Vis Sci 1999; 40:443–449.

60. Curcio CA, Millican CL, Bailey T et al. Accumulation of cholesterol with age in human Bruch's membrane. Invest Ophthalmol Vis Sci 2001; 42:265–274.

61. Starita C, Hussain AA, Patmore A et al. Localization of the site of major resistance to fluid transport in Bruch's membrane. Invest Ophthalmol Vis Sci 1997; 38:762–767.

62. Starita C, Hussain AA, Pagliarini S et al. Hydro-dynamics of ageing Bruch's membrane: implications for macular disease. Exp Eye Res 1996; 62:565–572.

63. Dallinger S, Findl O, Strenn K et al. Age dependence of choroidal blood flow. J Am Geriatr Soc 1998; 46:484–487.

64. Guymer R, Luthert P, Bird A. Changes in Bruch's membrane and related structures with age. Progr Retinal Eye Res 1999; 18:59–90.

65. Holz FG, Wolfensberger TJ, Piguet B et al. Macular drusen. Changes in the retinal pigment epithelium and angiographic characteristics as prognostic markers. Ophthalmol Z Dtsch Ophthalmol Gesellschaft 1994; 91:735–740.

66. Newsome DA, Huh W, Green WR. Bruch's membrane age-related changes vary by region. Curr Eye Res 1987; 6:1211–1221.

67. Loffler KU, Lee WR. Basal linear deposit in the human macula. Graefes Arch Clin Exp Ophthalmol 1986; 224:493–501.

68. Curcio CA, Saunders PL, Younger PW et al. Peripapillary chorioretinal atrophy: Bruch's membrane changes and photoreceptor loss. Ophthalmology 2000; 107:334–343.

69. Anderson DH, Mullins RF, Hageman GS et al. A role for local inflammation in the formation of drusen in the ageing eye 1. Am J Ophthalmol 2002; 134:411–431.

70. Alamouti B, Funk J. Retinal thickness decreases with age: an OCT study. Br J Ophthalmol 2003; 87:899–901.

71. Lovasik JV, Kergoat MJ, Justino L et al. Neuroretinal basis of visual impairment in the very elderly. Graefes Arch Clin Exp Ophthalmol 2003; 241:48–55.

72. Curcio CA, Drucker DN. Retinal ganglion cells in Alzheimer's disease and ageing. Ann Neurol 1993; 33:248–257.

73. Gao H, Hollyfield JG. Ageing of the human retina. Differential loss of neurons and retinal pigment epithelial cells. Invest Ophthalmol Vis Sci 1992; 33:1–17.

74. Curcio CA, Millican CL, Allen KA et al. Ageing of the human photoreceptor mosaic: evidence for selective vulnerability of rods in central retina. Invest Ophthalmol Vis Sci 1993; 34:3278–3296.

75. Bonnel S, Mohand-Said S, Sahel J. The ageing of the retina. Exp Gerontol 2003; 38:825–831.

76. Clarke G, Collins RA, Leavitt BR et al. A one-hit model of cell death in inherited neuronal degenerations. Nature 2000; 406:195–199.

77. Curcio CA, Medeiros NE, Millican CL. Photoreceptor loss in age-related macular degeneration. Invest Ophthalmol Vis Sci 1996; 37:1236–1249.

78. Medeiros NE, Curcio CA. Preservation of ganglion cell layer neurons in age-related macular degeneration. Invest Ophthalmol Vis Sci 2001; 42:795–803.

79. Marshall J, Grindle J, Ansell PL et al. Convolution in human rods: an ageing process. Br J Ophthalmol 1979; 63:181–187.

80. Ramirez JM, Ramirez AI, Salazar JJ et al. Changes of astrocytes in retinal ageing and age-related macular degeneration. Exp Eye Res 2001; 73:601–615.

81. Barron MJ, Johnson MA, Andrews RM et al. Mitochondrial abnormalities in ageing macular photoreceptors. Invest Ophthalmol Vis Sci 2001; 42:3016–3022.

82. Katz ML. Bernard Strehler – inspiration for basic research into the mechanisms of ageing. Mechanisms Ageing Dev 2002; 123:831–840.

83. Katz ML. Potential role of retinal pigment epithelial lipofuscin accumulation in age-related macular degeneration. Arch Gerontol Geriatr 2002; 34:359–370.

84. Bok D, Hall MO. The role of the pigment epithelium in the etiology of inherited retinal dystrophy in the rat. J Cell Biol 1971; 49:664–682.

85. LaVail MM, Mullen RJ. Role of the pigment epithelium in inherited retinal degeneration analyzed with experimental mouse chimeras. Exp Eye Res 1976; 23:227–245.

86. Dorey CK, Wu G, Ebenstein D et al. Cell loss in the ageing retina. Relationship to lipofuscin accumulation and macular degeneration. Invest Ophthalmol Vis Sci 1989; 30:1691–1699.

87. Marshall J. The ageing retina: physiology or pathology. Eye 1987;1:282–295.

88. Feeney-Burns L, Hilderbrand ES, Eldridge S. Ageing human RPE: morphometric analysis of macular, equatorial, and peripheral cells. Invest Ophthalmol Vis Sci 1984; 25:195–200.

89. Weiter JJ, Delori FC, Wing GL et al. Retinal pigment epithelial lipofuscin and melanin and choroidal melanin in human eyes. Invest Ophthalmol Vis Sci 1986; 27:145–152.

90. Boulton M, Docchio F, Dayhaw-Barker P et al. Age-related changes in the morphology, absorption and fluorescence of melanosomes and lipofuscin granules of the retinal pigment epithelium. Vision Res 1990; 30:1291–1303.

91. Katz ML, Robison J, Gerald W. What is lipofuscin? Defining characteristics and differentiation from other autofluorescent lysosomal storage bodies. Arch Gerontol Geriatr 2002; 34:169–184.

92. Terman A, Brunk UT. Lipofuscin. Int J Biochem Cell Biol 2004; 36:169–184.

93. Wihlmark U, Wrigstad A, Roberg K et al. Lipofuscin accumulation in cultured retinal pigment epithelial cells causes enhanced sensitivity to blue light irradiation. Free Radical Biol Med 1997; 22:1229–1234.

94. Wassell J, Davies S, Bardsley W et al. The photoreactivity of the retinal age pigment lipofuscin. J Biol Chem 1999; 274:23828–23832.

95. Boulton M, Dontsov A, Jarvis-Evans J et al. Lipofuscin is a photoinducible free radical generator. J Photochem Photobiol Biol 1993; 19:201–204.

96. Schutt F, Davies S, Kopitz J et al. Photodamage to human RPE cells by A2-E, a retinoid component of lipofuscin. Invest Ophthalmol Vis Sci 2000; 41:2303–2308.

97. Mata NL, Weng J, Travis GH. Biosynthesis of a major lipofuscin fluorophore in mice and humans with ABCR-mediated retinal and macular degeneration. Proc Natl Acad Sci USA 2000; 97:7154–7159.

98. Sparrow JR, Fishkin N, Zhou J et al. A2E, a byproduct of the visual cycle. Vision Res 2003; 43:2983–2990.

99. Brunk UT, Terman A. Lipofuscin: mechanisms of age-related accumulation and influence on cell function. 1. Free Radical Biol Med 2002; 33:611–619.

100. Sundelin SP, Nilsson SEG, Brunk UT. Lipofuscin-formation in cultured retinal pigment epithelial cells is related to their melanin content. Free Radical Biol Med 2001; 30:74–81.

101. Sundelin S, Wihlmark U, Nilsson SE et al. Lipofuscin accumulation in cultured retinal pigment epithelial cells reduces their phagocytic capacity. Curr Eye Res 1998; 17:851–857.

102. Marshall J. Radiation and the ageing eye. Ophthalm Physiol Optics 1985; 5:241–263.

103. Delori FC, Goger DG, Dorey CK. Age-related accumulation and spatial distribution of lipofuscin in RPE of normal subjects. Invest Ophthalmol Vis Sci 2001; 42:1855–1866.

104. Holz FG, Bellman C, Staudt S et al. Fundus autofluorescence and development of geographic atrophy in age-related macular degeneration. Invest Ophthalmol Vis Sci 2001; 42:1051–1056.

105. Delori FC, Fleckner MR, Goger DG et al. Auto-fluorescence distribution associated with drusen in age-related macular degeneration. Invest Ophthalmol Vis Sci 2000; 41:496–504.

106. Marmor MF, Sekuler R, Kline D, Dismukes K, eds. Ageing and the retina. In: Ageing and human visual function. New York: Alan R. Liss; 1982:59–78.

107. Owsley C. Contrast sensitivity. Ophthalmol Clin North Am 2003; 16:171–177.

108. Jackson GR, Owsley C. Visual dysfunction, neuro-degenerative diseases, and ageing. Neurol Clin 2003; 21:709–728.

109. Lovie-Kitchin JE, Brown B. Repeatability and intercorrelations of standard vision tests as a function of age. Optom Vision Sci 2000; 77:412–420.

110. Bergman B, Bergstrom A, Sjostrand J. Longitudinal changes in visual acuity and visual ability in a cohort followed from the age of 70 to 88 years. Acta Ophthalmol Scand 1999; 77:286–292.

111. Latham K, Barrett BT. No effect of age on spatial interval discrimination as a function of eccentricity or separation. Curr Eye Res 1998; 17:1010–1017.

112. Whitaker D, Elliott DB, MacVeigh D. Variations in hyperacuity performance with age. Ophthalm Physiol Optics 1992; 12:29–32.

113. Wright LA, Wormald RP. Stereopsis and ageing. Eye 1992; 6:473–476.

114. Kline DW, Culham JC, Bartel P et al. Ageing effects on Vernier hyperacuity: a function of oscillation rate but not target contrast. Optom Vision Sci 2001; 78:676–682.

115. Trick GL, Trick LR, Haywood KM. Altered pattern evoked retinal and cortical potentials associated with human senescence. Curr Eye Res 1986; 5: 717–724.

116. Trick LR. Age-related alterations in retinal function. Doc Ophthalmol Adv Ophthalmol 1987; 65:35–43.

117. Spear PD. Neural bases of visual deficits during ageing. Vision Res 1993; 33:2589–2609.

118. Porciatti V, Burr DC, Morrone MC et al. The effects of ageing on the pattern electroretinogram and visual evoked potential in humans. Vision Res 1992; 32:1199–1209.

119. Leventhal AG, Wang Y, Pu M et al. GABA and its agonists improved visual cortical function in senescent monkeys. Science 2003; 300:812–815.

120. Weale RA. The ageing population – changes in visual function with age. Optom Today 2003; 7:27–33.

121. Knoblauch K, Saunders F, Kusuda M et al. Age and illuminance effects in the Farnsworth-Munsell 100-hue test. Appl Optics 1987; 26:1441–1448.

122. Drance SM, Berry V, Hughes A. Studies on the effects of age on the central and peripheral isopters of the visual field in normal subjects. Am J Ophthalmol 1967; 63:1667–1672.

123. Drance SM, Berry V, Hughes A. The effects of age on the central isopter of the normal visual field. Can J Ophthalmol 1967; 2:79–82.

124. Haas A, Flammer J, Schneider U. Influence of age on the visual fields of normal subjects. Am J Ophthalmol 1986; 101:199–203.

125. Brenton RS, Phelps CD. The normal visual field on the Humphrey field analyzer. Int J Ophthalmol 1986; 193:56–74.

126. Johnson CA, Adams AJ, Lewis RA. Evidence for a neural basis of age-related visual field loss in normal observers. Invest Ophthalmol Vis Sci 1989; 30:2056–2064.

127. Johnson CA, Marshall D Jr. Ageing effects for opponent mechanisms in the central visual field. Optom Vision Sci 1995; 72:75–82.

128. Lakowski R. Age and color vision. Adv Sci 1958; 15:231–236.

129. Werner JS, Schefrin BE. Loci of achromatic points throughout the life span. J Opt Soc Am 1993; 10:1509–1516.

130. Sekuler R, Sekuler AB, Kazdin AE, eds. Age-related changes, optical factors, and neural processes. In: Encyclopedia of psychology. Washington DC: American Psychological Association/Oxford University Press; 2000:180–183.

131. Owsley C, Sekuler R, Siemsen D. Contrast sensitivity throughout adulthood. Vision Res 1983; 23:689–699.

132. Higgins KE, Jaffe MJ, Coletta NJ et al. Spatial contrast sensitivity. Importance of controlling the patient's visibility criterion. Arch Ophthalmol 1984; 102:1035–1041.

133. Burton KB, Owsley C, Sloane ME. Ageing and neural spatial contrast sensitivity: photopic vision. Vision Res 1993; 33:939–946.

134. Artal P, Ferro M, Miranda I et al. Effects of ageing in retinal image quality. J Opt Soc Am 1993; 10:1656–1662.

135. Morrison JD, McGrath C. Assessment of the optical contributions to the age-related deterioration in vision. Q J Exp Physiol 1985; 70:249–269.

136. Elliott DB. Contrast sensitivity decline with ageing: a neural or optical phenomenon? Ophthalm Physiol Optics 1987; 7:415–419.

137. Higgins KE, Jaffe MJ, Caruso RC et al. Spatial contrast sensitivity: effects of age, test–retest, and psychophysical method. J Opt Soc Am 1988; 5:2173–2180.

138. Sloane ME, Owsley C, Alvarez SL. Ageing, senile miosis and spatial contrast sensitivity at low luminance. Vision Res 1988; 28:1235–1246.

139. Whitaker D, Elliott DB. Simulating age-related optical changes in the human eye. Doc Ophthalmol Adv Ophthalmol 1992; 82:307–316.

140. Pardhan S, Gilchrist J, Elliott DB et al. A comparison of sampling efficiency and internal noise level in young and old subjects. Vision Res 1996; 36:1641–1648.

141. Sloane ME, Owsley C, Jackson CA. Ageing and luminance–adaptation effects on spatial contrast sensitivity. J Opt Soc Am 1988; 5:2181–2190.

142. Schefrin BE, Tregear SJ, Harvey LO Jr et al. Senescent changes in scotopic contrast sensitivity. Vision Res 1999; 39:3728–3736.

143. Weale RA. Stereoscopic acuity and convergence. J Opt Soc Am 1956; 46:907.

144. Pardhan S. A comparison of binocular summation in the peripheral visual field in young and older patients. Curr Eye Res 1997; 16:252–255.

145. Winn B, Gilmartin B, Sculfor DL et al. Vergence adaptation and senescence. Optom Vision Sci 1994; 71:797–800.

146. Bell B, Wolf E, Bernholtz CD. Depth perception as a function of age. Ageing Hum Dev 1974; 3:77–81.

147. Schneck ME, Haegerstrom-Portnoy G, Lott LA et al. Ocular contributions to age-related loss in coarse stereopsis. Optom Vision Sci 2000; 77:531–536.

148. Jackson GR, Owsley C. Scotopic sensitivity during adulthood. Vision Res 2000; 40:2467–2473.

149. Jackson GR, Owsley C, McGwin G Jr. Ageing and dark adaptation. Vision Res 1999; 39:3975–3982.

150. Sturr JF, Zhang L, Taub HA et al. Psychophysical evidence for losses in rod sensitivity in the ageing visual system. Vision Res 1997; 37:475–481.

151. Weleber RG. The effect of age on human cone and rod ganzfeld electroretinograms. Invest Ophthalmol Vis Sci 1981; 20:392–399.

152. Wright CE, Williams DE, Drasdo N et al. The influence of age on the electroretinogram and visual evoked potential. Doc Ophthalmol Adv Ophthalmol 1985; 59:365–384.

153. Martin DA, Heekenlively JR. The normal electroretinogram. Doc Ophthalmol Proc Ser 1982; 31:135–144.

154. Scilley K, Jackson GR, Cideciyan AV et al. Early age-related maculopathy and self-reported visual difficulty in daily life. Ophthalmology 2002; 109:1235–1242.

155. Werner JS, Steele VG. Sensitivity of human foveal color mechanisms throughout the life span. J Opt Soc Am 1988; 5:2122–2130.

156. Eisner A, Fleming SA, Klein ML et al. Sensitivities in older eyes with good acuity: cross-sectional norms. Invest Ophthalmol Vis Sci 1987; 28:1824–1831.

157. Johnson CA, Adams AJ, Twelker JD et al. Age-related changes in the central visual field for short-wavelength-sensitive pathways. J Opt Soc Am 1988; 5:2131–2139.

158. Zlatkova MB, Coulter E, Anderson RS. Short-wavelength acuity: blue-yellow and achromatic resolution loss with age. Vision Res 2003; 43:109–115.

159. Hammond BR Jr, Wooten BR, Snodderly DM. Preservation of visual sensitivity of older subjects: association with macular pigment density. Invest Ophthalmol Vis Sci 1998; 39:397–406.

160. Werner JS, Bieber ML, Schefrin BE. Senescence of foveal and parafoveal cone sensitivities and their relations to macular pigment density. J Opt Soc Am 2000; 17:1918–1932.

161. Coppinger NW. The relationship between critical flicker frequency and chronological age for varying levels of stimulus brightness. J Gerontol 1955; 10:48–52.

162. Mayer MJ, Kim CB, Svingos A et al. Foveal flicker sensitivity in healthy ageing eyes. I. Compensating for pupil variation. J Opt Soc Am 1988; 5:2201–2209.

163. Shadlen MN, Newsome WT. Motion perception: seeing and deciding. Proc Natl Acad Sci USA 1996; 93:628–633.

164. Sekuler R, Ball K. Visual localization: age and practice. J Opt Soc Am 1986; 3:864–867.

165. Wojciechowski R, Trick GL, Steinman SB. Topography of the age-related decline in motion sensitivity. Optom Vision Sci 1995; 72:67–74.

166. Gilmore GC, Wenk HE, Naylor LA et al. Motion perception and ageing. Psychol Ageing 1992; 7:654–660.

Chapter **4.3**

Dry-eye disorders

Frank Eperjesi

INTRODUCTION

Research has shown that up to 10% of the non-contact lens-wearing population who are under the age of 60 have dry-eye symptoms and these symptoms are even more common in older people and postmenopausal women.[1] Up to 25% of patients consulting an eye care clinician present with dry-eye symptoms[2] and some specialists have reported that up to 40% of contact lens wearers experience problems associated with dry eyes.[3] Dry eye has recently been defined as 'a disorder of the pre-corneal tear film due to tear deficiency or excessive evaporation of tears causing damage to the interpalpebral ocular surface associated with ocular discomfort'.[4]

TYPES OF DRY-EYE DISORDER

Two main types of dry-eye disorder have been identified. Tear-deficient dry eye occurs when there is a disorder of lacrimal gland function which results in reduced tear production and distribution; Farrell[5] considered the majority of dry-eye conditions to be of this type. Tear secretion may be decreased by any condition that decreases corneal sensation, such as diabetes, herpes zoster, long-term contact lens wear and surgery that involves corneal incisions or ablates corneal nerves.[6] Evaporative dry eye occurs when there is normal tear production but loss of tear constituents due to increased or excessive evaporation,[4] resulting in a decrease in the quality of tears. Increased tear evaporation may occur due to long-standing posterior blepharitis causing meibomian gland dysfunction or a large palpebral aperture width, which may occur naturally, secondary to surgery[7] or with thyroid eye disease.[8] Evaporation is proportional to palpebral aperture surface area, with widths greater than 10 mm placing significant evaporative stress on the tear film.[7] Inadequate tear quality may also occur when there is a deficiency in the basal mucous layer of the tear film.

Typical symptoms include photophobia, burning, itching, foreign-body sensation, chronic sandy-gritty irritation, eye fatigue and dryness.[9] The symptom pattern is often diurnal with symptoms becoming worse as the day progresses.[5] The most common ocular sign is a mildly red eye. Various strategies have been proposed to alleviate symptoms associated with dry eye. These include: changing lens material and cleaning solutions when symptoms are associated with contact lens wear,[10] using rewetting eye drops,[11] increasing the ambient humidity and reducing tear drainage by blocking the eye lid puncta with dissolvable or permanent plugs[12] and improved lid margin hygiene.[13]

MECHANISM

Central to nearly all types of dry-eye disorders is a reduction in the aqueous component of the tear film, which results in an increase of osmolarity above the normal limit of 311 mosmol/l.[14] Tear osmolarity increases when aqueous is lost from the tear film, while solutes such as sodium and potassium are not.[7] This loss of aqueous and increase in osmolarity may result from any condition which decreases tear production or increases tear evaporation. Increased tear osmolarity is the link between changes in the lacrimal glands and lids and disease of the ocular surface. Gilbard[7] proposed four milestones in dry-eye disease: (1) increased tear osmolarity; (2) decreased goblet cell density along with decreased corneal glycogen; (3) increased corneal epithelial desquamation; and (4) decreased corneal cell surface glycoproteins. Other investigators have put forward a neural feedback mechanism as a possible aetiology, whereby corneal damage leads to reduced tear production in the lacrimal gland which then leads to further corneal compromise.[15]

NUTRITION

There is considerable research that demonstrates the importance of a balanced diet in maintaining tear, conjunctival and corneal health. See Caffery[16] for a thorough review. Rask et al.[17] suggested that vitamin A is essential for the maintenance of the mucous membranes of the human eye and that vitamin A deficiency is probably the primary event of the mucous membrane breakdown that is associated with the subsequent dry eye (see Chapter 3.1 on the ocular effects of vitamin A deficiency associated with malnutrition). Goblet cells located on the conjunctival surface produce mucus which helps maintain a healthy tear film. These cells have been shown to increase in number with oral vitamin A therapy.[18] Sommer and Muhilal[19] have suggested that an intimate balance between vitamin A and protein status may determine the adequacy of vitamin A metabolism at the level of the target cells. Even when the diet provides substantial calories, conditions such as chronic liver disease that result in malabsorption can lead to reduced vitamin A levels.[20]

The evidence is unequivocal that sufficient dietary intake of protein is essential for the health of the tear film and ocular surface. Protein is required to deliver vitamin A (along with zinc) to the ocular surface and dietary amino acids are required at the lacrimal gland to allow proper production of proteins[16] and it is likely that ingested amino acids are used in more critical functions than lacrimal protein production during periods of malnutrition.[16] The average individual living in a developed country, however, is unlikely to have a deficiency in protein intake. Vitamin B_6 is involved in the metabolism of proteins[21] and therefore low intake could have an effect on localised protein production and vitamin A transport.[16] Also, a deficiency of potassium or vitamin C, because of their involvement with the cellular environment,[21] could result in a decrease in activity of the secretory cells of the lacrimal system, in particular lacrimal gland output.[16] Furthermore, Lane[22] correlated dietary factors of low vitamin C, B_6 and potassium intake with increased contact lens spoilage, while Hart et al.[23] noted a relationship between high protein and alcohol intake with excess lipid deposition on contact lenses.

The ocular surface is relatively unprotected and constantly exposed to radiation, atmospheric oxygen, environmental chemicals and physical insults, resulting in the generation of reactive oxygen species, which are thought to contribute to ocular damage.[24] Vitamin C (ascorbic acid) is found in high concentrations in the eye and is thought to be a primary substrate in ocular protection.[25] Diabetes mellitus is associated with a number of ocular complications that can lead to blindness. For example, 47–67% of diabetic patients have primary corneal lesions during their lifetime.[26] In addition many diabetic patients complain of dry-eye symptoms, indicating a clear role for tear film abnormalities.[27] Moreover, most studies have found that people with diabetes mellitus have circulating ascorbic acid concentrations at least 30% lower than people without diabetes mellitus.[28] Interestingly, Rubowitz et al.[29] have shown using a masked experimental protocol that followed phacoemulsification (a procedure involving the use of an ultrasound probe during cataract extraction in humans and which is known to produce large amounts of free radicals and ultraviolet radiation in both in vivo and in vitro environments[30]) in the rabbit model, postoperative endothelial cell counts were 70% higher in those rabbits where 0.001 mol/l ascorbic acid (a well-known free-radical scavenger found to occur naturally in the anterior chamber aqueous of the eye[31]) had been added to the irrigating solution. The investigators considered vacuoles in the endothelial cells to be an indicator of ruptured intracellular organelle membranes.

Data from a survey of over 32 000 female health professionals indicate that the higher the dietary ratio of omega-3 to omega-6 essential fatty acids, the lower the likelihood of dry eye.[32] Conversely lower ratios of omega-3 to omega-6 were more likely to be associated with dry eye. The best sources of omega-3s are dark, oily cold-water fish and flaxseed oil[7] while omega-6s are found in products such as beef, dairy and vegetable shortening and cooking oils. The recommended ratio of omega-3 to omega-6 is 1 : 2.3 while the consumption ratio has been estimated to be as low as

1 : 10.[33] Omega-3s block the formation of proinflammatory substances, are converted to anti-inflammatories that reduce the symptoms and signs of posterior blepharitis, prevent lacrimal gland proptosis and increase the response of lacrimal gland cells to innervation.[34]

According to Caffery,[16] because the indications are that a balanced diet is likely to have a positive effect on the tear film, individuals with dry eyes could be provided with the following dietary advice by their health/eye care practitioner:

- Balance the intake of macronutrients by lowering protein, total fat and cholesterol intake and increase complex carbohydrates.
- Increase vitamin A intake by eating red, orange, yellow and dark-green leafy vegetables.
- Increase zinc and folate intake by eating wholegrains, legumes and raw vegetables, especially spinach.
- Ensure sufficient B_6 and potassium intake by eating nuts, bananas and beans.
- Ensure sufficient vitamin C intake by eating citrus fruit.
- Eliminate alcohol and caffeine.
- Reduce sugar and salt intake.
- Drink six to eight glasses of water per day.

NUTRITIONAL SUPPLEMENTS

There is some evidence to suggest that dry-eye symptoms can be reduced with nutritional supplements. In a study without control subjects Shreeve[35] reported improved signs and symptoms for patients with dry eyes when treated with vitamins C and B_6 and linoleic acid (oil of evening primrose) while Silk[36] described good clinical results in dry-eye patients (no controls) using zinc supplements and oil of evening primrose. Patel et al.[37] measured the tear stability of 60 normal healthy subjects and repeated the measurement 10 days later. Using a double-masked protocol, during the interim period 66% of the subjects (the treatment group) took a commercially available daily dietary supplement and the remaining 33% acted as controls. The recommended daily dose was applied to the treatment group. Twenty of the treatment group took a daily dietary supplement of a mixture consisting of vitamins (e.g. A, B_1, B_2,

B_6, E) and trace elements (e.g. calcium, iron, manganese); the other 20 subjects took purely vitamin C tablets. The tear stability of both treated groups increased; however, the multivitamin and trace element group demonstrated the more consistent and individually predictable improvement. The tear stability of the control group individuals did not significantly change. These findings are of particular importance because low tear film stability is a common sign in tear film disorders but it has to be noted that none of the subjects suffered with dry eye. More recently, Blades et al.[38] used a prospective, randomised, placebo-controlled cross-over experimental protocol to assess the efficacy of an orally administered antioxidant dietary supplement in the management of marginal dry eye. Forty marginal dry-eye sufferers underwent baseline assessments of tear volume, quality, ocular surface status and dry-eye symptoms. Each subject was administered courses of active treatment, placebo and no treatment, in random order for 1 month each and the results were compared to baseline. Tear stability (tear thinning time) and ocular surface status (goblet cell density and conjunctival cell squamous metaplasia) were significantly improved following active treatment, although tear volume remained unchanged. No changes from baseline were detected for the placebo and no-treatment groups. The researchers proposed that these clinical improvements might have been promoted by sparing the tear film components from oxidative stress.

Nitric oxide (NO) has been implicated in ocular inflammatory diseases (uveitis, retinitis), degenerative diseases (glaucoma, retinal degeneration), allergic eye disease and diabetic retinopathy.[39] Peroxynitrite ($ONOO^-$) formed by the reaction between nitric oxide and superoxide (O_2^-) is a powerful oxidant capable of causing tissue injury.[40] Peponis et al.[41] studied the effect of oral vitamins C and E on NO levels and various clinical and cytological parameters of tear film and ocular surfaces in 50 patients diagnosed with non-insulin-dependent diabetes mellitus. Participants were given a combination of vitamin C (1000 mg/day) and E (400 IU/day) for a period of 10 days. Vitamin C is thought to enhance the activity of vitamin E by reducing the tocopheroxyl radical and thereby restoring the radical scavenging activity of vitamin E.[42] The results showed that vitamin C and E supplementation decreased NO levels in the lavage fluid from the ocular surface of diabetic patients towards normal levels. The antioxidant activity of these compounds results in a decrease in the oxidative burden in the ocular surface that could lead to elimination of NO and its cytotoxic effects. Interestingly, patients with proliferative diabetic retinopathy showed the greater reduction in nitrite levels. These patients had the greatest pretreatment values of nitrite and seemed to benefit more from vitamin supplementation. These findings demonstrate that the orally administered antioxidant supplements can improve the tear film stability, tear secretion and health of the ocular surface.

More recently the same group investigated the effect of supplementation with vitamin C and E on ocular surface cytology specimens and clinical tear film parameters in 60 diabetics, again using vitamin C (1000 mg/day) and vitamin E (400 IU/day) for 10 days.[43] There was a statistically significant increase in goblet cell densities (50–59 cells per field) after supplementation; in addition, increased values for the Schirmer test, tear break-up time and ocular ferning all reflect an improved tear film quality. The researchers concluded that supplementation with antioxidant vitamins C and E could play an important role in improving the ocular surface milieu.

SUMMARY

Dry-eye disorders are very common in the healthy population and are more likely to occur in contact lens wearers. There is considerable research that demonstrates the importance of a balanced diet in maintaining tear, conjunctival and corneal health. Vitamin A is particularly important, as it is essential for the maintenance of the mucous membranes of the eye. Vitamin B_6 is involved in the metabolism of proteins and a low intake could have an effect on protein production and vitamin A transport, while reduced levels of potassium and vitamin C could result in a decrease in activity of the secretory cells of the lacrimal system. Also, the higher the dietary ratio of omega-3 to omega-6 essential fatty acids, the lower the likelihood of dry eye. Nutritional supplements containing various combinations of vitamins, trace elements and essential fatty acids have been found to improve tear film characteristics in people with and without a dry-eye disorder, reduce the concentration of reactive oxygen species in the tear film, and generally improve corneal and conjunctival health.

References

1. Albietz JM. Prevalence of dry eye subtypes in clinical optometric practice. Optom Vis Sci 2000; 77:357–363.
2. Moss SE, Klein R, Klein BE. Prevalence and risk factors for dry eye syndrome. Arch Ophthalmol 2000; 118:1264–1268.
3. Patel S, Schwarz S. CLIDE in Germany: a preliminary survey and recommendations. Optician 2003; 225:20–22.
4. Lemp MA. Report of the national eye institute/industry workshop on clinical trials of dry eye. CLAO J 1995; 21:221–232.
5. Farrell J. Management of the dry eye in practice. Part 1: assessment and grading of dry eye conditions prior to CL fitting. Optician 2003; 225:20–29.
6. Gilbard JP, Gray KL, Rossi SR. A proposed mechanism for increased tear-film osmolarity in contact lens wearers. Am J Ophthalmol 1986; 102:505–507.
7. Gilbard JP. Nutrition and the eye: dry eye and the role of nutrition. Optom Today 2004; June 4:34–40.
8. Gilbard JP, Farris RL. Ocular surface drying and tear film osmolarity in thyroid eye disease. Acta Ophthalmol 1983; 61:108–116.
9. Ball GV. Symptoms in eye examination. London: Butterworth; 1982:114–116.
10. Efron N. Contact lens-associated tear film dysfunction. Optician 1998; 216:16–26.
11. Caffery BE, Josephson JE. Is there a better 'comfort drop'? J Am Optom Assoc 1990; 61:178–182.
12. Giovagnoli D, Graham SJ. Inferior punctual occlusion with removable punctual plugs in treatment of dry eye related contact lens discomfort. J Am Optom Assoc 1992; 63:481.
13. Paugh JR, Knapp LL, Martinson JR. Meibomian therapy in problematic contact lens wear. Optom Vis Sci 1990; 67:803–806.
14. Gilbard JP, Farris RL, Santamaria J. Osmolarity of tear microvenules in keratoconjunctivitis sicca. Arch Ophthalmol 1978; 96:677–681.
15. Murphy J. A new theory on dry eye: cornea and lacrimal gland function as a unit. Rev Optom 2002; October 15: 8.
16. Caffery B. Influence of diet on tear function. Optom Vis Sci 1991; 68:58–72.
17. Rask L, Geijer C, Bill A, Peterson PA. Vitamin A supply of the cornea. Exp Eye Res 1980; 31:201–211.
18. Sommer R, Green WR. Goblet cell response to vitamin A treatment for corneal xerophthalmia. Am J Ophthalmol 1982; 100:399–403.
19. Sommer A, Muhilal L. Nutritional factors in corneal xerophthalmia and keratomalacia. Arch Ophthalmol 1982; 100:399–403.
20. Sommer A. Effects of vitamin A deficiency on the ocular surface. Ophthalmology 1983; 90:592–600.
21. Linder MC. Nutrition and metabolism of vitamins. In: Linder MC, ed. Nutritional biochemistry and metabolism. New York: Elsevier; 1985:109.
22. Lane BC. Contact lens coating syndrome and dry eyes: strong metabolic and nutriture risk factors. Poster presented at the American Academy of Optometry meeting, December 1984.
23. Hart DE, Lane BC, Josephson JE et al. Spoilage of hydrogel contact lenses by lipid deposits. Ophthalmology 1987; 94:1315–1321.
24. Knight JA. Reactive oxygen species and the neurodegenerative disorders. Ann Clin Lab Sci 1997; 27:11–25.
25. Rose RC, Richer SP, Bode AM. Ocular oxidants and antioxidant protection. Proc Soc Exp Biol Med 1998; 217:397–407.
26. Schultz RO, Van Horn DL, Peters MA et al. Diabetic keratopathy. Trans Am Ophthalmol Soc 1981; 79:180–199.
27. Goebbels M. Tear secretion and tear film function in insulin dependent diabetics. Br J Ophthalmol 2000; 84:19–21.
28. Will JC, Byers T. Does diabetes mellitus increase the requirement for vitamin C? Nutr Rev 1996; 54:193–202.
29. Rubowitz A, Assia EI, Rosner M, Topaz M. Antioxidant protection against corneal damage by free radicals during phacoemulsification. Invest Ophthalmol Vis Sci 2003; 44:1866–1870.
30. Holst A, Rolfsen W, Svensson B et al. Formation of free radicals during phacoemulsification. Curr Eye Res 1993; 12:359–365.
31. Davson H. The aqueous humor and the intraocular pressure. In: Davson H, ed. Physiology of the eye, 5th edn. New York: Pergamon Press; 1990:3–95.
32. Trivedi KA, Dana MR, Gilbard JP et al. (2003). Dietary omega-3 fatty acid intake and risk of clinically diagnosed dry eye syndrome in women. Poster presented at Association for Research in Vision and Ophthalmology. Abstract available online at: www.arvo.org.
33. Kris-Etherton PM, Taylor DS, Yu-Poth S et al. Polyunsaturated fatty acids in the food chain in the United States. Am J Clin Nutr 2000; 71:179–188.
34. Zoukhri D, Kublen CL. Impaired neurotransmitter release from lacrimal and salivary gland nerves of a murine model of Sjögren's syndrome. Invest Ophthalmol Vis Sci 2001; 42:925–932.

35. Shreeve CM. Treating the dry eye. Ophthalm Opt 1982; 25:650–651.

36. Silk AA. Reducing grease. Optician 1989; 197:18.

37. Patel S, Plaskow J, Ferrier C. The influence of vitamins and trace element supplements on the stability of the pre-corneal tear film. Acta Ophthalmol (Copenh) 1993; 71:825–829.

38. Blades KJ, Patel S, Aidoo KE. Oral antioxidant therapy for marginal dry eye. Eur J Clin Nutr 2001; 55:589–597.

39. Becquet F, Courtois Y, Goureau O. Nitric oxide in the eye: multifaceted roles and diverse outcomes. Surv Ophthalmol 1997; 42:71–82.

40. Rösen P, Nawroth PP, King G et al. The role of oxidative stress in the onset and progression of diabetes and its complications: a summary of a Congress Series sponsored by UNESCO-MCBN, the American Diabetes Association and the German Diabetes Society. Diabetes Metabol Res Rev 2001; 17:189–212.

41. Peponis V, Papathanasiou M, Kapranou A et al. Protective role of oral antioxidant supplementation in ocular surface of diabetic patients. Br J Ophthalmol 2002; 86:1369–1373.

42. Packer L. Vitamin C and redox cycling antioxidants. In: Packer L, Fuchs J, eds. Vitamin C in health and disease. New York: Marcel Dekker; 1997:95–121.

43. Peponis V, Bonovas S, Kapranou A et al. Conjunctival and tear film changes after vitamin C and E administration in non-insulin dependent diabetes mellitus. Med Sci Monit 2004; 10: CR213-7. Epub 2004 Apr 28.

Chapter **4.4**

Glaucoma

Frank Eperjesi

CHAPTER CONTENTS

INTRODUCTION

'Glaucoma' is the name given to a group of eye conditions that cause damage to the optic nerve. The term covers a heterogeneous group of conditions, which have in common a non-reversible and progressive optic neuropathy characterised by distinctive patterns of structural change at the optic nerve head and by definite patterns of visual field loss. The most common type is primary open-angle glaucoma in which raised intraocular pressure (IOP) may or may not be a feature but there is always a degree of nerve damage.[1] IOP is the most important risk factor for the development of glaucomatous optic nerve head damage.[2]

OXIDATIVE STRESS

Oxidative stress and antioxidant status in eye tissues may be associated with glaucomatous damage. High levels of the antioxidant vitamin C,[3] and antioxidant enzymes such as superoxide dismutase, catalase and glutathione peroxidase, have been found in the aqueous humour and this has led to suggestions that chronic oxidative stress insult may result in compromised trabeculae meshwork function.[4] Conversely, Ferreira et al.[5] established the antioxidant status of the aqueous humour in people with primary open-angle glaucoma compared to those with cataract and found a significant reduction in the level of water-soluble antioxidants in the aqueous humour (glutathione, ascorbate and tyrosine). The investigators postulated that this decrease might be due to the occurrence of oxidative stress in the eye and that this makes this organ more susceptible to the damage associated with reactive oxygen species production. Also, the glaucomatous patients showed 57% greater antioxidant enzyme activity (in particular, superoxide dismutase and glutathione peroxidase) in the aqueous compared to the cataract group, which could be described as a compensatory upregulation as a direct consequence of oxidative stress.

A recent study[6] reported that 21 patients with primary open-angle glaucoma demonstrated reduced levels of glutathione in their blood when compared to an age- and gender-matched control group. The investigators proposed a general compromise to the antioxidant system to explain their findings and that this may be linked to a compromise in glutathione production. This takes place mainly in the liver in the presence of vitamins B_6, B_{12} and folate.

NUTRITION

Omega–3 fatty acids

There is some indirect evidence to suggest that a diet high in omega-3 fatty acids may reduce the prevalence of primary open glaucoma.[1] The prevalence of primary-angle glaucoma in a sample of 1686 Alaskan Eskimos was found to be 0.65%, which is much lower than that found in the general US population.[7] Eskimos are very likely to have a diet that is high in omega-3 fatty acids but there are many other differences between Eskimos (such as ocular anatomy) and the general US population that may account for the low prevalence of primary open-angle glaucoma and there is no strong evidence to suggest that omega-3 fatty acids have a useful role in the prevention or treatment of glaucoma.

NUTRITIONAL SUPPLEMENTS

Ginkgo biloba

Ginkgo biloba extract (GBE) is a powerful antioxidant for the retina and brain. Studies have reported that it increases retinal and brain circulation up to 30%.

Chung et al.[8] evaluated the possible therapeutic effect of GBE on glaucoma using a cross-over trial of GBE with placebo control in 11 healthy volunteers. Participants were treated with oral GBE 40 mg or placebo three times daily, for 2 days. A 2-week washout period was allowed between GBE and placebo treatment. GBE was found significantly to increase end-diastolic velocity in the ophthalmic artery, with no change seen in placebo (baseline versus GBE treatment). No side-effects related to GBE were found. This is important because reduced ocular blood flow may be an important factor in the aetiology of primary open-angle glaucoma.

In another study, researchers investigated the effect of GBE on pre-existing visual field damage in patients with normal-tension glaucoma (NTG) using a prospective, randomised, placebo-controlled, double-masked cross-over experimental design. NTG is a form of primary open-angle glaucoma in which damage of the optic nerve and visual field is present despite IOP measurements within statistically normal ranges.[9] Twenty-seven patients with bilateral visual field damage resulting from NTG took part. Participants received 40 mg GBE, administered orally, three times daily for 4 weeks, followed by a wash-out period of 8 weeks, then 4 weeks of placebo treatment (identical capsules filled with 40 mg fructose). Other subjects underwent the same regimen, but took the placebo first and the GBE last. Visual field tests, performed at baseline and at the end of each phase of the study, were evaluated for changes.

The main outcome measures were a change in visual field and any ocular or systemic complications. After GBE treatment, a significant improvement in visual fields indices was recorded while no significant changes were found in IOP, blood pressure or heart rate after placebo or GBE treatment. The researchers concluded that GBE administration appeared to improve pre-existing visual field damage in some patients with NTG.

However, when ginkgo biloba is combined with aspirin in certain instances, ocular complications can arise. An incidence of hyphaema in a 71-year-old man who was taking ginkgo and aspirin has been reported.[10] The hyphaema resolved once the man stopped taking the herb. The problem is that GBE inhibits platelet-activating factor; aspirin inhibits platelet adhesion factor, and a synergistic effect that can increase bleeding. Patients taking coumadin, warfarin or heparin should not take ginkgo because of a high risk of bleeding diathesis.

Vitamin C

Linner[11] investigated the effects of oral and topical vitamin C on IOP for a group of 25 and 19 subjects respectively, with ocular hypertension. The oral dose consisted of 0.5 g four times a day for 6 days while the topical dose was 10% aqueous solution administered in one eye three times a day for 3 days. An average reduction in IOP of 1.10 mmHg was found for the group taking vitamin C orally and 1.19 mmHg for the group where vitamin C was administered topically. Linner proposed that the fall in pressure could be explained by a reduction in the rate of aqueous flow or by increased outflow via the uveoscleral pathway. It is doubtful whether this level of reduction in IOP can be considered as clinically useful.

Vitamin B_{12}

A Japanese research group reported on the effects of long-term (at least 5 years) vitamin B_{12} supplementation on 24 patients with glaucoma.[12] Subjects had chronic open- or closed-angle glaucoma and were divided into age and glaucoma-type matched treatment and control groups. All participants were undergoing medical treatment with topical or systemic IOP-lowering drugs. The treatment group exhibited stable or improved visual fields and visual acuity when compared to the control group. In addition, subjects in the treated group had better IOP control, although vitamin B_{12} did not lower IOP per se. It is not clear from their report whether the subjects or investigators were masked and whether the placebo effect was controlled for; these omissions weaken the conclusion drawn from the findings. The investigators theorised that the long-term administration of vitamin B_{12} may improve optic nerve metabolism and prevent optic nerve atrophy in glaucoma sufferers, as it has been proposed that vitamin B_{12} has an affinity for nerve cells[13] and a relationship with lipid and nucleic acid metabolism.[14] Vitamin B_{12} deficiency has also been shown to cause myelin degeneration in the monkey model.[15]

SUMMARY

Glaucoma is a common sight-threatening ocular disorder. Currently there is very little evidence to suggest that dietary factors play a role in its onset. However, administration of GBE has been shown to reverse the visual field loss in NTG and vitamin C in oral and topical formats has been shown to have an IOP-lowering effect, although it remains doubtful as to whether this effect is clinically significant. Furthermore, oral vitamin B_{12} administration has been shown to result in myelin regeneration in an animal model and stabilise visual field loss in glaucomatous human subjects.

References

1. Bennett D. Nutrition and glaucoma: do supplements reduce IOP? Optom Today 2004; May 7: 32–39.
2. Sommer A. Intraocular pressure and glaucoma. Am J Ophthalmol 1989; 107:186–188.
3. Garland DL. Ascorbic acid and the eye. Am J Clin Nutr 1991; 54:1193–1202.
4. Kahn M, Giblin F, Epstein D. Glutathione in calf trabecular meshwork and its relation to aqueous humor outflow facility. Invest Ophthalmol Vis Sci 1983; 24:1283–1287.
5. Ferreira SM, Lerner SF, Brunzini R et al. Oxidative stress markers in aqueous humor of glaucoma patients. Am J Ophthalmol 2004; 137:62–69.
6. Gherghel D, Griffiths HR, Hilton EJ et al. Systemic reduction in glutathione levels occurs in patients with primary open-angle glaucoma. Invest Ophthalmol Vis Sci 2005; 46:877–883.
7. Arkell SM, Lightman DA, Sommer A et al. The prevalence of glaucoma among Eskimos of northwest Alaska. Arch Ophthalmol 1987; 105:482–485.
8. Chung HS, Harris A, Kristinsson JK et al. Ginkgo biloba extract increases ocular blood flow velocity. J Ocul Pharmacol Ther 1999; 15:233–240.
9. Levene RZ. Low tension glaucoma: a critical review and new material. Surv Ophthalmol 1980; 24:621–664.

10. Rosenblatt M, Mindel J. Spontaneous hyphema associated with ingestion of ginkgo biloba extract (letter). N Engl J Med 1997; 336:1108.

11. Linner E. The pressure lowering effect of ascorbic acid in ocular hypertension. Acta Ophthalmol 1969; 47:685–689.

12. Sakai T, Murata M, Amemiya T. Effect of long term treatment of glaucoma with vitamin B_{12}. Glaucoma 1992; 14:167–170.

13. Cardinale GJ, Dreyfus PM, Auld P, Abeles RH. Experimental vitamin B_{12} deficiency: its effect on tissue vitamin B_{12}-coenzyme levels and on the metabolism of methylmalonyl-CoA. Arch Biochem Biophys 1969; 131:92–99.

14. Cox EV, White AM. Methylmalonic acid excretion: an index of vitamin-B_{12} deficiency. Lancet 1962; 2:853–856.

15. Agamanolis DP, Chester EM, Victor M et al. Neuropathology of experimental vitamin B12 deficiency in monkeys. Neurology 1976; 26:905–914.

Chapter **4.5**

Cataract

Frank Eperjesi

INTRODUCTION

The crystalline lens is a vital organ for the visual process. Together with the cornea, the lens has two main optical functions: (1) transparency; and (2) refractive power.[1] The progressive opacification of the crystalline lens with age, which produces a reduction in visual acuity, is defined as a cataract.[2] There are many different mechanisms involved in the aetiology of age-related cataract, which include changes to the proteins, including enzymes and membrane proteins, metabolic changes and ionic changes.[3]

There are many different types of cataract depending on the location or aetiological classification. Based on the location in the lens there are three main types: (1) nuclear; (2) cortical; and (3) posterior subcapsular (PSC) cataract. Cataract of a mixed morphology can also be present, especially in an eye with fairly advanced cataract.

Age-related cataract is a multifactorial disease and many risk factors have been identified, ageing being the most common. In addition, heavy smoking has an increased risk,[4] while sunlight (ultraviolet irradiation),[5] diabetes,[6] female gender,[2] corticosteroids,[7] dehydration, renal failure[8] and hypertension[9] have all been found to have an increased risk. The various types of cataract have also been found to possess different risk factors.

It is thought that if the onset of cataract could be delayed by 10 years it would reduce the need for cataract surgery by 50%.[10] Surgery alone will not eradicate blindness from cataract, so the elimination of certain causes of cataract seems reasonable. Another approach is through nutritional intervention for the prevention of cataract. Cell-free, in vitro and animal research together with epidemiological and clinical studies have suggested a protective role for certain nutrients and medications in the development of age-related cataract, as they are potentially modifiable. The discussion here will revolve around evidence from epidemiological studies and clinical trials involving human participants.

OXIDATIVE STRESS

There are several reasons for suspecting that nutrition may play a role in the formation of cataracts. With ageing, lens constituents sustain extensive photo-oxidative damage. The long-lived lens proteins and the enzymes that might otherwise recognise and remove these proteins are themselves damaged with ageing. It has been hypothesised that this results in the accumulation and precipitation of proteins in cataracts.

Oxidation of the lens proteins and lipids plays an important role in the pathogenesis of age-related cataract.[11] The human crystalline lens and the aqueous humour are isolated from the blood supply and contain few cells to provide repair mechanisms when oxidative damage occurs. Suggestions about how micronutrients may protect the lens from oxidative damage have stimulated interest in the relationship between micronutrient intake and age-related cataract.

Oxygen intermediates such as hydrogen peroxide, superoxide and hydroxide free radicals, which may be produced by a variety of external insults or may be products of normal metabolism, are very noxious due to their strong oxidising properties.[12] However, the damaging effects of oxygen are combated by an inbuilt system of enzymatic and non-enzymatic defence mechanisms.[13]

A high concentration of reduced glutathione (GSH) protects the lens from the damaging effects of certain oxidants.[11] It also protects the certain protein groups, preventing soluble protein cross-linking and the formation of insoluble protein aggregates,[11] as well as preserving normal permeability and transport functions of the cell membranes.[14] Reduced levels of glutathione have been linked with the presence of cortical opacities.[12]

Hydrogen peroxide is present in human aqueous humour,[15] which can give rise to activated forms of oxygen, and it has been reported to be increased in the aqueous humour of eyes with age-related cataracts. Hydrogen peroxide disrupts the function of the sodium–potassium pump of the anterior lens epithelium, which can give rise to cortical[16] and PSC[17] cataracts.

The breakdown of hydrogen peroxide and other potential oxidising agents is carried out by enzyme systems that originate from glutathione. Glutathione peroxidase is involved in scavenging hydrogen peroxide, and levels of this enzyme begin to reduce from the age of 40 years.[18] Catalase is another enzyme that can also degrade hydrogen peroxide.[12] Superoxide dismutase (SOD) scavenges superoxide free radicals and converts them into hydrogen peroxide and oxygen, which in turn can be broken down by glutathione peroxidase and catalase respectively.[12] There is evidence of reduced SOD activity in nuclear and cortical cataracts.[19] In addition, naturally occurring non-enzymatic antioxidants such as vitamin C, vitamin E and possibly carotenoids, also act against oxidative species, and may act together or in combination with the antioxidant enzymes.[13]

NUTRITION

Epidemiological studies have indicated that age-related cataractous changes in the lens may be modulated by dietary factors, and there are many nutrients that are rendered to be protective against age-related cataract. These include vitamin C, vitamin E, carotenoids and the B-vitamins.

The Lens Opacities Case-Control Study concluded that individuals with higher levels of an antioxidant index that was rich in the dietary intake of riboflavin, vitamin C, vitamin E and carotene resulted in a 50% reduction in nuclear, cortical and mixed cataracts.[20] The India–US Case-Control Study of Cataract found similar results in that lower levels of an antioxidant index (composed of red blood cell levels of glutathione peroxidase, glucose-6-phosphate dehydrogenase and plasma levels of vitamin C and E) increased the risk of PSC and mixed cataracts, in analyses after adjusting for a number of cataract risk factors.[9] The role of antioxidants is supported by a study using biochemical markers, which reported an association of cataract with an antioxidant index, which included plasma levels of vitamin C, vitamin E and carotenoids. There was a reduced risk of cataract in people with high serum levels of two or more of these antioxidants.[21]

In contrast, Vitale et al.[22] found no association of the overall antioxidant status to the risk of nuclear opacities, in a study of individuals of the Baltimore Longitudinal Study on Aging. The Italian–American Cataract Study also failed to find an association between any cataract type and an antioxidant index (consisting of plasma vitamin E, selenium and red blood cell glutathione peroxidase).[23]

NUTRITIONAL SUPPLEMENTS

Vitamin C

Vitamin C is a small, water-soluble molecule that can penetrate the onion-like layers of the lens, providing the body with a means of delivering chemical protection into this isolated area.[24] The accumulation of vitamin C in the lens and aqueous humour is striking: vitamin C concentrations here are 20 times higher than those found in plasma.[25] Only very high or very low vitamin C intakes appear to change the concentration in the lens notably, whereas intakes in the range of those usually found in the diet may not have much effect.

The use of vitamin C supplements, for more than 10 years, was reported to be associated with a lower prevalence of mild (77% lower) and moderate (83% lower) lens opacities in a subsample of the Nurses' Health Study.[26] Women who took vitamin C supplements for less than 10 years displayed no evidence of a reduced occurrence of early opacities. This study suggested that the long-term supplementation of vitamin C might reduce the development of age-related opacities. Also, the prevalence of early nuclear opacities was lower in women who consumed vitamin C supplements for more than 10 years and none of the women who consumed vitamin C supplements for more than 10 years presented with any moderate nuclear opacities. In the larger cohort study of this group, vitamin C from food sources was unrelated to cataract extraction after adjusting for confounding variables. However, women who used supplemental vitamin C for more than 10 years had a 45% lower risk of cataract severe enough for extraction.[27]

In another study on antioxidant vitamins, Jacques and Chylack[28] reported that subjects with low and moderate levels of plasma vitamin C had an increased risk of any form of cataract, particularly PSC cataract, compared to subjects with high plasma vitamin C levels. There was also an increased risk of cataract in subjects with a low vitamin C intake, of which the occurrence of PSC cataract was the strongest. However, in contrast to plasma vitamin C, moderate levels of vitamin C intake did not show an increased cataract risk. This may mean that only a moderate amount of nutrient intake is necessary to prevent cataract formation. However, in the Blue Mountains Eye Study, Cumming and colleagues[29] reported that vitamin C intake was not associated with a reduction in nuclear, cortical or PSC cataract prevalence.

A study of individuals from the Beaver Dam Eye Study reported a protective effect of the past intake of vitamin C against nuclear sclerosis in men and was strengthened after including the contributions from supplements. Also, the inverse relationship with the intake of vitamin C from food persisted regardless of whether or not multivitamins were being taken. However, vitamin C intake was unrelated to the severity of nuclear sclerosis in women.[30] In another study,[31] it was reported that moderate intake levels of supplemental vitamin C 10 years in the past reduced the risk for nuclear sclerosis, but increased the risk for cortical opacities. No significant relations were observed between PSC and moderate or high intakes of vitamin C.

In an investigation of supplementary vitamin intake, there was a 70% lower risk of cataract in persons consuming vitamin C supplements over 5 years.[32] This was in contrast to the findings of a study consisting of participants from the Physicians' Health Study.[33] There was no correlation between vitamin C supplementation and a reduced risk of cataract or cataract extraction. Nonetheless, the sample size of this group was very small. This study did not suggest a protective role of vitamin C used either alone or in combination with multivitamins.

A study by Jacques et al.[34] concluded that persons with cataract might have a lower level of blood plasma vitamin C. In particular, individuals with a high level of plasma vitamin C had a significantly reduced risk of PSC cataract. The results also indicated a protective effect of vitamin C on cortical cataract but they were not statistically significant. This was in contrast to a study in Italy that showed no correlation between plasma vitamin C and cataract.[35] Vitale and co-workers[22] measured the plasma levels of three antioxidants in 660 subjects in the Baltimore Longitudinal Study on Aging and also observed no association between plasma vitamin C and nuclear or cortical cataract after adjusting for risk factors.

The consumption of vitamin C was not associated with cataract extraction in a study by Tavani et al.[36] However, high intakes of citrus fruits that are rich in vitamin C had a significant association with a lower risk of cataract extraction. The Italian–American Cataract Study also reported no significant association between the dietary intake of vitamin C and any form of cataract.[23]

In another trial of persons recruited from the Beaver Dam Eye Study,[37] it was demonstrated that nuclear cataract was not significantly related to the intake of vitamin C from supplements and the intake combined in the distant past or at the time of the examination. However, an inverse trend was observed between vitamin C intake and opacities in individuals with risk factors for nuclear cataracts.

Another study compared the self-reported consumption of supplementary vitamins and the risk of cataract.[38] The findings indicated that patients with cataract were only 30% likely to have taken supplementary vitamin C compared to the control group. Hence, individuals with clear lenses tended to consume more supplemental vitamin C. This is comparable to a large nutritional study with a follow-up of 5 years,[39] which revealed a 60% reduction in the risk of any type of cataract in individuals who used vitamin C supplements for more than 10 years.

Although the study by Mohan et al.[9] suggested an increased risk of nuclear and PSC cataract with increasing plasma vitamin C, they showed a significantly reduced risk of cataract with increasing antioxidant levels that contained plasma vitamin C as one of the antioxidant components.

Jacques et al.[34] found that persons with 90 mmol of ascorbate per litre of plasma had less chance of developing cataract than those with lower amounts. To achieve these high levels of plasma ascorbate, it has been suggested by Jacob et al.[40] that daily doses of more than 500 mg of ascorbate would need to be consumed. However, this has been disputed by Olson and Hodges,[41] who stated that increased levels of ascorbate do not increase the body's ascorbate levels to a level that is beneficial. This is supported by another study which concluded that supplements of 250 mg or more of vitamin C did not lead to a further increase in plasma and aqueous humour ascorbate levels, indicating that a greater amount would not be advantageous.[42]

Podmore et al.[43] questioned the antioxidant nature of vitamin C. It was found that supplementation of more than 500 mg/day of vitamin C resulted in an increase in a marker for damage mediated by oxygen radicals, hence promoting a pro-oxidant role of vitamin C. However, doses of vitamin C below 500 mg/day may retain this antioxidant role.

Vitamin E

Vitamin E (α-tocopherol is the most biologically active vitamin E compound) is also found in the lens but is present at similar concentration levels to that of the plasma. It is a lipid-soluble antioxidant and is mainly found in the lens fibre membranes.[44] Vitamin E is believed to protect against cataract by preventing the free radical attack on the lens lipid membranes.[45] Vitamin E has been suggested to act together with glutathione peroxidase to prevent oxidative damage.[46]

In a study by Jacques and Chylack,[28] there did not appear to be a relationship between plasma vitamin E levels and age-related cataract development. However, it was noted that subjects with low and moderate dietary vitamin E intakes had an increased risk of all types of cataract, especially cortical cataract, compared to those with high intakes.

In a trial of the Beaver Dam cohort study,[30] it was reported that the past intake (10 years before the examination) of dietary vitamin E significantly reduced the risk of nuclear cataract in men, and was more evident after including the contribution from supplements. There was also a strengthening of this relationship in men who had a high vitamin E intake and regularly used multivitamins, that is, the odds ratios were significantly lower for nuclear opacities. In contrast, vitamin E intake was not associated with nuclear cataract in women.

Another investigation of persons in the Nutritional Factors in Eye Disease Study as part of the Beaver Dam Eye Study[30] concluded that there was a negative correlation between the intake of moderate levels of vitamin E supplements and the risk of nuclear sclerosis, after adjusting for confounding variables. This review also found a positive correlation between moderate levels of vitamin E supplements and cortical cataract, after adjusting for confounding variables. In addition, subjects consuming multivitamins with a low and high dietary intake of vitamin E had reduced risks of nuclear cataract that were of a similar magnitude in low- and high-intake groups. Therefore, the relationship between multivitamin supplement use and nuclear sclerosis appeared to be independent of dietary intake of vitamin E. For cortical opacities, the positive association was strongest in individuals with a high intake of vitamin E compared to those with a low intake.

In the Longitudinal Study of Cataract,[47] in which subjects were followed for 5 years, regular users of vitamin E supplements and individuals with increased plasma vitamin E levels had a reduced risk of nuclear opacities by approximately a half. Similarly, biochemical data of individuals from the Lens Opacities Case-Control Study revealed that high plasma levels of vitamin E were associated with a significantly decreased risk of cataract, in particular, nuclear opacities.[48] These results were similar to those of the earlier Lens Opacities Case-Control Study,[20] where a high dietary intake of vitamin E was protective for nuclear, cortical and mixed types of cataract.

Hankinson et al.[27] carried out a nutritional analysis on 50 000 US nurses with a follow-up period of 8 years. The results indicated that the intake of vitamin E was not correlated to cataract extraction after adjusting for multiple risk factors. This was in contrast to a case-control study by Tavani et al.,[36] where the relationship between cataract extraction and diet was assessed. It was found that there were lower risks for cataract extraction in patients with a high intake of vitamin E compared to those with a low intake.

A large cohort study of participants in the Physicians' Health Study did not find a reduced cataract risk in individuals taking vitamin E supplements, alone or in addition to multivitamins. However, the numbers of individuals in this group were small.[33] This was similar to the findings of an analysis that was conducted in 112 individuals of some biochemical markers of nutritional status and age-related cataract.[34] The results indicated that there was no overall association between blood vitamin E levels and overall cataract risk. However, there was a slight inverse correlation of blood vitamin E levels and PSC cataract.

A smaller case-control study in Finland[49] showed that low serum concentrations of vitamin E predicted a higher risk for age-related cataract, after adjusting for several risk factors. However, a study in Italy demonstrated no correlation between plasma vitamin E levels and cataract risk.[35]

Another trial of subjects in the Beaver Dam Eye Study,[50] on nuclear and cortical cataracts, found no inverse relationships between the level of vitamin E in the serum or the dietary intake of vitamin E and the severity of nuclear or cortical opacities. Higher levels of vitamin E were actually associated with a higher risk for nuclear opacities, particularly in women. In contrast, a study incorporating a random sample of 400 adults from the Beaver Dam Eye Study[51] revealed that serum vitamin E was associated with age-related nuclear cataract. The incidence of nuclear cataract was significantly and inversely related to the total serum vitamin E levels. Subjects with a high serum vitamin E concentration had less than half the risk of developing a severe nuclear cataract over the 5-year follow-up period compared to those with a low concentration.

A similar pattern was observed in the Baltimore Longitudinal Study on Aging,[22] in which higher plasma vitamin E concentrations were associated with a lower risk of nuclear opacities in persons who had serum concentrations measured 2–4 years before the assessment of the lens status. However, the associations were not as strong for those persons whose blood samples and lens status were examined at the same time. These results were comparable to another study,[52] which involved participants of the Kuopio Atherosclerosis Study, where a low plasma vitamin E level was associated with a 3.7-fold excess risk of the progression of early cortical cataracts. No significant association with nuclear opacities was found. Another review reported that there was a 55% reduction in cataract risk in persons receiving supplemental vitamin E over 5 years.[32] In the Linxian Cataract Study,[53] there were differing results, in which the administration of supplements containing vitamin E for 5 years did not influence the incidence of age-related cataract.

In a sample of 1828 participants of the Alpha-tocopherol, Beta-carotene Cancer Prevention Study, long-term supplementation of vitamin E for 5–8 years did not influence the cataract prevalence among middle-aged men.[54] Another recent trial of the Beaver Dam Eye Study group also demonstrated no correlation between the intakes of vitamin E from dietary nutrients or supplements and nuclear cataract. However, vitamin E was inversely associated with nuclear opacities in individuals susceptible to nuclear cataract due to the presence of other risk factors.[37]

A study involving individuals from the Vitamin E and Cataract Prevention Study reported that prior vitamin E supplementation may be protective against cortical cataract but not against nuclear cataract regardless of the level, regularity or duration of supplementation.[55] Similarly, a study[39] of over 3000 individuals over 5 years reported that the risk of any type of cataract was 60% lower in individuals who used vitamin E supplements for over 10 years.

Plasma vitamin E was not significantly associated with any cataract type in the Italian–American Cataract Study,[23] the India–US Case-Control Study[9] and also in a study of 685 Hong Kong fishermen.[56]

Carotenoids

β-Carotene, which is the main carotenoid, is a lipid-soluble antioxidant thought to play a role in retaining membrane integrity.[44] It is also thought to prevent cataract development by serving as a free-radical-trapping antioxidant under low partial pressures of oxygen, such as those found in the lens.[28] There have been no suggested mechanisms for any of the other carotenoids.

Jacques and Chylack[28] found that subjects with moderate and high plasma carotenoid levels had a reduced risk of cataract, of which the odds ratios were of a similar magnitude. This is consistent with the antioxidant properties of β-carotene. In contrast, dietary carotene intake was unrelated to cataract risk.

Relations between diet and nuclear opacities were investigated in 1919 participants of the Beaver Dam Eye Study.[30] There was an inverse relationship between the past α-carotene intake and the severity of nuclear sclerosis in men. This was consistent with a reduced prevalence of nuclear sclerosis with many food sources of α-carotene, e.g. green salad, green beans and vegetables. There were inverse relations with intakes of α-carotene, β-carotene and lutein in men who consumed multivitamins regularly. However, this relationship persisted regardless of whether or not multivitamins were regularly used. Men in the highest intake group for β-carotene who used multivitamins had a significantly reduced risk for nuclear sclerosis. There was a progressive reduction in the risk of nuclear sclerosis in individuals with an increasing lutein intake. This inverse association reflected food sources of lutein as well such as spinach, green salad and green beans, which all had reduced odds ratios. Women with large intakes of lycopene were much more likely to have severe nuclear sclerosis. Lycopene is a carotenoid provided mainly by tomatoes.[57] This direct relationship was maintained with all food sources of this carotenoid.

This is consistent with findings described by Mares-Perlman et al.,[50] who reported that high serum levels of lycopene were related to more severe nuclear cataract. In contrast, a high intake of tomatoes had a decreased risk of cataract extraction in a study by Tavani et al.[36] In this study there was no association of β-carotene with cataract extraction after adjusting for confounding variables. However, an increased spinach intake showed an inverse relationship with cataract extraction.

In a large cohort study by Hankinson et al.[27] of US female nurses with a follow-up of 8 years, the total carotene intake of women with the highest intake was associated with a 27% lower risk of cataract extraction compared to those with the lowest intake. Among food items, carrots that contain the richest source of β-carotene[58] were unrelated to cataract extraction. However, high intakes of spinach were associated with a reduced risk of cataract extraction.

Jacques et al.[34] analysed the relationship between some biochemical markers of antioxidant status and age-related cataract in 112 subjects. It was concluded that there was a greater incidence of cortical cataract in individuals with reduced carotenoid levels. The odds ratio of the presence of a cataract for subjects with the highest carotenoid intake relative to subjects with the lowest intake was 0.18. This was similar to the results of Jacques and co-workers,[21] who found a specific protective effect of moderate or high plasma carotenoid levels against cortical or any type of cataract. A beneficial effect was also observed for PSC cataract but it was not statistically significant. A smaller case-control study in Finland with a 15-year follow-up period also reported that low serum concentrations of β-carotene had an increased risk of age-related cataract relative to high serum concentrations.[48] However, plasma β-carotene was unrelated to nuclear opacities in the Baltimore Longitudinal Study on Aging.[22]

In another report from the Beaver Dam Eye Study,[37] it was concluded that, out of five carotenoids examined, only lutein was associated with nuclear cataracts. Persons with a high intake of lutein in the distant past were half as likely to have nuclear cataracts than those with a low intake. The recent intake of lutein also showed an inverse association but the relationship was weaker. Spinach and other dark leafy greens, which are sources of lutein, had a negative associ-

ation with nuclear cataract in persons with the highest intakes.

In a further investigation of a subsample from the Beaver Dam Eye Study, concentrations of serum carotenoids (α-carotene, β-carotene, lutein, lycopene and cryptoxanthin) were unrelated to nuclear cataract after a 5-year follow up. However, there were weak non-significant inverse relations with lutein and cryptoxanthin in older participants so a protective effect of these carotenoids cannot be totally ruled out.[51]

These findings were in contrast with the more severe nuclear cataracts in women with a high level of serum carotenoids.[50] In men, higher levels of β-carotene in the serum had lower odds ratios for nuclear and cortical cataracts. Nonetheless, nuclear and cortical opacities were not consistently inversely related to the same five carotenoids overall.

Cumming et al.[29] found that β-carotene and carotenoids were associated with a lower incidence of nuclear cataract. Individuals who ate spinach more than four times a week also had a lower incidence of nuclear cataract risk. In contrast, a study by Teikari et al.[54] found that supplementation with β-carotene (20 mg/day) for 5–8 years did not influence cataract prevalence among middle-aged men.

Two large recent studies, one of female nurses,[59] over a 12-year period and the other of males[60] with an 8-year follow-up period, both showed similar results. Those individuals with the highest intake of lutein and zeaxanthin had a 20% decreased risk of cataract extraction compared to those with the lowest intakes. Foods rich in these carotenoids such as spinach and broccoli also followed this inverse relationship. However, other carotenoids, such as α- or β-carotene, lycopene and β-cryptoxanthin, were not associated with cataracts severe enough for extraction.

Vitamin B

Several of the B-vitamins are thought to limit age-related cataract development, including thiamin (B$_1$), riboflavin (B$_2$), nicotinamide (B$_3$), pantothenic acid (B$_5$) and pyridoxine (B$_6$). The use of these vitamins appears to be based on their ability to serve as enzyme cofactors.[45]

Riboflavin is the most common B vitamin that has received much attention in its ability to protect against cataract formation or progression. Riboflavin is a water-soluble vitamin and is thought to be a precursor for flavin adenine dinucleotide (FAD) synthesis.[10] FAD is a cofactor for glutathione reductase (an antioxidant enzyme that replenishes the supply of reduced glutathione), which is essential for preventing damage to the lens proteins by scavenging free radicals.[61] The protective effects of niacin and thiamin can be attributed to their strong association with riboflavin.[29] Sources of riboflavin, thiamin and niacin include liver, fish and eggs and the recommended daily allowances are 1.6, 1.4 and 20 mg respectively.[62]

The Linxian Study in China[53] concluded that there was a 44% lower prevalence of nuclear cataract in subjects aged between 65 and 74 years, receiving a riboflavin (3 mg)/niacin (40 mg) supplementation for 5–6 years. No effect was observed on cortical cataract of any vitamin or mineral combination. There was a slight increase in PSC cataract associated with the supplementation of riboflavin/niacin, but the numbers of these cases were very few.

There was a strong inverse association for high intakes of thiamin, niacin and riboflavin and the incidence of nuclear cataract in a recent study.[29] There was also a significant inverse association of the intake of niacin with cortical cataract. Another study[31] also reported that moderate intakes of vitamin B supplements (vitamin B_6, riboflavin, niacin and thiamin) had a reduced risk of nuclear cataract. Higher intakes of these vitamin supplements did not yield reduced odds ratios for nuclear cataract. However, moderate intakes of these vitamin supplements resulted in an increased prevalence of cortical cataract, of which higher intakes strengthened the relationship.

In a subsequent study on nuclear cataract,[30] it was reported that there was a reduced prevalence of nuclear cataract in men who previously consumed dietary B-vitamins riboflavin and niacin even after the contributions from supplements had been accounted for. Women who had diets high in riboflavin also had a reduced risk of severe nuclear sclerosis. The inverse pattern with riboflavin persisted in women who did not use multivitamins. The intake of niacin and thiamin was unrelated to nuclear cataract in women. While the consumption of the most concentrated sources of riboflavin (liver or cheese) was unrelated to the severity of nuclear sclerosis, drinking milk was related to a reduced risk of nuclear sclerosis. Food sources of niacin and thiamin were also unrelated to nuclear sclerosis.

An epidemiological study[21] found little evidence of a protective role of riboflavin on overall cataract formation, but the results do suggest some function of riboflavin on PSC cataract development (odds ratio 0.18). Thiamin was also unrelated to cataract formation. Low blood vitamin B_6 levels were found to be protective against PSC cataract. This result was found to be unusual as vitamin B_6 is essential to many enzymes and no mechanism has been identified as to how high levels would increase the risk of PSC cataract.

A prospective study of nutritional status and cataract extraction of females from the Nurses' Health Study[27] concluded that the intake of riboflavin from food sources was not associated with cataract extraction. These results were similar to another study,[61] where no association was found between riboflavin deficiency and cataract formation. However, there was no sign of riboflavin deficiency in older patients with clear lenses, but the numbers in this category were very small.

In a large case-control study of the Lens Opacities Case-Control Study population,[48] individuals who had a high glutathione reductase activity (with FAD) from red blood cell analysis indicated that there was a higher demand for riboflavin, which in turn suggested that there was a low riboflavin level which resulted in an increase in the risk of opacities. However, a study in India failed to find an association between cataract and blood glutathione reductase stimulation by FAD, which is riboflavin-dependent. No relationship between cataract and thiamin was found.[9]

A review by Bunce[63] stated that excess riboflavin supplements to that required for glutathione reductase saturation would not offer any extra benefit and may actually be considered to be detrimental.

Multivitamins

Mares-Perlman and co-workers[31] evaluated the relationship of the self-reported supplemental vitamin and mineral use and various types of lens opacities of subjects in the Nutritional Factors in Eye Disease Study. Regular multivitamin and mineral supplement users 10 years in the past had a 40% reduced prevalence of nuclear cataract, but a 60% increased risk of cortical cataract. No significant association was observed for multivitamin use and PSC cataract, or for the current use of multivitamins and any type of cataract. The Lens Opacities Case-Control Study[20] also verified that all types of opacities were less likely in frequent users of multivitamin supplements for at least 1 year.

The Linxian intervention trials demonstrated that there was a significant reduction (36%) in the prevalence of nuclear cataract in those subjects aged between 65 and 74 years receiving multivitamin and mineral supplements at doses 1.5–3 times the recommended daily allowance. Younger individuals showed no benefit of supplementation. Treatment with these supplements had no effect on cortical or PSC cataract.[53] In contrast, Hankinson et al.[27] reported no correlation between the long-term use of multivitamins and cataract severe enough for extraction in a study of US nurses, with an 8-year follow-up period. Similar results were found by two other studies.[22,32]

In the Physicians' Health Study of over 17 000 participants, men who took multivitamin supplements experienced a decreased risk of cataract and cataract extraction after 5 years of follow-up, compared to physicians who used no supplements, after adjusting for various cataract risk factors. The risk of cataract reduced with an increasing duration of multivitamin use.[33] Mares-Perlman et al.[39] also reported a 60% lower risk in nuclear and cortical but not PSC cataract in subjects who used multivitamins for greater than 10 years in a recent study of participants from the Beaver Dam Eye Study. These findings coincided with those of the Longitudinal Study of Cataract,[47] where the risk of progression of nuclear opacification was reduced by approximately one-third in regular users of multivitamin supplements. In addition, there was a progressive reduction in the risk of nuclear cataract with an increasing duration of multivitamin use.

The Barbados Eye Study reported that regular users of nutritional supplements, including multivitamins had a one-fourth lower risk of all types of cataract, particularly cortical opacities in individuals under the age of 70 years. However, the protective effect on lens opacities was not stronger in long-term supplement users (greater than 2 or 5 years).[64]

Another epidemiological study[30] suggested that the use of multivitamin supplements was associated with a reduced risk of age-related nuclear cataract. There was a strengthening of the inverse relations of some nutrients such as vitamin E and β-carotene in men who used multivitamins. In contrast, the Italian–American Cataract Study of 1500 individuals found no significant associations between any cataract type and multivitamin supplementation.[23]

The Roche European American Cataract Trial (REACT)[65] was a multicentred, prospective, double-masked, randomised, placebo-controlled 3-year trial in which half the subjects were given antioxidant vitamins daily: vitamin A (β-carotene) 18 mg, vitamin C 750 mg, vitamin E 600 mg. Cataract severity was documented with serial digital retroillumination imagery of the lens; progression was quantified by image analysis assessing increased area of opacity. There were no statistically significant differences between the treatment groups at baseline. After 2 years of treatment, there was a small positive treatment effect in US patients; after 3 years a positive effect was apparent in the US and the UK groups. The positive effect in the US group was even greater after 3 years. There was no statistically significant benefit of treatment in the UK group. The investigators concluded that daily use of the aforementioned micronutrients for 3 years produced a small deceleration in progression of age-related cataract.

The 11-centre Age-Related Eye Disease Study (AREDS) was a double-masked clinical trial.[66] Participants were randomly assigned to receive daily oral tablets containing antioxidants (vitamin C, 500 mg; vitamin E, 400 IU; and β-carotene, 15 mg) or no antioxidants. Participants with more than a few small drusen were also randomly assigned to receive tablets with or without zinc (80 mg zinc as zinc oxide) and copper (2 mg copper as cupric oxide) as part of the age-related macular degeneration trial. Baseline and annual (starting at year 2) lens photographs were graded at a reading centre for the severity of lens opacities. The investigators concluded that use of a high-dose multivitamin and β-carotene formulation in a relatively well-nourished older adult cohort had no apparent effect on the 7-year risk of development or progression of age-related lens opacities or visual acuity loss.

In a randomised trial involving 22 071 male US physicians, β-carotene (50 mg on alternate days for 12 years) had no influence in comparison with placebo on the overall incidence of cataract or cataract extraction. There was a reduction in the numbers of cases of cataracts in smokers in the β-carotene group compared with placebo. Among non-smokers there were no differences.[67]

In the most recent nutrition intervention trial (Vitamin E, Cataract and Age-Related Maculopathy Trial), there was no effect of vitamin E on cataract. In this randomised study, 1193 subjects with early or no cataract aged 55–80 years were enrolled and followed up for 4 years. Subjects were assigned to receive 500 IU of natural vitamin E or placebo. After 4 years of follow-up, there was no difference in the incidence or progression of nuclear, cortical or subscapular cataracts.[68]

OTHER NUTRIENTS

There have been many studies on the role of other nutrients being protective against age-related cataract development but this is outside the scope of this review. Higher levels of vitamin A (retinol),[31] protein and fibre[29] and minerals such as iron,[48] magnesium[21] and zinc[69] have all been shown to be protective against age-related cataract progression.

A Spanish group investigated the effect of long-term antioxidant supplementation (lutein and α-tocopherol) on serum levels and visual performance in patients with cataracts.[70] Seventeen patients clinically diagnosed with age-related cataracts were randomised in a double-masked study involving dietary supplementation with lutein (15 mg; $n = 5$), α-tocopherol (100 mg; $n = 6$), or placebo ($n = 6$) three times a week for up to 2 years. Serum carotenoid and α-tocopherol concentrations were determined and visual performance (visual acuity and glare sensitivity) and biochemical and haematological indexes were monitored every 3 months. Serum concentrations of lutein and α-tocopherol increased with supplementation, although statistical significance was only reached in the lutein group. Visual performance improved in the lutein group, whereas there was a trend toward the maintenance of and decrease in visual acuity with α-tocopherol and placebo supplementation, respectively. The researchers concluded that higher intake of lutein, through lutein-rich fruit and vegetables or supplements, may have beneficial effects on the visual performance of people with age-related cataracts.

FREE-RADICAL SCAVENGERS

A number of sulphur-containing reducing agents are available as anticataract agents. Anticataract action arises from reduction of the oxidised sulfhydryl components in the lens that are thought to accumulate during cataract formation.[45]

There is a reduction in GSH in the lens during cataract formation.[12] GSH has been thought to protect sulfhydryl groups in the lens through its ability to serve as a reducing agent.[71] As glutathione levels are reduced in cataract formation, it is reasonable to prevent or delay cataractogenesis by directly increasing the GSH levels within the lens. This can be done by adding GSH to the medium, by inhibiting the breakdown of GSH or by stimulating its production by supplementing the medium with its constituent amino acids.[72]

Preparations such as phakan that contains the three individual amino acids of GSH (glutamic acid, glycine and cysteine) have been formulated to increase the lenticular levels of GSH.[73] A randomised study of 140 patients has been carried out with phakan over a 9-month period. Subjects were administered with phakan twice daily in 20-day cycles with 10 days of relief in between the cycles. The results showed only slight, if any, beneficial effects of phakan on cortical, nuclear and mixed cataracts. However, these results are disputable as there was a high drop-out rate of participants in the study.[74] A review by Creighton and Trevithick[75] claimed that a mixture of vitamin E and GSH could have a protective effect on cortical cataract.

Tiopronin is another drug that can act as a reducing agent, converting dehydroascorbic acid to ascorbic acid and cystine to cysteine,[73] which can act as a free-radical scavenger and can be used to produce GSH respectively. In a controlled study, tiopronin was administered three times daily for 12 months to 150 individuals. There was a larger increase of visual acuity in the tiopronin-treated group (29% increase) than in the control group. Slit-lamp microscopy revealed that a 26% reduction in the opacities in the tiopronin group, which was greater than the increase in the control group. Also, the combined evaluation of visual acuity and slit-lamp findings indicated a 40% improvement of cataract regression in the tiopronin-treated group.[76] There were also no reported side-effects. These results are consistent with the findings of Matsuura et al.,[77] who concluded that there was a protective effect of tiopronin on age-related cataract.

Taurine, a sulphur-containing agent, is found in high concentrations in the lens and has been found to be reduced in patients with age-related cataracts.[78] Vodovozov and Glotova[79] suggested the use of taurine as an anticataract agent to supplement the loss. In this study, 100 patients were given 4% taurine solution and another 50 patients were given vitamin drops over a 6-month period. There was an increase in the visual acuity in subjects receiving taurine, thereby supporting the use of taurine as an anticataract drug.

SOD is an enzyme that acts as a scavenger of the superoxide radical, and has also been considered as an anticataract agent.[80] Indirect evidence for the importance of SOD in the maintenance of good vision has been provided by Chinese researchers who reported that people with age-related cataract have less SOD in their blood serum than those with healthy eyes.[81]

SUMMARY

Currently, there is no firm evidence to support that nutritional intervention, early or late in life, may reduce the incidence and severity of age-related cataracts. Nevertheless, the protective effect of the antioxidant vitamins seems extremely promising. It is also unclear as to whether dietary intake or supplemental nutrients have the greater effect. It is possible that some of the anticataract medications such as aspirin-like analgesics and bendazac together with new agents will be shown to be effective in the future.

References

1. Stafford MJ. The histology and biology of the lens. Optom Today 2001; 41:23–29.
2. Hammond C. The epidemiology of cataract. Optom Today 2001; 41:24–28.
3. Harding JJ. Pharmacological treatment strategies in age-related cataracts. Drugs Aging 1992; 2:287–300.
4. Flaye DE, Sullivan KN, Cullinan TR et al. Cataracts and cigarette smoking. The City Eye Study. Eye 1989; 3:379–384.
5. Taylor HR, West SK, Rosenthal FS et al. Effect of ultraviolet radiation on cataract formation. N Engl J Med 1988; 319:1429–1433.
6. Sperduto RD, Hiller R. The prevalence of nuclear, cortical and posterior subcapsular lens opacities in a general population sample. Ophthalmologica 1984; 91:815–818.
7. Hodge WG, Witcher JP, Santariano W. Risk factors for age related cataracts. Epidemiol Rev 1995; 17:336–346.
8. van Heyningen R, Harding JJ. A case-control study of cataract in Oxfordshire: some risk factors. Br J Ophthalmol 1988; 72:804–808.
9. Mohan M, Sperduto RD, Angra SK et al. India–US case-control study of age-related cataract. Arch Ophthalmol 1989; 107:670–676.
10. Taylor A. Associations between nutrition and cataract. Nutr Rev 1989; 47:225–233.
11. Ottonello S, Foroni C, Carta A et al. Oxidative stress and age-related cataract. Ophthalmologica 2000; 214:78–85.
12. Hurst MA. Lens structure, biochemistry and transparency. In: Douthwaite WA, Hurst MA, eds. Cataract-detection, measurement and management in optometric practice. Oxford: Butterworth-Heinemann; 1993:4–12.
13. Sperduto RD, Ferris FL, Kurinij N. Do we have a nutritional treatment for age-related cataract or macular degeneration? Arch Ophthalmol 1990; 108:1403–1405.

14. Walsh S, Paterson JW. Effects of oxidants on lens transport. Invest Ophthalmol Vis Sci 1991; 32:1648–1658.

15. Spector A, Wanchao M, Wang RR. The aqueous humor is capable of generating and degrading H_2O_2. Invest Ophthalmol Vis Sci 1998; 39:1188–1197.

16. Spector A. The search for a solution to senile cataracts. Invest Ophthalmol Vis Sci 1984; 25:130–146.

17. Phillipson BT, Fagerholm PP. Lens changes responsible for increased light scattering in some types of senile cataract. In: The human lens in relation to cataract. Ciba Foundation Symposium 19. London: Elsevier; 1973: 45–58.

18. Bron AJ, Vrenson GFJM, Koretz J et al. The ageing lens. Ophthalmologica 2000; 214:86–104.

19. Augestyn RC. Protein modification in cataract: possible oxidative mechanisms. In: Duncan G, ed. Mechanisms of cataract formation in the human lens. London: Academic Press; 1981:71–116.

20. Leske MC, Chylack LT, Wu SY et al. The Lens Opacities Case-Control Study: risk factors for cataract. Arch Ophthalmol 1991; 109:244–251.

21. Jacques PF, Chylack LT, McGandy RB, Hartz SC. Antioxidant status in persons with and without senile cataract. Arch Ophthalmol 1988; 106:337–340.

22. Vitale S, West S, Hallfrisch J. Plasma antioxidants and risk of cortical and nuclear cataract. Epidemiology 1993; 4:195–203.

23. The Italian–American Cataract Study Group. Risk factors for age-related cortical, nuclear and posterior subcapsular cataracts. Am J Epidemiol 1991; 133:541–553.

24. Seddon JM. Nutrition and age-related eye disease. Vitamin Nutrition Information Service. Backgrounder 2 (2).

25. Taylor A, Jacques PF, Nadler D et al. Relationship in humans between ascorbic acid consumption and levels of total and reduced ascorbic acid in lens, aqueous humor, and plasma. Curr Eye Res 1991; 10:751–759.

26. Jacques PF, Taylor A, Hankinson SE et al. Long term vitamin C supplement use and prevalence of early age-related lens opacities. Am J Clin Nutr 1997; 66: 911–916.

27. Hankinson SE, Stampfer MJ, Seddon JM et al. Nutrient intake and cataract extraction in women – a prospective study. Br Med J 1992; 305:335–339.

28. Jacques PF, Chylack LT. Epidemiologic evidence of a role for the antioxidant vitamins and carotenoids in cataract prevention. Am J Clin Nutr 1991; 53:S352–S355.

29. Cumming RG, Mitchell P, Smith W. Diet and cataract – the Blue Mountains Eye Study. Ophthalmologica 2000; 107:450–456.

30. Mares-Perlman JA, Brady WE, Klein BEK et al. Diet and nuclear lens opacities. Am J Epidemiol 1995; 141:322–334.

31. Mares-Perlman JA, Klein BE, Ritter LL. Relation between lens opacities and vitamin and mineral supplement use. Ophthalmologica 1994; 101:315–325.

32. Robertson JM, Donner AP, Trevithick JR. Vitamin E intake and risk of cataracts in humans. Ann NY Acad Sci 1990; 503:372–382.

33. Seddon JM, Christen WG, Manson JE et al. The use of vitamin supplements and the risk of cataract among US male physicians. Am J Public Health 1994; 84: 788–792.

34. Jacques PF, Hartz SC, Chylack LT et al. Nutritional status in persons with and without senile cataract: blood vitamin and mineral levels. Am J Clin Nutr 1988; 48:152–158.

35. Mariani G, Pasquini P, Sperduto RD. Risk factors for age-related cortical, nuclear and posterior subcapsular cataracts. Am J Epidemiol 1991; 133:541–553

36. Tavani A, Negri E, La Vecchia C. Food and nutrient intake and risk of cataract. Ann Epidemiol 1996; 6:41–46.

37. Lyle BJ, Mares-Perlman JA, Klein BEK, Greger JL. Antioxidant intake and risk of incident age-related nuclear cataracts in the Beaver Dam Eye Study. Am J Epidemiol 1999; 149:801–809.

38. Robertson JM, Donner AP, Trevithick JR. A possible role for vitamins C and E in cataract prevention. Am J Clin Nutr 1991; 53:346S–351S.

39. Mares-Perlman JA, Lyle BJ, Klein R et al. Vitamin supplement use and incident cataracts in a population-based study. Arch Ophthalmol 2000; 118:1556–1563.

40. Jacob RA, Otradovec CL, Russell RM. Vitamin C status and nutrient interactions in a healthy elderly population. Am J Clin Nutr 1988; 48:1436–1442.

41. Olson JA, Hodges RE. Recommended dietary intakes (RDI) of vitamin C in humans. Am J Clin Nutr 1987; 45:693–703.

42. Taylor A, Jacques PF, Nowell T. Vitamin C in human and guinea pig aqueous, lens and plasma in relation to intake. Curr Eye Res 1997; 16:857–864.

43. Podmore ID, Griffiths HR, Herbert KE et al. Vitamin C exhibits pro-oxidant properties (letter). Nature 1998; 392:559.

44. Christen WG, Glynn RJ, Hennekens CH. Antioxidants and age-related eye disease – current and future perspectives. Ann Epidemiol 1996; 6:60–66.

45. Young S. The medical treatment of cataract. In: Douthwaite WA, Hurst MA, eds. Cataract-detection, measurement and management in optometric practice. Oxford: Butterworth-Heinemann; 1993:128–136.

46. Chow CK, Reddy K, Tappel AL. Effect of dietary vitamin E on activities of glutathione peroxidase system in rat tissue. J Nutr 1973; 103:618–624.

47. Leske MC, Chylack LT, He Q et al. Antioxidant vitamins and nuclear opacities: the Longitudinal Study of Cataract. Ophthalmologica 1998; 105:831–836.

48. Leske MC, Wu SY, Hyman L et al. Biochemical factors in the Lens Opacities Case-Control Study. Arch Ophthalmol 1995; 113:1113–1119.

49. Knekt P, Heliovaara M, Rissanen A et al. Serum antioxidant vitamins and risk of cataract. Br Med J 1992; 305:1392–1394.

50. Mares-Perlman JA, Brady WE, Klein BEK et al. Serum carotenoids and tocopherols and severity of nuclear and cortical opacities. Invest Ophthalmol Vis Sci 1995; 36:276–288.

51. Lyle BJ, Mares-Perlman JA, Klein BEK et al. Serum carotenoids and tocopherols and incidence of age-related nuclear cataract. Am J Clin Nutr 1999; 69:272–277.

52. Rouhiainen P, Rouhiainen H, Salonen JT. Association between low plasma vitamin E concentration and progression of early cortical lens opacities. Am J Epidemiol 1996; 144:496–500.

53. Sperduto RD, Hu TS, Milton RC et al. The Linxian Cataract Studies: two nutrition intervention trials. Arch Ophthalmol 1993; 111:1246–1253.

54. Teikari JM, Virtamo J, Routalahti M et al. Long-term supplementation with alpha-tocopherol and beta-carotene and age-related cataract. Acta Ophthalmol Scand 1997; 75:634–640.

55. Nadalin G, Robman LD, McCarty CA et al. The role of past intake of vitamin E in early cataract changes. Ophthalm Epidemiol 1999; 6:105–112.

56. Wong L, Ho SC, Coggon D. Sunlight exposure, antioxidant status, and cataract in Hong Kong fishermen. J Epidemiol Commun Health 1993; 47: 46–49.

57. Chug-Ahuja JK, Holden JM, Forman MR. The development and application of a carotenoid database for fruits, vegetables and selected multicomponent foods. J Am Diet Assoc 1993; 93:318–323.

58. Romieu I, Stampfe MJ, Stryker WS et al. Food predictors of plasma beta-carotene and alpha-tocopherol: a validation of a food frequency questionnaire. Am J Epidemiol 1990; 131:864–876.

59. Chasan-Taber L, Willett WC, Seddon JM et al. A prospective study of carotenoid and vitamin A intakes and risk of cataract extraction in US women. Am J Clin Nutr 1999; 70:509–516.

60. Brown L, Rimm EB, Seddon JM et al. A prospective study of carotenoid intake and risk of cataract extraction in US men. Am J Clin Nutr 1999; 70:517–524.

61. Skalka HW, Prchal JT. Cataracts and riboflavin deficiency. Am J Clin Nutr 1981; 34:861–863.

62. Brown NAP, Bron AJ, Harding JJ, Dewar HM. Nutrition supplements and the eye. Eye 1998; 12:127–133.

63. Bunce E. Evaluation of the impact of nutrition intervention on cataract prevalence in China. Nutr Rev 1994; 52:99–101.

64. Leske MC, Wu SY, Connell AMS et al. Lens opacities, demographic factors and nutritional supplements in the Barbados Eye Study. Epidemiology 1997; 26: 1314–1322.

65. Chylack LT Jr, Brown NP, Bron A et al. The Roche European American Cataract Trial (REACT): a randomized clinical trial to investigate the efficacy of an oral antioxidant micronutrient mixture to slow progression of age-related cataract. Ophthalm Epidemiol 2002; 9:49–80.

66. Age Related Eye Disease Study Research Group. A randomized, placebo-controlled, clinical trial of high-dose supplementation with vitamins C and E and beta-carotene for age-related cataract and vision loss. AREDS report no. 9. Arch Ophthalmol 2001; 119:1439–1452.

67. Christen WG, Manson JE, Glyn RJ et al. A randomized trial of beta carotene and age-related cataract in US physicians. Arch Ophthalmol 2003; 121:372–378.

68. McNeil J, Robman L, Tikellis G et al. Vitamin E supplementation and cataract Ophthalmology 2004; 111:75–84.

69. Bhat KS. Plasma calcium and trace metals in human subjects with mature cataract. Nutr Rep Int 1988; 37:157–163.

70. Olmedilla B, Granado F, Blanco I et al. Lutein in patients with cataracts and age-related macular degeneration: a long term supplementation study. J Sci Food Agric 2001; 81:904–909.

71. Kinoshita JH. Selected topics in ophthalmic biochemistry. Arch Ophthalmol 1964; 72:554–572.

72. Harding JJ. Cataract – biochemistry, epidemiology and pharmacology. London: Chapman & Hall; 1991:218–324.

73. Kador PF. Overview of the current attempts toward the medical treatment of cataract. Ophthalmologica 1983; 90:352–364.

74. Hockwin O, Wiegelin E. Medical treatment of senile cataract in man. A controlled study on the efficacy of a preparation. In: Regnault F, ed. Symposium of the lens. Amsterdam: Excerpta Medica; 1981:78–101.

75. Creighton MO, Trevithick JR. Cortical cataract formation prevented by vitamin E and glutathione. Exp Eye Res 1979; 29:689–693.

76. Ichikawa H, Imaizumi K, Tazawa Y et al. Effect of tiopronin on senile cataracts. A double-blind clinical study. Ophthalmologica 1980; 180:293–298.

77. Matsuura H, Watanabe T, Kurimoto S. Clinical effect of 2-mercaptopropionylglysine (Thiola) for senile cataracts. Jpn J Clin Ophthalmol 1971; 25:1875–1884.

78. Reddy VN. Studies on intraocular transport of taurine. II. Accumulation in the rabbit lens. Invest Ophthalmol Vis Sci 1970; 9:206–219.

79. Vodovozov AM, Glotova NM. Results of treating senile cataracts with taurine. Vestn Oftalmol 1981; 2:44–45.

80. Varma SD, Srivastava VK, Richards RD. Photoperoxidation in lens and cataract formation: preventative role of superoxide dismutase, catalase and vitamin C. Ophthalm Res 1982; 14:167–175.

81. Yang W, Yu W, Li Z. The study on superoxide dismutase and trace elements in patients with senile cataracts. Yan Ke Xue Bao 2000; 16:246–248.

Chapter **4.6**

Age-related macular degeneration

Rasha Al Taie, John Nolan and Kumari Neelam

INTRODUCTION

The late stage of age-related maculopathy (ARM), known as AMD, is the commonest cause of visual impairment in the western world. Importantly, the prevalence of AMD is expected to rise as a result of increasing longevity. For the purpose of this chapter, we have adopted and modified the International Classification System of Age-Related Maculopathy and Age-Related Macular Degeneration.[1] In brief, early ARM is characterised by the presence of any of the following findings in persons aged > 50 years: soft drusen; areas of increased pigment associated with drusen; or areas of hypopigmentation of the RPE associated with drusen. Late ARM is diagnosed in the presence of geographic atrophy (GA) within 3000 μm of the fovea, an RPE detachment or choroidal neovascularisation (CNV) (and/or its sequelae), and is henceforth known as AMD.[2]

INCIDENCE AND PREVALENCE

Visual loss due to AMD rises exponentially with increasing age, reflected in the finding that individuals of 75 years or older have a higher incidence of large drusen, soft indistinct drusen, RPE abnormalities, exudative macular degeneration and GA than younger age groups. The prevalence of ARM is 18% in the population aged 65–74 years, and 30% in the population older than 74 years.[3,4]

HISTORICAL BACKGROUND

ARM was first described in 1855 by Bessig, and this is relatively recent compared to the first description of other ocular diseases such as glaucoma and cataract, prompting speculation that ARM is a relatively new disease.[5]

RISK FACTORS FOR ARM/AMD

Risk factors for ARM are generally classed as established or putative.

Established risk factors

Age

Age is the strongest risk factor for ARM and AMD. The prevalence, incidence and progression of all forms of ARM rise exponentially with advancing age.[6]

Race and ethnicity

The prevalence of ARM and AMD is higher in white populations than amongst other races. For example, large drusen are seen in 15% of white people in comparison with only 9% of black people. Pigmentary changes are seen in 7.9% and 0.4% of white and black populations, respectively. The difference in melanin content of the choroid may underlie, in part, the differences in risk for AMD between races.[7–13]

Genetics

There is a compelling and growing body of evidence in support of the role of genetics in ARM. Familial aggregation studies have shown an increased prevalence of ARM in first-degree relatives of sufferers when compared with first-degree relatives of a control proband, with odds ratios ranging between 2.4 and 19.8 depending on the stage of disease under investigation. The Beaver Dam Eye and Framingham Eye Studies also identified a genetic contribution to ARM through population-based segregation analyses. Meyers has shown concordance of ARM in 23 of 23 monozygotic, compared with 2 of 8 dizygotic twin pairs.[14–17]

Smoking

Smoking has now been established as a risk for ARM and AMD, by at least one of several mechanisms. The postulated mechanisms include: (1) its role as a pro-oxidant; (2) its association with hypoxia; and (3) its contribution to reduced choroidal blood flow.[18–23]

Putative risk factors

Adiposity

Adiposity, defined as an excess of body fat, has been shown to increase the risk of progression to advanced AMD. Body mass index (BMI) reflects adiposity, and it is defined as weight in kilograms divided by height in metres squared (kg/m^2).[24–26]

The mechanisms underlying the putative link between adiposity and ARM include: inflammation; hypertension; cardiovascular disease; and oxidative stress. Of these, oxidative stress, which is independently associated with adiposity and ARM, is the most plausible explanation (see Chapter 2.7). Macular pigment, composed of the carotenoids lutein and zeaxanthin, is believed to protect against ARM by blue light filtration and/or its antioxidant properties (see Chapter 3.4). Body fat is of particular interest in this respect, because adipose tissue is a major storage organ for carotenoids, and some investigators have suggested that adipose tissue acts as a sink and a reservoir for lutein and/or zeaxanthin.[27,28] In other words, a person's body fat may influence carotenoid levels in serum and retina. Further, adiposity results in reduced high-density lipoprotein cholesterol,[29] which is known to be the primary carrier of lutein and zeaxanthin,[30] thereby impairing transport and delivery of the macular carotenoids to the retina in obese individuals. Finally, it is also possible that a relative lack of macular pigment in obese subjects simply reflects a poor diet amongst these individuals, as it has been demonstrated that adiposity is associated with reduced dietary intake of the carotenoids that comprise the macular pigment.

It is unsurprising, therefore, that an inverse relationship between macular pigment and various measures of adiposity has been demonstrated in two recently published studies.[27,28] It is important to note that, in both of these studies, the inverse relationship between macular pigment and adiposity persisted even after the dietary intake of the relevant carotenoids was factored into the analyses.

Cardiovascular disease

Cardiovascular disease has been linked to ARM and/or AMD in several population-based studies. A positive association has also been found between ARM (and AMD) and the following cardiovascular conditions: (1) hypertension; (2) atherosclerosis; (3) plasma fibrinogen level; and (4) cerebrovascular accident. It has been hypothesised that choroidal circulation is compromised in these conditions, and that this contributes to ARM and/or AMD.[31]

Diabetes and hyperglycaemia

The majority of studies that have investigated the relationship between diabetes and ARM and/or AMD have found no significant association.[18]

Reproductive and related factors

The role of oestrogens, which protect against peri-oxidative damage of cell membranes, has also been investigated, and early menopause is associated with increased risk of AMD. Women who have been pregnant (parity = 1) have been shown to be at reduced risk of ARM when compared with nulliparous women.[32]

Alcohol consumption

There are conflicting reports regarding the effect of alcohol intake on the development of ARM. Some investigators have reported a positive association, whereas others have reported a negative association.

Iris colour

A number of studies have reported an increased risk of ARM in people with blue or light-coloured irides, compared with those of darker iris colour.

However, this association has not been consistently demonstrated.

Cataract and cataract surgery

The association between ARM and cataract has not been consistently reported. A positive association between nuclear sclerosis and ARM has been identified by some investigators, but no relationship between other types of lens opacity and onset (or progression) of ARM has been demonstrated. The risk of progression of ARM is increased following cataract surgery, possibly due to increased light transmission or inflammatory changes.[33–35]

Refractive error

Some investigators have found that hyperopic eyes are at greater risk of ARM when compared with emmetropic eyes.[35–39]

Cup-to-disc ratio

Large horizontal and vertical cup-to-disc ratios have been associated with reduced risk of AMD, but this has not been consistently demonstrated.

PATHOGENESIS

In order to understand the changes that occur in AMD, an overview of the structures and functions of the elements that are involved in its pathogenesis is required. Although the pathogenesis of ARM and/or AMD is poorly understood, and is probably multifactorial, there is a growing body of evidence to support the view that ARM and/or AMD occurs in the presence of changes which are both physiological and pathological.[39]

Retinal pigment epithelium

The retina is composed of two laminar structures: the inner, neurosensory layer, which is in contact with the vitreous body; and the outer, RPE layer, which is in contact with Bruch's membrane. The RPE is composed of a single layer of epithelial cells located between the highly vascular choriocapillaris and the outer segment of the photoreceptors

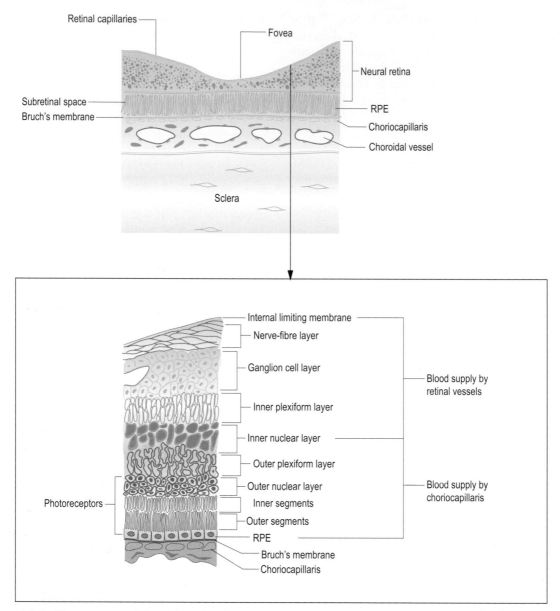

Figure 4.6.1   The structure of the retina, showing the location of the retinal pigment epithelium (RPE).

(Figure 4.6.1). The functions of the RPE include: vitamin A metabolism; maintenance of the outer blood–retina barrier; phagocytosis of the photoreceptor outer segments; reduction of light scatter; heat exchange; and production of the mucopolysaccharide matrix which surrounds photoreceptor outer segments.

Bruch's membrane

Bruch's membrane consists of a connective tissue sheet that is highly permeable to small molecules. It has five elements: (1) the basal lamina of the RPE; (2) an inner collagen layer; (3) a thicker porous band of elastic fibres; (4) an outer collagen

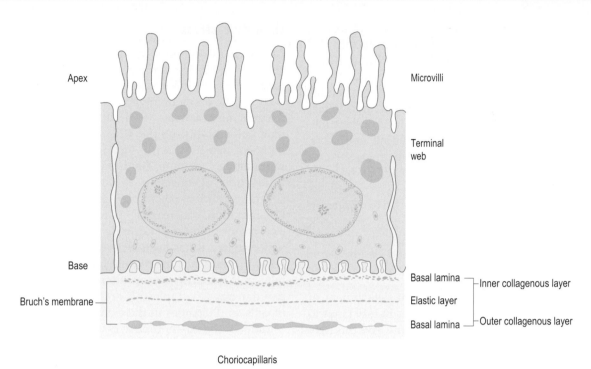

Apex

Microvilli

Terminal web

Base

Basal lamina — Inner collagenous layer

Bruch's membrane — Elastic layer

Basal lamina — Outer collagenous layer

Choriocapillaris

Figure 4.6.2   Bruch's membrane.

layer; and (5) the basal lamina of the choriocapillaris (Figure 4.6.2).

Pathogenesis of ARM

Drusen

Drusen are usually the first clinically detectable feature of ARM, and are large periodic acid–Schiff-positive deposits between the basement membrane of the RPE and Bruch's membrane.

RPE changes

In ARM, the RPE cells may lose their pigment, but may also become hyperplastic with thickened Bruch's membrane.

Pathogenesis of AMD

The lesions that lead to loss of central vision in AMD include CNV, retinal pigment detachment and GA. Their pathogenesis is as follows.

Choroidal neovascular membrane (CNVM)

A choroidal neovascular membrane (CNVM) consists of fibrovascular tissue which grows from the choriocapillaris, through defects in Bruch's membrane, into the sub-RPE space (type 1) or subretinal space (type 2), or both the sub-RPE and subretinal spaces (combined). There is some evidence that the angiographic appearance of a CNVM correlates with its growth pattern: in type 1 CNVM, the membrane starts with multiple growth sites, and tufts of CNV extend laterally in a horizontal fashion under the RPE after breaking through Bruch's membrane. In type 2, or subretinal CNVM, the growth pattern most likely occurs with a single, or a few, in-growth site(s).

There is a growing body of evidence which suggests that CNVM is the result of an imbalance between growth factors derived from the RPE (vascular endothelial growth factor (VEGF) which stimulates vasculogenesis, and pigment epithelium-derived factor (PEDF) which suppresses vasculogenesis). During the growth phase of a CNVM, increased and decreased levels of VEGF and PEDF, respectively, have been observed; however, the situation is reversed in the involution phase. In addition to VEGF and PEDF, recent studies indicate that angiopoietin 1 and 2, and their receptor Tie-2, play a role in the genesis of a CNVM. Angiopoietin 1 acts as an agonist, promoting vascular integrity and maturation, reducing permeability and inhibiting apoptosis. Conversely, angiopoietin 2 is an antagonist of angiopoietin 1, thus promoting VEGF-induced angiogenesis. The receptor Tie-2, as well as angiopoietin 1 and 2, has been shown to be present in choroidal neovascular tissue.[40]

RPE detachment

There is evidence to suggest that detachment of the RPE may be related to changes in resistance to water flow in the Bruch's membrane, and this may be largely due to lipid accumulation in the Bruch's membrane from the RPE with advancing age. It has been hypothesised that reduction of hydraulic conductivity of the Bruch's membrane would hamper movement of water toward the choroid, thus causing it to accumulate in the subretinal space, resulting in RPE detachment.[41,42]

Geographic atrophy (GA)

In GA there is loss of the outer neurosensory retina, RPE and choriocapillaris without preceding retinal detachment. Until recently little was known about the aetiology of GA, but it is now believed that GA is preceded by accumulation of lipofuscin (autofluorescent material) in the RPE, and a possible causal relationship between the two has been postulated. It is understood that the accumulation of lipofuscin in the RPE is an index of defective recycling of degradation products from the photoreceptor cells, and that this reflects ageing in the RPE.[41,43–45]

CURRENT CONCEPTS IN THE AETIOLOGY OF ARM AND AMD

The following concepts have been putatively linked to the development of ARM and AMD.

Oxidative stress

Ageing is associated with, and possibly attributable to, oxidative damage. Oxidative damage refers to tissue injury caused by the interaction between the tissue involved and unstable reactive oxygen intermediates (ROI). It has been shown that vulnerability of the RPE cells to oxidative damage increases with ageing, and this may represent a common final pathway for ARM. Production of unstable ROI is stimulated by several conditions, including: irradiation; ageing; inflammation; increased partial pressure of oxygen; air pollutants; cigarette smoke; and reperfusion injury. It has been shown that ROI interact with nucleic acids, membrane lipids, surface proteins and integrity glycoproteins, causing oxidative damage to cytoplasmic and nuclear elements of cells, and changes in the extracellular matrix.[46]

Indeed, the susceptibility of the RPE to oxidative damage increases with age. The retina is an ideal site for generation of, and damage by, unstable ROI for the following reasons:

- The retina is exposed to high levels of cumulative irradiation throughout life.
- The retina and RPE contain several photosensitisers (rhodopsin, lipofuscin, cytochrome c oxidase).
- The RPE phagocytoses photoreceptor outer segments, thus producing hydrogen peroxide.
- The retina has a very high consumption of oxygen.
- The photoreceptor outer-segment membranes contain very high levels of polyunsaturated fatty acids, which are an ideal substrate for oxidative damage.

Reduced foveal choroidal circulation

Reduced foveal choroidal circulation has been consistently demonstrated in the presence of ARM and AMD, but whether the nature of this relationship is causal or chronological has yet to be established. Some investigators have postulated that an age-related increase in scleral rigidity contributes to a reduction in foveolar choroidal circulation, thereby (possibly) contributing to ARM and AMD.

Light damage

It has been hypothesised that excessive exposure to visible light results in damage to the RPE and/or the neurosensory retina through photo-oxidative injury, and that such injury may contribute aetiologically to ARM and/or AMD. Several studies investigated the relationship between sunlight exposure and the risk of ARM and/or AMD, but the results have been inconsistent. Cohort studies, however, did detect a significantly increased risk of AMD in association with higher cumulative lifetime exposure to sunlight.[47]

RPE dysfunction

RPE function deteriorates with increasing age. The reduction of the RPE capability to pump the waste products leads to the accumulation of debris in Bruch's membrane, thus altering its composition (i.e. increased lipid and protein content) and permeability (e.g. decreased permeability to water-soluble constituents); these changes reduce the hydraulic conductivity of Bruch's membrane, resulting in RPE detachment.

With ageing, the capability of RPE cells to phagocytose the outer segment of the photoreceptors becomes impaired, resulting in accumulation of lipofuscin with possible eventual GA. In response to this metabolic stress, the RPE probably produces substances such as VEGF and basic fibroblast growth factor, which may act synergistically to stimulate new blood vessel growth, forming a CNVM.

CLINICAL FEATURES OF ARM

Drusen

These are round, dull, yellow lesions at the level of the outer retina (Figure 4.6.3). There are several different types:

1. Hard drusen: discrete and well-demarcated. They are not a feature of ARM.
2. Soft drusen: amorphous and poorly demarcated.
3. Confluent drusen: contiguous boundaries between drusen.

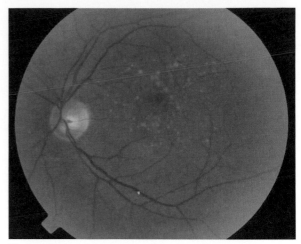

Figure 4.6.3   Fundus photograph of the left eye, showing small drusen in age-related maculopathy.

Drusen are also categorised according to size, as follows:

Small: < 64 μm in diameter
Intermediate: 64–125 μm in diameter
Large: =125 μm in diameter.

Pigmentary changes

Pigmentary changes include hypopigmentation and hyperpigmentation of the RPE.

CLINICAL FEATURES OF AMD

These are divided into two main types: (1) atrophic AMD is a slowly progressive disease, which accounts for 90% of cases; and (2) exudative AMD, which is less common, may occur in isolation or in combination with atrophic AMD. Important features of exudative AMD are CNV and detachment of the RPE (Figure 4.6.4).

Choroidal neovascularisation

Symptoms

Distortion or blurring of central vision in a patient with drusen may indicate the onset of leakage from CNV. Signs of CNV may be detected ophthalmoscopically as an elevation of the neurosen-

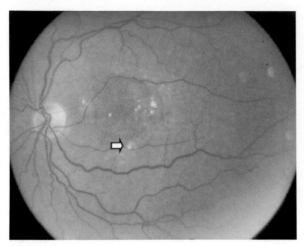

Figure 4.6.4 Exudative age-related maculopathy, showing exudation and retinal pigment epithelial detachment (the raised dome area).

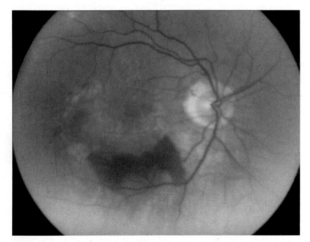

Figure 4.6.5 Colour fundus photograph of right subretinal blood due to choroidal neovascularisation.

sory retina, and may be associated with subretinal blood or exudation (Figure 4.6.5).

Angiography

Fluorescein and indocyanine green (ICG) angiography play a very important role in the detection and precise localisation of CNV. The following characteristics may be seen on fluorescein angiography.

Classic CNV is characterised by an area of bright, well-demarcated hyperfluorescence identified in the early phase of the angiogram with progressive dye leakage into the overlying sub-sensory retinal space in the late phase of the angiogram. These membranes are also classed according to anatomical location, and are described as extrafoveal, subfoveal or juxtafoveal.

Occult CNV is a poorly-defined membrane which has less precise features on early-phase angiography but which gives rise to late leakage. There are two types of occult CNV:

1. Fibrovascular pigment epithelial detachment comprises areas of irregular elevation of the RPE consisting of speckled hyperfluorescence that is not as bright or discrete as classic CNV 1–2 minutes after fluorescein injection, and with persistence of staining or leakage of dye 10 minutes after injection.

2. Late leakage of undetermined source comprises areas of leakage at the level of the RPE in the late phase of the angiogram, without classic CNV discernible in the early mid-phase of the angiogram to account for the leakage. By definition, these cannot be well demarcated.

ICG angiography may also be useful in the detection of occult or poorly defined CNV, and to distinguish a serous RPE detachment from a vascularised portion of a fibrovascular pigment epithelial detachment. Further, ICG angiography is essential if idiopathic polypoidal choroidal vasculopathy is suspected (Figures 4.6.6 and 4.6.7).

Subsequent course of CNV

The sequelae of CNV include:

- haemorrhagic RPE detachment
- haemorrhagic neurosensory retinal detachment
- vitreous haemorrhage
- disciform scar (Figure 4.6.8)
- massive exudation
- exudative retinal detachment.

RPE detachment

RPE detachment is thought to be caused by a reduction in the hydraulic conductivity of the thickened

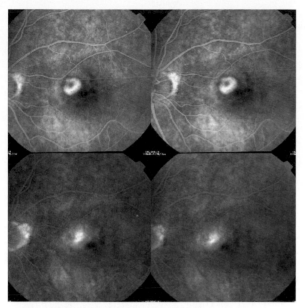

Figure 4.6.6 Classical choroidal neovascularisation on angiogram, showing a bright, well-demarcated hyperfluorescent lesion.

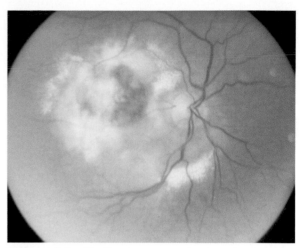

Figure 4.6.8 Disciform scar secondary to advanced age-related macular degeneration.

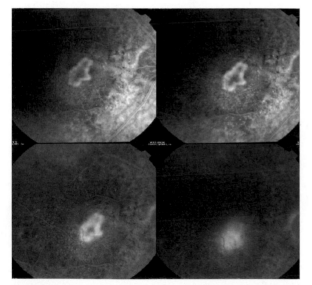

Figure 4.6.7 Classic choroidal neovascular membrane on fluorescein angiogram.

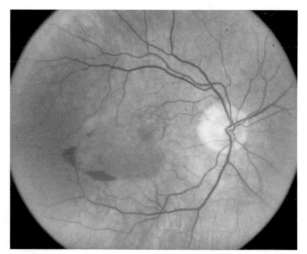

Figure 4.6.9 Retinal pigment epithelial detachment with subretinal blood.

Bruch's membrane, thus impeding the movement of fluid from the RPE towards the choroid. The diagnosis of an RPE detachment (Figure 4.6.9) can be made using slit-lamp biomicroscopy, and confirmed on fluorescein angiography.

Free fluorescein, which has leaked through the fenestrated choriocapillaris, pools in the sub-RPE space, giving rise to an area of hyperfluorescence. The early phase of the angiogram shows the extent of the detachment. The late phase shows that the margins of the detachment are well circumscribed, but there is no increase in the area of hyperfluorescence (Figure 4.6.10).

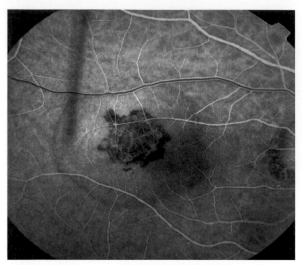

Figure 4.6.10   Early phase of fluorescein angiogram showing large retinal pigment epithelial detachment.

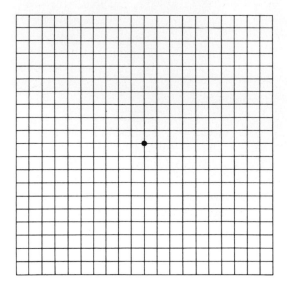

Figure 4.6.11   Amsler chart.

ICG angiography

A well-defined area of hypofluorescence is seen beneath the RPE detachment, and a ring of hyperfluorescence staining the margins becomes more prominent in the later phase.

The subsequent course of an RPE detachment includes:

- spontaneous resolution
- GA
- development of occult CNV
- tear in the RPE.

MANAGEMENT OF ARM

Education and Amsler chart

Patients with drusen or abnormalities in the RPE, in one or both eyes, should be educated on how to recognise symptoms of AMD, and be advised to contact their ophthalmologist promptly if such symptoms arise. An Amsler chart is given for this purpose (Figure 4.6.11).

Nutrition

Antioxidants

Macular pigment originates entirely from diet, and thus can be augmented following dietary modification and/or supplementation. Other noteworthy antioxidants include vitamins C and E, and the trace element zinc, which support the enzymatic systems in the retina and RPE, and are crucial to maintain the health of the macula.

Results from various observational studies linking antioxidants with AMD in humans have been inconsistent. Recently, the findings of the AREDS have indicated that disease progression can be altered with supplementation of antioxidants (vitamins C, E, β-carotene and zinc) (see Chapter 5.1).[48] Similarly, the Lutein Antioxidant Supplementation Trial (LAST) has demonstrated an improvement in visual function with lutein alone, or together with other antioxidants, in patients with atrophic AMD (see Chapter 5.3).[49] Furthermore, a prospective follow-up study in 77 562 females and 40 866 males has observed a protective role for fruit intake on the risk of neovascular AMD.[50]

Currently, there is no evidence from randomised trials that healthy people and/or people with early signs of ARM will benefit from antioxidant supplementation. Although antioxidant vitamins and mineral supplementation may delay the progression of moderate and severe AMD, vitamin E alone is unlikely to have a protective effect. Patients at high risk of developing ARM/AMD and patients with established ARM/AMD should be encouraged to eat a diet rich in fruit and vegetables. Further well-designed randomised controlled trials are required to investigate the influence of nutrition on the onset and progression of ARM/AMD.

Dietary fat

There is a growing body of evidence that suggests that high fat intake is associated with an increased risk of ARM and AMD. The mechanism underlying the association between dietary intake of saturated fat (and cholesterol) with ARM/AMD is unknown. One possibility is that a high dietary intake of fats increases the risk for systemic vascular disease, which in turn promotes the process of degenerative changes in the macula and elsewhere. Also, a high dietary intake of saturated fat may be associated with an augmentation of direct deposition of fat in the Bruch's membrane, with consequent impairment in the flow of metabolites in and out of the RPE, thus predisposing to ARM/AMD. Smith et al.[51] reported significantly increased risk for AMD associated with high-energy-adjusted intake of cholesterol, and borderline increased risk for ARM associated with a high intake of total and monounsaturated fat, in a cross-sectional study. Seddon et al.[52] observed a significant and positive association between progression of ARM and a high dietary intake of fat.

Although the putative beneficial effects of dietary fat restriction in terms of risk for ARM/AMD occurrence and progression has not been investigated, it would seem prudent to recommend appropriate dietary modification in patients with ARM, or in subjects at high risk for this condition.

Ω-3 fatty acids

The human retina contains a high proportion of Ω-3 long-chain polyunsaturated fatty acids (Ω-3 LCPUFA), in particular docosahexaenoic acid (DHA), which is a major structural lipid of retinal photoreceptor outer-segment membranes. Ω-3 LCPUFA, in particular DHA, which is synthesised from α-linoleic acid or obtained directly from fish oils, may prevent RPE lipofuscin accumulation, and hence RPE oxidative damage, thereby protecting against ARM/AMD.[53]

Three population-based studies have examined the relationship between dietary intake of fish and ARM/AMD. The third National Health and Nutrition Examination Survey (NHANES) reported a reduced risk of ARM/AMD with increasing frequency of fish consumption among people aged 60 years or older. Seddon et al.[52] reported a significantly reduced risk for AMD in subjects with a high dietary intake of Ω-3 LCPUFA and fish, where intake of linoleic acid was low. However; AMD was not found to be significantly associated with dietary intake of fish in the Beaver Dam Eye Study (BDES) or the Blue Mountains Eye Study (BMES).

However, the putative beneficial effects of supplementation with Ω-3 LCPUFAs, in terms of risk for ARM/AMD occurrence and progression have not been investigated.

Vitamin B₁₂ and folate

Homocysteine is an active amino acid, and high serum levels of homocysteine are toxic to the vascular endothelium, causing vascular occlusion and neovascularisation. Indeed, hyperhomocysteinemia has been positively associated with neovascular AMD.[54] Dietary factors have been shown to influence serum levels of homocysteine in adults. In particular, low serum levels of folate and vitamin B_{12} are associated with hyperhomocysteinaemia. In other words, there is a biologically plausible rationale for recommending supplemental vitamin B_{12} and folate in an attempt to reduce the risk of neovascular AMD.

MANAGEMENT OF AMD

Management of geographic AMD and RPE detachment includes dietary advice, as described above. Management of a CNVM is more complex, and a case-by-case therapeutic approach is required.

Argon laser

Laser treatment has been used for classic CNV, or classic CNV with an occult component with well-demarcated boundaries. Photocoagulation is of proven benefit for extrafoveal and juxtafoveal lesions where the central fovea will be spared from photocoagulation, although the aim of laser treatment is not to improve vision but to limit the size of the inevitable scotoma. However, despite the use of photocoagulation for juxtafoveal or extrafoveal lesions, the vision continues to deteriorate in some cases because of persistent or recurrent CNVM which may extend subfoveally.[55,56]

Photodynamic therapy

Photodynamic therapy (PDT) involves the systemic administration of a photosensitising drug followed by application of light of a particular wavelength (689 nm diode) to the affected tissue to incite a localised photochemical reaction. This causes damage to, and closure of, the CNVM. A variety of photosensitising drugs have been used in PDT, including verteporfin (Visudyne), tin ethyl etiopurpurin ($SnET_2$, or purlytin), and lutetium (Lu-Tex). These are all being actively evaluated in the management of subfoveal CNVM due to AMD. The Treatment of Age-Related Macular Degeneration with Photodynamic Therapy (TAP) study concluded that verteporfin therapy can safely reduce the risk of moderate and severe vision loss in patients with subfoveal, predominantly classic, CNV secondary to AMD. At 2-year follow-up, 41% of eyes with predominantly classic CNV lost at least 15 letters versus 69% in the control group.

The advantage of PDT rests on its selectivity for choroidal neovascular tissue, with minimal collateral damage to the overlying photoreceptors. Adverse effects of this treatment have been published, and these include extravasal injection of verteporfin with painful skin lesions (including necrosis), transient visual disturbances and back pain.[57]

Transpupillary thermotherapy

The use of transpupillary thermotherapy (TTT) for subfoveal CNVM has been associated with some success in the treatment of classic and occult CNVM, using diode laser at wavelength 810 nm with a large spot size to induce hyperthermia and apoptosis of the choroidal neovascular tissue. This wavelength is mainly absorbed by melanin at the level of the RPE and choroid, thus selectively treating choroidal lesions. Diode laser has a theoretical advantage over other wavelengths of light because there is little absorption in the xanthophyll layer and, therefore, damage to the nerve fibre layer is minimised. Additionally, compared with argon laser, diode laser is poorly absorbed by haemoglobin, thus enabling the operator to treat through preretinal and subretinal haemorrhage. Although TTT is relatively safe and does not require the same time and financial commitment as PDT, its role in the treatment of CNV is still unclear because a treatment benefit has yet to be definitively shown.[58]

Macular translocation surgery

Macular translocation surgery is a new technique for the treatment of subfoveal CNVM. Originally described by Machemer and Steinhorst in 1993,[59] macular translocation moves the neurosensory retina from the subfoveal abnormality to a new site of healthier RPE and choriocapillaris with the goal of maintaining or recovering visual function. The theoretical aim of this surgery is to preserve the foveal photoreceptor function. Initial case series of limited macular translocation and macular translocation with 360° peripheral retinectomy have demonstrated that the central vision can be preserved, and even improved in some patients, with subfoveal CNVM secondary to AMD.[60]

Antiangiogenic therapy

Therapy aimed at blocking one or more of the pathways in the angiogenic process responsible for the growth and development of CNV could, in theory, treat all forms of CNV. Various clinical trials evaluating these therapies are currently in progress. These include anti-VEGF approaches with antibody fragments capable of inhibiting the action of VEGF. Also, and based on the observation that the concentration of PEDF is reduced in patients with CNV, gene therapy using intravitreal injection of adenovirus containing a PEDF construct has been proposed.

SUMMARY

The identification of risk factors for AMD is particularly important, as treatment options for the condition are limited. The main factor in the development of the condition is age, but smoking and genetic predisposition are also linked with a higher prevalence of the condition. AMD is a complex condition and it is likely that several genes are involved. Although factors such as alcohol intake, sunlight exposure, BMI, dietary fat intake and hypertension have not been consistently linked with increased risk of developing the condition, it may be that, in those with genetic predisposition for AMD, the condition manifests itself according to exposure to these and other relevant risk factors. The evidence determined in favour of a relationship between cardiovascular disease, hypertension, BMI and dietary fat intake lends support for the vascular-insufficiency hypothesis for pathogenesis of AMD. Results from studies investigating these risk factors have not been conclusive. There is inconsistency between trials investigating the role of race and iris colour in AMD. Evidence for a reduced risk of the condition in blacks and those with dark irides supports the hypothesis that ocular melanin plays a role in the reduction of oxidative stress. However, the lack of evidence in support of sunlight exposure as a risk factor suggests that further investigation is required to clarify the role of these factors in the development of AMD. Smoking cessation is one important step in reducing the risk of developing AMD.

The maintenance of a well-balanced diet is advised in general, but research into lutein and zeaxanthin will hopefully provide a definitive answer as to their role in the promotion of retinal health. Future research may also provide the opportunity genetically to identify those at risk, so that they can control their exposure to risk factors. The main aim of genetic and biological studies is not to find a cure for the condition but to focus on its prevention or delay. Determination of the pathogenic mechanisms of the disease will allow the development of preventive measures as well as safer and more successful treatments.

References

1. The International ARM Epidemiology Study Group. An international classification and grading system for age-related maculopathy and age-related macular degeneration. Surv Ophthalmol 1995; 39:367–374.

2. Bressler NM, Bressler SB, West SK et al. The grading and prevalence of macular degeneration in Chesapeake Bay watermen. Arch Ophthalmol 1989; 107:847–852.

3. Klein R, Klein BE, Linton K. Prevalence of age-related maculopathy. The Beaver Dam Eye Study. Ophthalmology 1992; 99:933–943.

4. Vingerling JR, Dielemans I, Hofman A et al. The prevalence of age-related maculopathy in the Rotterdam Study. Ophthalmology 1995; 102:205–210.

5. Lewin Altschuler E. Is age-related macular degeneration a new disease? Ophthalm Res 2001; 33:121–122.

6. Klein R, Klein BE, Jenson SC, Meure SM. The five-year incidence and progression of age-related maculopathy. The Beaver Dam Eye Study. Ophthalmology 1997; 104:7–21.

7. Vingerling JR, Klaver CCW, Hofman A, de Jong PT. Epidemiology of age-related maculopathy. Epidemiol Rev 1995; 17:347–360.

8. Klein R, Klein BE, Jenson SC et al. Age-related maculopathy in a multiracial United States population. The National Health and Nutrition Examination Survey III. Ophthalmology 1999; 106:1056–1065.

9. Schachat AP, Hyman L, Leske C et al. Features of age-related macular degeneration in a black population. Barbados Eye Study Group. Arch Ophthalmol 1995; 113:728–735.
10. Gregor Z, Joff L. Senile macular changes in black Africans. Br J Ophthalmol 1978; 62:547–550.
11. Sommer A, Tielsch JM, Katz J et al. Racial difference in the cause-specific prevalence of blindness in East Baltimore. N Engl J Med 1991; 325:1412–1417.
12. Friedman DS, Katz J, Bressler NM et al. Racial difference in the prevalence of age-related macular degeneration. The Baltimore Eye Survey. Ophthalmology 1999; 106:1049–1055.
13. Klein R, Rowland ML, Harris MI. Racial/ethnic differences in age-related maculopathy. Third National Health and Nutrition Examination Survey. Ophthalmology 1995; 102:371–381.
14. Heiba IM, Elston RC, Klein BE, Klein R. Sibling correlation and segregation analysis of age-related maculopathy. The Beaver Dam Eye Study. Genet Epidemiol 1994; 11:51–67.
15. Gorin M, Breitner J, De Jong PTVM et al. The genetics of age-related macular degeneration. Mol Vision 1999; 5:29.
16. Klaver C, Wolf R, Assink J et al. Genetic risk of age-related maculopathy. Population based familial aggregation study. Arch Ophthalmol 1998; 116:1646–1651.
17. Meyers SM. The twin study on age-related macular degeneration. Trans Am Ophthalmol Soc 1994; XCII:776–843.
18. The Eye Disease Case-Control Study Group. Risk factors for neovascular age-related macular degeneration. Arch Ophthalmol 1992; 110:1701–1708.
19. Evans JR. Risk factors for age-related macular degeneration. Progr Retina Eye Res 2001; 20:227–253.
20. Delcourt C, Diaz J-L, Ponton-Sanchez A. The POLA Study. Smoking and age-related macular degeneration. Arch Ophthalmol 1998; 116:1031–1035.
21. Smith W, Mitchell P, Leedere S. Smoking and age-related maculopathy. The Blue Mountain Eye Study. Arch Ophthalmol 1996; 114:1518–1523.
22. Vingerling J, Hofman A, Grobbee D et al. Age-related macular degeneration and smoking. The Rotterdam Study. Arch Ophthalmol 1996; 114:1193–1196.
23. Klein R, Klein BE, Linton KL, DeMets DL. The relationship of age-related maculopathy to smoking. The Beaver Dam Eye Study. Am J Epidemiol 1993; 137:190–200.
24. Schaumberg D, Christen W, Hankinson S, Glynn R. Body mass index and the incidence of visually significant age-related maculopathy in men. Arch Ophthalmol 2001; 119:1259–1265.
25. Klein BE, Klein R, Lee K, Jensen S. Measures of obesity and age-related eye disease. Ophthalm Epidemiol 2001; 8:251–262.
26. Snow K, Cote J, Yang W et al. Association between reproductive and hormonal factors and age-related maculopathy in postmenopausal women. Am J Ophthalmol 2002; 134:842–848.
27. Hammond BR, Ciulla TA, Snodderly DM. Macular pigment density is reduced in obese subjects. Invest Ophthalmol Vis Sci 2002; 43:47–50.
28. Nolan J, O'Donovan O, Kavanagh K et al. Macular pigment and percentage of body fat. Invest Ophthalmol Vis Sci 2004; 45:3940–3950.
29. Viroonudomphol D, Pongpaew P, Tungtrogchitr R et al. The relationship between anthropometric measurement, serum vitamin A, and E concentration and lipid profile in overweight and obese subjects. Asia Pacific J Clin Nutr 2003; 12:73–79.
30. Clevidence BA, Bieri JG. Association of carotenoids with human plasma lipoproteins. Methods Enzymol 1993; 214:33–46.
31. Sperduto R, Hiller R. Systemic hypertension and age-related maculopathy in the Framingham Study. Arch Ophthalmol 1986; 104:216–219.
32. Klein BE, Klein R, Jenson SC, Ritter LL. Are sex hormones associated with age-related maculopathy in women? The Beaver Dam Eye Study. Trans Am Ophthalmol Soc 1994; 92:289–295.
33. Gibson JM, Shaw DE, Rosenthal AR. Senile cataract and senile macular degeneration: an investigation into possible risk factors. Trans Ophthalmol Soc UK 1986; 105:463–468.
34. Hiller R, Sperduto RD, Ederer F. Epidemiologic association with nuclear, cortical and posterior subcapsular cataract. Am J Epidemiol 1986; 124:916–925.
35. Taylor HR, West SK, Munoz B et al. The long-term effects of visible light on the eye. Arch Ophthalmol 1992; 110:99–104.
36. Delcourt C, Carriere I, Ponton-Sanchez A et al. Light exposure and the risk of cortical, nuclear, and posterior subcapsular cataracts. Arch Ophthalmol 2000; 118:385–392.
37. Chaine G, Hullo A, Sahel J et al. Case-control study of the risk factors for age-related macular degeneration. Br J Ophthalmol 1998; 82:996–1002.
38. Klein R, Klein BE, Jensen SC, Cruickshanks KJ. The relationship of ocular factors to the incidence and progression of age-related maculopathy. Arch Ophthalmol 1998; 116:506–513.
39. Zabrin MA. Current concepts in the pathogenesis of age-related macular degeneration. Arch Ophthalmol 2004; 122:598–611.
40. Hangai M, Murata T, Miyawaki N et al. Angiopoietin-1 upregulation by vascular endothelial growth factor in human retinal pigment epithelial cells. Invest Ophthalmol Vis Sci 2001; 42:1617.
41. Holz FG, Pauleikhoff D, Klein R, Bird A. Pathogenesis of lesions in late age-related macular disease. Am J Ophthalmol 2004; 137:504–510.
42. Witmer AN, Vresen GF, Van Noorden CJ, Schlinemann RO. Vascular endothelial growth factors and angiogenesis in eye disease. Progr Retina Eye Res 2003; 22:1–29.

43. Ramrattan RS, Van der Schaft TL, Mooy CM et al. Morphometric analysis of Bruch's membrane, the choriocapillaris and the choroid in aging. Invest Ophthalmol Vis Sci 1994; 35:2857–2864.

44. Kennedy CJ, Rakoczy PE, Constable IJ. Lipofuscin of the retinal pigment epithelium: a review. Eye 1995; 9:763–771.

45. Moor DJ, Hussain AA, Marshall J. Age-related variation in the hydraulic conductivity of Bruch's membrane. Invest Ophthalmol Vis Sci 1995; 36:1290–1297.

46. Beatty S, Koh H-H, Henson D, Boulton M. The role of oxidative stress in the pathogenesis of age-related macular degeneration. Surv Ophthalmol 2000; 45:115–134.

47. Tomany S, Cruickshanks K, Klein R et al. Sunlight and the 10-year incidence of age-related maculopathy. Beaver Dam Eye Study. Arch Ophthalmol 2004; 122:750–757.

48. Age-Related Eye Disease Study Research Group. A randomised, placebo-controlled clinical trial of high dose supplementation with vitamin C and E, beta-carotene, and zinc for age-related macular degeneration and vision loss. AREDS report no 8. Arch Ophthalmol 2001; 119:1417–1436.

49. Richer S, Stiles W, Statkute L et al. Double masked, placebo-controlled, randomised trial of lutein and antioxidant supplementation in the intervention of atrophic age-related macular degeneration: the Veterans LAST study (Lutein Antioxidant Supplementation Trial). Optometry 2004; 75:216–230.

50. Cho E, Seddon JM, Rosner B et al. Prospective study of intake of fruits, vegetables, vitamins, and carotenoids and risk of age-related maculopathy. Arch Ophthalmol 2004; 122:883–892.

51. Smith W, Mitchell P, Leeder S. Dietary fat and fish intake and age-related maculopathy. Arch Ophthalmol 2000; 118:401–404.

52. Seddon JM, Rosner B, Sperduto R et al. Dietary fat and risk for advanced age-related macular degeneration. Arch Ophthalmol 2001; 119:1191–1199.

53. Elner VM. Retinal pigment epithelial acid lipase activity and lipoprotein receptors: effect of dietary omega-3 fatty acids. Trans Am Ophthalmol Soc 2002; 100:301–338.

54. Macular Photocoagulation Study Group. Argon laser photocoagulation for neovascular maculopathy. Three-year results from randomized clinical trials. Arch Ophthalmol 1986; 104:503–512.

55. Axer-Siegel R, Bourla D, Ehrlich R et al. Association of neovascular age-related macular degeneration and hyperhomocysteinemia. Am J Ophthalmol 2004; 137:84–89.

56. Macular Photocoagulation Study Group. Laser photocoagulation for juxtafoveal choroidal neovascularization. Five-year results from randomized clinical trials. Arch Ophthalmol 1994; 112:500–509.

57. Bressler NM, for Treatment of Age-related macular degeneration with Photodynamic therapy (TAP) study group. Photodynamic therapy of subfoveal choroidal neovascularization in age-related macular degeneration with verteporfin: two-year results of 2 randomized clinical trials. Arch Ophthalmol 2001; 119:198–207.

58. Thach AB, Sipperley JO, Dugel PU et al. Large-spot size transpupillary thermotherapy for treatment of occult choroidal neovascularization associated with age-related macular degeneration. Arch Ophthalmol 2003; 121:817–820.

59. Machemer R, Steinhorst UH. Retinal separation, retinotomy, and macular relocation I. Experimental studies in the rabbit eye. Graefes Arch Clin Exp Ophthalmol 1993; 231:591–594.

60. Submacular Surgery Study Group. Submacular surgery trials randomized pilot trial of laser photocoagulation versus surgery for recurrent choroidal neovascularisation secondary to age-related macular degeneration: I Ophthalmic outcomes submacular surgery trials pilot study report number 1. Am J Ophthalmol 2000; 130:387–407.

SECTION 5

Recent advances in research into nutrition-related eye health

Chapter **5.1**

Age-Related Eye Disease Study (AREDS)

Ruth Hogg and Usha Chakravarthy

INTRODUCTION

The Age-Related Eye Disease Study (AREDS) was initially conceived as a long-term, multicentre, prospective study designed to assess the clinical course of, and risk factors for, age-related macular degeneration (AMD) and age-related cataract.[1] In addition, it was decided to incorporate a clinical trial of vitamin and mineral supplements for progression of AMD and cataract, using high doses of these antioxidants because of the widespread use of pharmacological doses by the public in the USA (in the absence of definitive studies on the safety and efficacy of such supplements).

RISK FACTORS FOR AMD, NUCLEAR AND CORTICAL CATARACT[2,3]

The primary aim of these studies was to explore the relationship between baseline macular and lens status and prior or concurrent potential non-nutritional risk factors. Since AMD and cataract are of huge public health significance, it was hoped that identification of risk factors for either may lead to the identification of modifiable risk factors for these conditions, or possible strategies for interventions.

In AREDS, data were collected on potential risk factors as putatively determined by earlier laboratory and clinical studies. For AMD, these included smoking, cardiovascular disease, hypertension, sunlight exposure and dietary intake of various micronutrients. For cataract, attention was directed towards educational status, smoking, diabetes, sunlight exposure, body mass index, drug use, oestrogen replacement therapy and dietary intake of various micronutrients.

STUDY POPULATION

Eleven retinal speciality clinics enrolled 4757 participants from 1992 to 1998, and subjects were aged between 55 and 80 years.

Inclusion and exclusion criteria

- Best corrected visual acuity of 20/32 or better in at least one eye.
- Media sufficiently clear to obtain stereoscopic fundus pictures of the macula, of adequate quality, in the study eye.
- At least one eye free of ocular pathology that could complicate assessment of AMD or lens opacity progression (e.g. optic atrophy, acute uveitis).
- The study eye could not have undergone previous ocular surgery (except cataract surgery or unilateral photocoagulation for AMD).
- Participants were excluded for illnesses or disorders that would make long-term follow-up, or compliance with the study protocol, unlikely or difficult.

Recruitment strategies

Sources of subjects included: persons identified through the medical records of patients seen at AREDS clinics; referring physicians; patient lists from hospitals and health maintenance organisations; screening at malls, fairs, senior citizen centres and other gathering places; public advertisements; friends and family of participants; and clinic centre staff.

Case-control definitions for AMD

See Table 5.1.1.

Case-control definitions for cataract

See Table 5.1.2.

Table 5.1.1 Grading of age-related macular degeneration for Age-Related Eye Disease Study, based on the better eye

Group 1	Absence of drusen or non-extensive small drusen in both eyes
Group 2	Extensive small drusen, non-extensive intermediate drusen or pigment abnormalities in at least one eye
Group 3	Large drusen, extensive intermediate drusen in either eye
Group 4	At least one eye with geographic atrophy
Group 5	Evidence suggesting choroidal neovascularisation or retinal pigment epithelial detachment in one eye

Table 5.1.2 Grading of cataract for Age-Related Eye Disease Study

Type of cataract	Grading	
Posterior subcapsular cataract (PSC)	Ignored in the analysis as they were so uncommon in the study cohort (2.5%)	
Nuclear lens opacity (ignoring cortical opacity)	Group 1	Moderate nuclear: ≥4 in at least one eye
	Group 2	Mild nuclear: grade <4 in each eye, and >2 in at least one eye
	Group 3	Controls: nuclear grade ≤2 in each eye
Cortical lens opacity	Group 1	Moderate cortical: >5% in at least one eye
	Group 2	Mild cortical: cortical ≤5% in each eye, and >0% in at least one eye
	Group 3	Controls: cortical = 0% in each eye

Risk factor definitions

Each case group was compared with a control group. The baseline variables were classed into one of the following four categories: (1) demographic; (2) medical history; (3) use of oral medication; and (4) ocular factors.

Demographic data

Demographic data included age; race; gender; education; smoking status (current, past or never); body mass index; weight change since age 20; sunlight exposure.

Medical history

The medical history covered hypertension; angina; diabetes; skin cancer; and arthritis.

Use of oral medication

Oral medications included diuretics; aspirin; antacids; hydrochlorothiazide; non-steroidal anti-inflammatory drugs; thyroid hormones; β-blockers; oestrogen and progesterone (women only).

Ocular factors

Ocular factors included iris colour and refractive error.

RESULTS

AMD

Risk factors for AMD identified in AREDS are given in Table 5.1.3.

Table 5.1.3   Risk factors for age-related macular degeneration (AMD) identified in the Age-Related Eye Disease Study

Group	Grading of AMD	Risk factors significantly associated with AMD
Group 1	Absence of drusen, or non-extensive small drusen, in both eyes	
Group 2	Extensive small drusen, non-extensive intermediate drusen or pigment abnormalities in at least one eye	More likely to be female More likely to have a history of arthritis Less likely to have angina
Group 3	Large drusen, extensive intermediate drusen, in either eye	More likely to use hydrochlorothiazide diuretics More likely to have arthritis More likely to have completed fewer years at school More likely to be a smoker Associated with hypertension, hyperopia, presence of lens opacities and white race
Group 4	At least one eye with geographic atrophy	More likely to use thyroid hormones and antacids More likely to have completed fewer years at school or to be smokers
Group 5	Evidence suggesting choroidal neovascularisation or retinal pigment epithelial detachment in one eye	Associated with increased body mass index More likely to have completed fewer years at school More likely to be smokers Associated with hypertension, hyperopia, presence of lens opacities and white race

Cataract groups

Participants with moderate nuclear opacities were more likely to be female, non-white, smokers and to have large drusen. These lens opacities were less common in persons with higher educational status, a history of diabetes and among those taking non-steroidal anti-inflammatories.

Moderate cortical opacities were associated with dark iris colour, large drusen, weight change and (at borderline significance) higher levels of sunlight exposure and use of thyroid hormones. These cataracts were less common in those of higher educational status.

AREDS REPORT NO. 8[4]

Introduction

This randomised clinical trial was designed to evaluate the effect of high levels of zinc and selected antioxidant vitamins (5–15 times the recommended daily allowance) on the development of advanced AMD in a cohort of older persons. There were four treatment interventions:

1. antioxidants (500 mg vitamin C, 400 IU vitamin E and 15 mg β-carotene)
2. zinc (80 mg zinc as zinc oxide and 2 mg copper as cupric oxide)
3. antioxidants + zinc
4. placebo.

Two tablets were taken, morning and evening, with food.

Randomisation

A total of 3640 patients aged between 55 and 80 years were enrolled. Participants were categorised at baseline according to morphological features noted in fundus photographs into one of four severity groups accordingly, as follows:

1. Category 1 subjects had a total drusen area of fewer than five small drusen (<63 μm), and visual acuity of 20/32 or better in both eyes.
2. Category 2 subjects exhibited multiple small drusen, single or non-extensive intermediate drusen (64–124 μm), pigment abnormalities or any combination of these in one or both eyes,

and a visual acuity of 20/32 or better in both eyes.
3. Category 3 subjects demonstrated the absence of advanced AMD in both eyes, and at least one eye had a visual acuity 20/32 or better with at least one large druse (125 μm), extensive intermediate drusen (measured by drusen area), or geographic atrophy that did not involve the centre of the macula, or any combination of these.
4. Category 4 participants had visual acuity of 20/32 or better, and no advanced AMD, in the study eye, with the fellow eye exhibiting either lesions of advanced AMD or visual acuity less than 20/32 (and with AMD abnormalities sufficient to explain the reduced visual acuity). Advanced AMD was defined as the presence of geographic atrophy within the centre of the macula, or features of choroidal neovascularisation.

Categories 2, 3 and 4 participants were assigned with a probability of one-quarter to each treatment group, whereas category 1 participants were assigned with a probability of one-half to either antioxidants or placebo.

Outcomes

Primary

1. Progression to advanced AMD (this was defined as follows: photocoagulation or other treatment for choroidal neovascularisation (clinic centre reports) or photographic documentation of any of the following: geographic atrophy involving the centre of the macula; non-drusenoid retinal pigment epithelial detachment; serous or haemorrhagic retinal detachment; haemorrhage under the retina or retinal pigment epithelium; and/or subretinal fibrosis (reading centre reports).
2. At least 15-letter decrease in visual acuity score.

Secondary

Secondary outcome included worsening of category 2 in AMD classification to either category 3 or 4 during follow-up. Secondary visual acuity outcomes included a decrease of 30 letters or more in the study eye, and progression to visual acuity worse than 1/100 in one or both eyes.

Results

Natural history

AREDS categories 1 and 2 were least likely to progress, whereas categories 3 and 4 were at greatest risk of progression.

Randomised controlled trial of supplemental antioxidants

The results demonstrated a statistically significant odds reduction for the development of advanced AMD for subjects in categories 3 and 4 when supplemental antioxidants plus zinc (odds ratio, 0.72; 99% confidence interval, 0.54–0.99) were used. The odds ratios for zinc alone and antioxidants alone were 0.75 and 0.80, respectively.

The results of AREDS, therefore, represent an evidence base upon which recommendations have been made that subjects with a diagnosis of AMD, and high-risk features of disease progression, should consider taking a supplement.

AREDS REPORT NO. 9[5]

Introduction

This was a double-masked clinical trial where participants were either assigned to receive antioxidants (vitamin C 500 mg, vitamin E 400 IU, β-carotene 15 mg) or no antioxidants. Participants with more than a few drusen were also randomly assigned to receive tablets with or without zinc and copper. Baseline and annual lens photographs were taken. No statistically significant effect was seen for any of the main outcome measures, which were development or progression of age-related lens opacities, or moderate visual acuity loss. No statistically significant serious adverse effect was associated with treatment.

AREDS REPORT NO. 10[6]

Assessment of health-related quality of life (HRQL) is important to obtain a more complete understanding of the effect of treatments, ageing and the natural history of disease on individuals' daily routines. The National Eye Institute Visual Function Questionnaire (NEI-VFQ) was designed to measure areas of functioning and well-being that have been identified as important by persons with eye disease. The questionnaire was designed to evaluate the level of disability on HRQL across several common eye conditions (age-related cataracts, AMD, diabetic retinopathy, primary open-angle glaucoma and cytomegalovirus retinitis). Field testing has shown that the NEI-VFQ is valid and reliable, and that the type or severity of the underlying eye disease does not affect the underlying psychometric properties of the NEI-VFQ.

Within AREDS, study patients were stratified according to AMD category, lens opacity category and visual acuity following protocol refraction, all of which were determined at the time of the NEI-VFQ administration. NEI-VFQ-25 plus appendix (containing 39 items and 12 subscales) was administered to 86.6% of the entire cohort at the 5-year annual clinic visit.

The results demonstrated that all multi-item subscales showed a moderately strong internal consistency and reliability. Vision-targeted HRQL scores assessed with NEI-VFQ-25 (plus appendix) were lower for participants with progressive manifestations of AMD, nuclear opacity, cataract surgery in one eye or progressive degrees of visual impairment. These results demonstrate that the NEI-VFQ questionnaire is sensitive to the effect of age-related nuclear cataract and macular degeneration, and support the construct validity of the questionnaire.

AREDS REPORT NO. 11[7]

AREDS has created considerable controversy, with some practitioners feeling that there is insufficient evidence to ask patients to take expensive high-dose micronutrient supplements indefinitely. Therefore, it is important to look at the big picture and assess the public health impact of the AREDS results.

The potential impact of the recommendations can be assessed by estimating the number of people at least 55 years old for whom supplementation treatment has been recommended, and applying progression rates to advanced AMD for this population, thereby estimating the numbers of persons in whom the progression to visually disabling AMD will have been prevented.

An estimated 8 million individuals have monocular or binocular intermediate AMD, or monocular advanced AMD. Of these, 1.3 million would develop advanced AMD if no treatment was given to reduce their risk. But, if all of these people at risk were to receive supplementation, more than 300 000 (95% confidence interval, 158 000–487 000) would avoid advanced AMD, and any associated vision loss, during the next 5 years.

SUMMARY

On the whole, AREDS has made a significant contribution to a growing body of evidence which suggests that enhancement of antioxidant defences protects against progression of AMD. Further study of a similar nature is required to confirm these findings, and to explore the possibility that the inclusion of lutein and zeaxanthin to antioxidant formulations may augment the beneficial effect.

References

1. The Age-Related Eye Disease Study (AREDS). Design implications AREDS report no. 1. Controlled Clin Trials 1999; 20:573–600.
2. Age-Related Eye Disease Study Group. Risk factors associated with age-related macular degeneration 1: a case-control study in the Age-Related Eye Disease Study: Age-Related Eye Disease Study report number 3. Ophthalmology 2000; 107:2224–2232.
3. Age-Related Eye Disease Study Group. Risk factors associated with age-related nuclear and cortical cataract: a case-control study in the Age-Related Eye Disease Study. AREDS report no. 5. Ophthalmology 2001; 108:1400–1408.
4. Age-Related Eye Disease Study Research Group. A randomized, placebo-controlled, clinical trial of high-dose supplementation with vitamins C and E, beta carotene, and zinc for age-related macular degeneration and vision loss: AREDS report no. 8. Arch Ophthalmol 2001; 119:1417–1436.
5. Age-Related Eye Disease Study Research Group. A randomized, placebo-controlled, clinical trial of high-dose supplementation with vitamins C and E and beta carotene for age-related cataract and vision loss: AREDS report no. 9. Arch Ophthalmol 2001; 119:1439–1452.
6. Clemons TE, Chew EY, Bressler SB et al. National Eye Institute visual function questionnaire in the Age-Related Eye Disease Study (AREDS): AREDS report no. 10. Arch Ophthalmol 2003; 121:211–217.
7. Bressler NM, Bressler SB, Congdon NG et al. Potential public health impact of Age-Related Eye Disease Study results: AREDS report no. 11. Arch Ophthalmol 2003; 121:1621–1624.

Chapter **5.2**

Carotenoids in Age–Related Eye Disease Study (CAREDS)

Ruth Hogg and Usha Chakravarthy

INTRODUCTION

Carotenoids in Age-Related Eye Disease Study (CAREDS) is a multicentre observational study, which forms a component of the National Institutes of Health-sponsored Women's Health Initiative (WHI). Its primary purpose is to investigate potential and specific dietary protective factors for age-related macular degeneration (AMD) and nuclear cataract.[1]

The WHI is a major 15-year research programme designed to address the most common causes of death, disability and poor quality of life in postmenopausal women, namely cardiovascular disease, cancer and osteoporosis. It comprises three components:

1. a randomised control trial of promising, but unproven, approaches to prevention
2. an observational study to identify predictors of disease
3. a study of community approaches to developing healthful behaviours.

Women who were ineligible or unwilling to participate in the clinical trial were offered the opportunity to enrol in a concurrent long-term observational study. Over 93 000 subjects, aged between 50 and 79 years, have enrolled for this observational study, and have been monitored over an average period of 9 years. The CAREDS is being carried out in a cohort of women who are enrolled in the WHI Observational Study (WHI-OS) at three sites – (1) Madison, Wisconsin; (2) Portland, Oregon; and (3) Iowa City.

CAREDS has a number of aims, which are outlined below:[1]

1. To determine whether women in the WHI-OS with sustained dietary levels of lutein (L) which are in the lowest versus highest quintile have:
   - a lower density of macular pigment
   - a higher prevalence of early ARM and, in particular, specific macular lesions that increase the risk of developing late ARM (large soft indistinct drusen and pigmentary abnormalities)
   - more severe nuclear sclerosis of the lens.
2. To identify dietary, lifestyle, health history and physiological determinants of macular pigment density in women.

THE REFERENCE SAMPLE[1]

The WHI is a large, multicentre investigation of strategies for the prevention and control of the most common causes of morbidity among postmenopausal women. Over 160 000 women have been enrolled at 40 clinical centres across the USA since its initiation in 1993. Women were enrolled into two main study components: (1) the clinical trials (low-fat diets or hormone replacement therapy (HRT)); or (2) the observational study (which comprised those women unwilling or unable to enrol in the clinical trials). Subjects in the WHI-OS underwent physical examinations at baseline and at 3 years, and completed a study questionnaire yearly.

ELIGIBILITY CRITERIA FOR ENROLMENT IN OBSERVATIONAL STUDY OF WHI[1]

Women ranged in age from 50 to 79 years at entry into the study (1994–1998). They had the ability and willingness to provide written informed consent and an expectation of being resident in the study recruitment area for at least 3 years following enrolment. Subjects were excluded if they had medical conditions predictive of a survival time of less than 3 years, if they were known to have conditions or characteristics inconsistent with study participation and adherence (alcoholism, drug dependency, mental illness, dementia) or if they were active participants in another randomised controlled clinical trial. The eligibility criteria were purposely broad in order to enhance the generalist ability of the study's conclusions.

RESULTS

In total, 2005 women participated in CAREDS (1894 underwent all study evaluations, while 111 failed to undergo every study assessment), and study visits were completed in January 2004 (personal communication, JA Mares). Peer-reviewed publications are pending, and preliminary information is available from oral presentations and abstracts submitted to key international meetings and personal communication with the principal investigators. Data concerning macular pigment optical density (MPOD) and dietary intake of L and zeaxanthin (Z) on a sample of 1512 CAREDS subjects at baseline (1994–1997) form the basis of the following discussion, and no results are currently available concerning nuclear cataract.

MACULAR PIGMENT DENSITY MEASUREMENTS[2,3]

On a one-way analysis of variance, the strongest predictors of MPOD were dietary L, body mass index (BMI), waist-to-hip ratio (WHR: an indicator of abdominal adiposity) and diabetes. An analysis of variance, which accounted for the key variables, demonstrated a clear dose–response relationship between MPOD and dietary intake of L (Table 5.2.1).

Other putative determinants of MPOD identified in smaller studies (e.g. smoking, iris colour) were unrelated to MPOD in CAREDS. A small but significant difference was found between study sites with lower MPOD at Madison (0.30) than the other two sites (0.35–0.36, $P < 0.01$), and this difference persisted following adjustment for dietary L and Z, body mass index and diabetes.[3]

DIETARY PATTERNS AND ARM IN CAREDS[4]

Cluster analysis was employed to identify women who had reported high or low intakes of L and Z at baseline, but dietary patterns were not found to

Table 5.2.1 Relationship between dietary intake of lutein and macular pigment optical density

Dietary intake of lutein	Macular pigment optical density
Quintile 1 (median intake 677 μg/day)	0.31
Quintile 2	0.34
Quintile 3	0.39
Quintile 4	0.39
Quintile 5 (median intake 4796 μg/day)	0.40

be related to specific lesions of early ARM or late AMD, thus suggesting that self-selected dietary patterns of older women in the recent past do not appear to be strongly associated with prevalence of ARM. However, further work is needed to investigate whether dietary intakes over longer periods in an individual's past are related to ARM.

In CAREDS, although total dietary intake of fat was not associated with early ARM, the type of dietary fat was related to risk for this condition with diets high in polyunsaturated fatty acids associated with increased risk of drusen, pigmentary abnormalities and retinal pigment abnormalities, whereas monounsaturated fats were protective against these lesions. Dietary intake of long-chain omega-3 fatty acid was not associated with early ARM in CAREDS.

BODY FAT LEVEL AND DISTRIBUTION AND ARM IN CAREDS[5,6]

BMI (kg/m²) and WHR at CAREDS baseline were used to determine body fat level and distribution, respectively. High BMI was positively related to pigmentary abnormalities at the macula, whereas high WHR was associated with retinal pigment epithelial abnormalities, suggesting that adiposity represents a risk for ARM.

SUPPLEMENT USE AND ARM IN CAREDS[7]

Eighty-eight per cent of women in CAREDS used vitamin and mineral supplements. Three types of supplement were identified, as follows: multivitamins; high-dose antioxidants (at least two of the following: >10 000 IU/day of β-carotene; >120 mg/day vitamin C; or >60 IU/day of vitamin E); and high-dose zinc (>15 mg/day). Interestingly, use of high-dose antioxidant supplements for a prolonged duration (>10 years) was associated with lower risk for early stages of ARM, whereas use of multivitamins or high-dose zinc supplements was unrelated to ARM.

Forty-eight per cent of subjects had consumed supplements containing L, although the median intake of supplemental L was only 250 μg. Preliminary analysis has revealed that supplement use is more common with higher dietary intake of L and Z, and may therefore confound relationships. Consequently, the investigators have emphasised that they will evaluate the relationships between supplement use over time and the ophthalmic end-points, and adjust for dietary intake.

MENOPAUSAL HORMONE THERAPY AND ARM[8]

The profile of the CAREDS sample provided an excellent opportunity to investigate previous reports indicating a reduced risk of ARM among women who used HRT. Past use of HRT was found, in CAREDS, to be associated with reduced risk of soft drusen, although the protective effect was not related to the duration of HRT use.

Current HRT use was marginally associated with increased risk of late ARM, suggesting that such therapy use may have a different impact on ARM pathogenesis or progression depending on the stage of the disease at the time of exposure to HRT.

CONCLUSION

CAREDS has the potential to investigate a number of other important relationships, including those between serum concentrations of L and Z and

MPOD. Also, factors contributing to a relative lack of MPOD and/or serum levels of the xanthophylls (in spite of adequate dietary intake of the macular carotenoids), if any, will be identified. Further, the relationship between MPOD and ARM will be investigated.

CAREDS is the largest cohort study of the relationships between dietary carotenoids and the two major age-related eye diseases, ARM and cataract. It will help to determine whether intake of these carotenoids is essential to eye health in middle and older age, and, if so, will suggest a level of intake that is associated with a reduction in risk for such ocular morbidity, and will help to identify factors that may modify these relationships.

References

1. Carotenoids and Age-related Eye Disease Study Research Group. CAREDS manual. Madison, WI: University of Wisconsin, Madison.
2. Snodderly M, Mares JA, Wooten BR et al. Macular pigment density of women in the Carotenoids in Age-Related Eye Disease Study (CAREDS). ARVO Abstract 2004; B605.
3. Mares-Perlman JA, Snodderly D, Gruber M et al. Determinants of macular pigment density in the Carotenoids in Age-Related Eye Disease Study (CAREDS), an ancillary study of the Women's Health Initiative. ARVO Abstract 2004; B601.
4. Moeller SM, Tinker LF, Blodi B et al. Relationship between dietary patterns and age-related maculopathy in the Carotenoids in Age-Related Eye Disease Study (CAREDS), an ancillary study of the Women's Health Initiative. ARVO Abstract 2004; B729.
5. LaRowe TL, Mares JA, Wallace RB et al. Relationships of body fat level and distribution to age-related maculopathy in the Carotenoids in Age-Related Eye Disease Study (CAREDS), an ancillary study of the Women's Health Initiative. ARVO Abstract 2004; 2244.
6. Mehta NR, Blodi B, Ritenbaugh C et al. Relationship between dietary fat and age-related maculopathy in the Carotenoids in Age-Related Eye Disease Study (CAREDS), an ancillary study of the Women's Health Initiative. ARVO Abstract 2004; B759.
7. Gruber MJ, LaRowe T, Moeller SM et al. Relationship of supplement use to age-related maculopathy in the Carotenoids in Age-Related Eye Disease Study (CAREDS), an ancillary study to the Women's Health Initiative (WHI). ARVO Abstract 2004; B766.
8. Wallace RB. Association of menopausal hormone therapy to age-related maculopathy in the Carotenoids in Age-Related Eye Disease Study (CAREDS), an ancillary study of the Women's Health Initiative. ARVO Abstract 2004; B764.

Chapter **5.3**

Lutein Antioxidant Supplementation Trial (LAST)

Frank Eperjesi

INTRODUCTION

The objective of the Lutein Antioxidant Supplementation Trial (LAST) was to determine whether nutritional supplementation with lutein (L) or L together with antioxidants, vitamins, and minerals improved visual function and symptoms in atrophic AMD.

LAST PROTOCOL

The study was a well-organised prospective, 12-month, randomised, double-masked, placebo-controlled trial. This type of protocol is often described as the 'gold standard ' in experimental design for clinical trials. Ninety patients with atrophic AMD were referred by ophthalmologists at two Chicago-area veterans medical facilities and were then randomised into three groups.

Subjects in Group 1 received 10 mg non-esterified L per day; in Group 2, a non-esterified L 10 mg/antioxidants/vitamins and minerals broad-spectrum supplementation formula (L/A) per day (see reference 1 for details of the antioxidants); and in Group 3, a maltodextrin placebo (P) per day, all over 12 months. The outcome measures were MPOD measured using heterochromic flicker, distance Snellen equivalent visual acuity (converted to logMAR), near visual acuity using low- and high-contrast Smith-Kettlewell Institute low-luminance (SKILL) test targets, contrast sensitivity using single large-letter charts of varying contrasts, Amsler grid result and glare recovery symptoms determined via a questionnaire. These were measured at baseline, 4 months, 8 months and 12 months. The seven-increment Lens Opacity Cataract Scale was used to evaluate subjectively lens opacification at baseline and the final examination. Compliance was assessed by telephone. Fourteen subjects failed to complete the study, but 96% of subjects took nearly 92% of their assigned capsules.

At the end of the trial when the groups were unmasked, in groups 1 (L) and 2 (L/A), MPOD increased by approximately 0.09 log units from baseline, Snellen equivalent visual acuity improved by 5.4 letters for group 1 (L) and 3.5 letters for group 2 (L/A); contrast sensitivity also improved for groups 1 and 2. There was a net subjective improvement in Amsler grid for group 1 (L) only and there was a subjective improvement in glare recovery after 4 months of supplementation for group 2 (L/A); this finding is very likely to relate to the increase in MPOD. Subjects in group 3, who received the placebo, had no significant changes in any of the measured findings. Interestingly, there was no progression in AMD retinopathy or lens opacification for any subject, irrespective of their group, and there were no significant between-group differences in minor side-effects among groups 1 (L) and 2 (L/A) and 3 (P). None of the subjects in group 2 (L/A) experienced a minor cardiovascular event or died during the trial, whereas 4 subjects in group 1 (L) and 3 subjects in group 3 (P) underwent cardiovascular surgery or died.

CONCLUSIONS

The investigators concluded that visual function improved with L alone or L together with other nutrients. However, they also noted that the results should be considered as preliminary given the small number of subjects, the short time period of observation and the lack of statistical significance among the three groups. Nevertheless, this is an important study, which showed that atrophic AMD is a nutrition-responsive disorder and that improvements in visual function can be obtained over a short period of time. The research team went on to suggest that further studies were needed with more patients, of both genders, and for longer periods of time to assess long-term effects of L or L together with a broad spectrum of antioxidants, vitamins and minerals in the treatment of atrophic AMD.

Reference

1. Richer S, Stiles W, Statkute L et al. Double-masked, placebo-controlled, randomized trial of lutein and antioxidant supplementation in the intervention of atrophic age-related macular degeneration: the Veterans LAST study (Lutein Antioxidant Supplementation Trial). Optometry 2004; 75:216–230.

Chapter **5.4**

The Aston Randomised Controlled Trial (Aston RCT)

Hannah Bartlett and Frank Eperjesi

Age-related macular disease is the leading cause of blind registration in the developed world. One aetiological hypothesis involves oxidation, and the intrinsic vulnerability of the retina to damage via this process. This has prompted interest in the role of antioxidants, particularly the carotenoids lutein and zeaxanthin, in the prevention and treatment of this eye disease.

Randomised controlled trials (RCTs) are considered to be the 'gold standard' in clinical research.[1,2] They involve random assignment of participants into treatment and placebo groups. They have the ability to reduce, by masking, the influence of confounding variables by random assignment of the treatment (intervention), and the ability to reduce bias or the possibility that any observed effect is due to other factors. The term 'double-masked' or 'double-blinded' refers to the fact that neither participants nor investigators know who is in the treatment or placebo group. In RCTs designed to investigate the effect of nutritional supplements, this is usually achieved by coding the tablet containers. At the end of the trial period the code is broken and the gathered data analysed.

In summary, any RCT will involve the following steps:[3]

1. sample selection from the population
2. baseline variables measured
3. participants randomised
4. interventions applied (one will be a placebo)
5. follow-up of the cohort
6. outcome variables measured
7. results analysed.

PURPOSE

The purpose of the Aston RCT is to determine the effect of 18 months of daily lutein and antioxidant supplementation on measures of visual function in subjects with and without age-related macular disease. At the time of writing the study is ongoing.

INCLUSION/EXCLUSION CRITERIA

For inclusion participants have to present with no ocular pathology in one eye, or no ocular pathology other than dry age-related macular degeneration in one eye. A cataract-grading system consisting of grades 1, 2 and 3 for each of cortical, nuclear and posterior subcapsular cataracts has been developed. Participants presenting with lens opacities precluding fundus photography are excluded. Throughout the trial period, progression of any type of cataract to the successive grade will require the participant to withdraw. Participants also have to provide written informed consent, and have to be available for three visits to Aston University, Birmingham.

Exclusion criteria include type 1 and 2 diabetes because vitamin E has been shown to affect glucose tolerance[4–8] and diabetic retinopathy may confound the results. Those taking warfarin medication are excluded as zinc may decrease the absorption and activity of warfarin,[9] as are those who use nutritional supplements that potentially raise vitamin and mineral intake above safe limits. The most recent guidelines for upper limits of nutritional supplementation are set out in the UK Food Standards Agency report.[10] Neovascular age-related macular degeneration and other ocular disease that could potentially interfere with the results are excluded.

RANDOMISATION

The random number-generator function in Microsoft Excel is being used to allocate participants to μ and λ groups. Even numbers are allocated to the λ group.

MASKING

The study formulation and placebo tablets have been produced by Quest Vitamins, Aston Science Park, Birmingham B7 4AP, and are identical in external and internal appearance, and taste. The tablets are packaged in identical, sealed, white containers; the only difference is the symbol on the label. The manufacturer has allocated distinguishing symbols, μ and λ. Investigators and participants do not know which symbol represents the placebo tablets, and which represents the active formulation.

STUDY FORMULATION

The study formulation contains the following nutrients in each tablet:

Lutein	6 mg
Vitamin A	750 μg
Vitamin C	250 mg
Vitamin E	34 mg
Zinc	10 mg
Copper	0.5 mg

Participants in both groups are instructed to take one tablet, at the same time every day, with food.

BASELINE DATA

On application, participants complete a food frequency questionnaire, a food diary and a health questionnaire. The food questionnaire and diary ask for information about diet for analysis using Foodbase 2000 software (Institute of Brain Chemistry and Human Nutrition, London N7 8DB).

The health questionnaire provides information about general health, ocular health, nutritional supplementation, medication, smoking history and time spent living abroad.

OUTCOME MEASURES

The investigation of several measures of visual function is required, as age-related macular disease can produce varying signs and symptoms.

FUNDUS PHOTOGRAPHY

Fundus photographs of the macula will be assessed using colour and edge analysis software.

Macular Mapping Test

The Macular Mapping (MM) test (Smith-Kettlewell Research Institute, 2318 Fillmore Street, San Francisco, CA 94115, USA) was developed to map visual defects caused by macular disease. It was developed by MacKeben and Colenbrander[11] and differs from conventional field analysis in that the stimuli are single letters rather than spots of light. This is a novel piece of equipment and each participant is given a practice run to eliminate learning effects. At the end of the test a single figure score is presented.

Glare recovery

Eger Macular Stressometer (EMS) (Gulden Ophthalmics, Elkins Park, PA 19027, USA) is used to assess photostress recovery time (PSRT). This is the time taken for the regeneration of photo-pigments in bleached photoreceptors. Resynthesis of the photopigments is dependent upon the integrity of the photoreceptors and retinal pigment epithelium;[12] it follows that the PSRT may be extended in those with diseases affecting these structures.

VISUAL ACUITY

Distance and near visual acuity are measured using Bailey–Lovie logMAR charts. LogMAR charts have five letters and 0.1 logMAR progression per line. The advantage of using these charts is that they provide an equal-interval scale, and there are five letters per line. Standard Snellen charts do not provide a linear scale and have a decreasing number of letters per line as the letter size increases.

CONTRAST SENSITIVITY

Contrast sensitivity is measured using a Pelli–Robson chart (Clement Clarke International, Edinburgh Way, Harlow, Essex CM20 2TT, UK) and provides additional information about vision. The Pelli–Robson chart determines the contrast required to read large letters and is designed to test mid to low spatial frequencies.

COLOUR VISION

Colour vision measured using the PV-16 quantitative colour vision test (Precision Vision, 944 First Street, La Salle, IL 61301, USA). Macular disease can cause a deficiency in blue-yellow colour vision as the short-wavelength photoreceptors are concentrated around the fovea.

FOLLOW-UP

Data collection will take place at baseline and 9 and 18 months. Data collection takes place in a standard consulting room at Aston University. Enrolment, randomisation and data collection are carried out by HB. HB and FE are masked to group assignment.

DISCUSSION

There is evidence for selective deposition of lutein in the retina, increase of retinal and serum levels of lutein with supplementation, and an increased risk of age-related macular disease with reduced retinal lutein levels. This RCT will provide further information regarding the effect of lutein and antioxidant supplementation on specific measures of visual function in people with and without age-related macular disease.

Randomised masked trials differ from observational studies in that they have the ability to demonstrate causality. Masking reduces the influence of investigator bias, and the influence of confounding variables is reduced by random assignment of participants to intervention groups. The current paucity of treatment modalities for this condition has prompted research into the development of prevention strategies. A positive effect of the supplementation on normals may be indicative of its potential role in preventing or delaying the onset of age-related macular disease. This may be particularly important for those with a positive family history, or exposure to other risk factors. A positive effect in age-related macular disease-affected eyes may suggest a role of nutritional supplementation in prevention of progression of the disease, or even in reversal of symptoms.

References

1. Muir Gray J. Appraising the quality of research. In: Richardson P, ed. Evidence-based healthcare. How to make health policy and management decisions. London: Churchill Livingstone; 1997:117–168.
2. Huwiler-Muntener K, Juni P, Junker C, Egger M. Quality of reporting randomized trials as a measure of methodologic quality. J Am Med Soc 2002; 287:2801–2804.
3. Cummings S, Grady D, Hulley S. Designing an experiment: clinical trials I. In: Hulley S, Cummings S, Browner W et al., eds. Designing clinical research. Philadelphia: Lippincott/Williams & Wilkins; 2001: 143–155.
4. Bierenbaum M, Noonan F, Machlin L. The effect of supplemental vitamin E on serum parameters in diabetics, post coronary and normal subjects. Nutr Rep Int 1985; 31:1171–1180.
5. Paolisso G, D'Amore A, Giugliano D. Pharmacologic doses of vitamin E improve insulin action in healthy subjects and non-insulin dependent diabetic patients. Am J Clin Nutr 1993; 57:650–656.
6. Paolisso G, D'Amore A, Galzerano D. Daily vitamin E supplements improve metabolic control but not insulin secretion in elderly type II diabetic patients. Diabetes Care 1993; 16:1433–1437.
7. Tütüncü N, Bayraktar M, Varli K. Reversal of defective nerve condition with vitamin E supplementation in type 2 diabetes. Diabetes Care 1998; 21:1915–1918.
8. Skrha J, Sindelka G, Kvasnicka J, Hilgertova J. Insulin action and fibrinolysis influenced by vitamin E in obese type 2 diabetes mellitus. Diabetes Res Clin Pract 1999; 44:27–33.
9. Pinto J. The pharmacokinetic and pharmacodynamic interactions of foods and drugs. Top Clin Nutr 1991; 6:14–33.
10. Expert Group on Vitamins and Minerals. Safe upper limits for vitamins and minerals. Food Standard Agency 2003. Available online at: www.foodstandards.gov.uk/multimedia/pdfs/vitamins2003.pdf (accessed 2003).
11. MacKeben M, Colenbrander A. The assessment of residual vision in patients with maculopathies. Non-invasive assessment of the visual system. Tech Dig 1993; 3:274–277.
12. Brindley G. Physiology of the retina and visual pathways. Baltimore, MD: Williams & Wilkins, 1970.

Chapter 5.5

Celtic Age–Related Maculopathy Arrestation (CARMA) study

Stephen Beatty and Usha Chakravarthy

The CARMA study is a multicentre study investigating the potential beneficial effects of antioxidant supplements, including lutein (L) and zeaxanthin (Z), on the course of age-related maculopathy (ARM). Recruitment started in July 2004, and preliminary results will be available in 2007. The following is a description of the CARMA protocol.

INTRODUCTION

There is general consensus that cumulative blue light damage and/or oxidative stress play important roles in the pathogenesis of ARM and its late stage, AMD. Macular pigment, composed of the carotenoids L and Z, is a blue light filter and powerful antioxidant and is thought to protect against AMD. A recent randomised placebo-controlled trial of 4757 subjects, the AREDS,[1] demonstrated a reduction in the risk of progression to AMD in eyes with ARM after long-term supplementation with high doses of naturally occurring antioxidants (vitamin C, vitamin E, β-carotene and zinc). AREDS was not designed to detect subtle differences in visual function in the short term between the various intervention groups as its principal aim was to identify a protective role in the prevention of progression to advanced AMD. AREDS also did not use L and Z which were unavailable at the time of inception of that study.

The CARMA investigators therefore designed a pilot randomised controlled clinical trial of parallel-group design, where patients at high risk of developing advanced AMD are invited to participate. Subjects are randomised to receive an antioxidant cocktail containing vitamins, minerals and L + Z or placebo, and undergo tests of macular function at baseline and at 6-monthly intervals. Differences between groups in the rate of deterioration of visual function in response to antioxidant supplements, if observed, will strengthen the argument for screening for ARM and the use of dietary modification with or without supplementation. This study will also provide insight into the potential role that antioxidants play in maintaining macular health.

The primary hypothesis is that progression from early ARM to late AMD may be delayed or prevented through supplementation with key antioxidants (vitamins, minerals and carotenoids) which are either known to be present in high concentrations in healthy neural retina–retinal pigment epithelium–choroidal interface, or are free radical scavengers and thus have potential protective roles in minimising oxidative stress.

OBJECTIVES

- To study the effect of supplemental antioxidants on macular psychophysical function in eyes at very high risk of AMD within the context of a randomised controlled clinical trial.
- To measure macular pigment in vivo by resonance Raman spectroscopy and to assess serum levels of the biochemical constituents of macular pigment in subjects participating in the above trial.

TEST AND CONTROL ARTICLES

Study medications

- test article: L + Z+ vitamins C, E and zinc: 2 tablets per day (to be known as Carmavite)
- the test article and placebo will be supplied in sealed containers.

LABELLING

The container labelling will consist of the following particulars:

1. protocol number
2. production lot number of the test articles
3. investigator number
4. patient number
5. expiry date of the test and placebo articles
6. storage conditions
7. caution.

ROUTE OF ADMINISTRATION

Patients will be randomised to receive by mouth two tablets of Carmavite daily, or two tablets of the placebo during the 12-month study period. Masking of the patient, study coordinator, visual acuity examiner, photographer and examining ophthalmologist is maintained throughout the 12-month study period.

PATIENTS

Number and source

Approximately 500 patients who meet the inclusion/exclusion criteria will be enrolled in this study.

Inclusion criteria

- Patients must be willing to give written informed consent, make the required study visits and follow instructions.
- Patients must be at least 50 years of age.
- Patients may be of any race and either sex.
- Two categories of ARM patients may be included: category 1 and category 2.

Category 1

- If there is choroidal neovascularisation or geographic atrophy in one eye, any level of ARM is permissible in the fellow eye provided that visual acuity is equal to or better than logMAR 0.3.

Category 2

- clinical diagnosis of severe ARM in at least one eye
- ≥20 soft distinct or soft indistinct drusen

- or if <20 soft drusen, focal hyperpigmentation must be present
- visual acuity ≥6/12 or 0.3 logMAR in the study eye (which may be both eyes).

Exclusion criteria

- any retinal laser therapy in the study eye
- history of any unstable medical condition that would preclude scheduled study visits or completion of the study
- history of ophthalmic disease in the study eye (other than ARM) that would compromise the visual acuity of the study eye
- patients currently on supplements containing the antioxidants vitamins C, E, Zn, L and Z will be asked to discontinue them. After a washout period of 3 months they may be eligible for randomisation into the study.

STUDY PROCEDURE

General study design

General information

CARMA is a two-arm double-masked trial of an antioxidant preparation versus placebo given orally in subjects with ARM. Approximately 500 patients enrolled in two centres, Belfast and Waterford, Ireland, fulfilling the eligibility criteria will be randomised to receive either Carmavite or placebo. Outcomes will be monitored by measuring psychophysical retinal functions, Raman spectroscopy and serological levels of antioxidants.

Duration of the trial

The trial will last 2 years, with recruitment being undertaken in the first 12 months.

Frequency of follow-up

Patients will undergo periodic ophthalmic and serological evaluations at baseline, 6 and 12 months after study entry.

Arrangements for allocating participants to trial groups

The investigator or study staff will enrol eligible patients into the study. A computer-generated randomisation will secure the randomisation code. The ready-prepared masked test articles will be kept in the hospital pharmacy and released by the pharmacist on randomisation of each patient in a sequential manner by patient number, beginning with the first number in the numerical series assigned to each site.

Protecting against sources of bias

Subjects can only be entered into the study following a reading-centre grading of ARM status. In order to minimise potential bias toward the outcome of this study by patients, investigators and study personnel regarding the safety or efficacy of the test articles, the study will be double-masked. Patients will be randomly assigned to receive either Carmavite or the placebo. Allocation of treatment status is concealed from investigators and the study medication will be dispensed in appropriately labelled containers. The hospital pharmacist will hold the key to the randomisation code. A sealed envelope containing the identification of the test article will be provided for each patient and, in the event that it becomes necessary to know which test article the patient received, this will be made available to the principal investigator.

Study population

The study population includes patients of either sex, of any race, aged 50 years and over, fulfilling the inclusion criteria (see above).

CLINICAL EXAMINATIONS/PROCEDURES TO BE PERFORMED DURING THE STUDY

A full ophthalmic examination will be performed at each study visit. This will include:

- slit-lamp examination and biomicroscopy of the anterior segment
- dilated fundus examination to include an evaluation of the posterior segment

- best corrected logMAR visual acuity following refraction.

Contrast sensitivity

Evaluations of contrast sensitivity will be conducted using Pelli–Robson charts.

Colour photography

Colour stereo pair fundus photographs will be taken of both eyes.

General physical examination

A general physical examination will be performed at baseline and will include the following:

- recording of anthropomorphic measurements
  - height and body weight
  - blood pressure
  - heart rate
- routine evaluation of other organ systems.

Masking of study personnel

Procedures for maintaining masking of study personnel must be observed throughout the 12-month study.

The following study personnel must be masked to participant study status:

- the examining ophthalmologist(s)
- the study coordinator(s)
- the study photographer(s)
- the study visual acuity examiner(s)
- the photographic graders.

STUDY VISITS AND EVALUATIONS

Visit 1: screening visit

This will include:

- informed consent form signed and dated by the patient and the investigator
- documentation of the patient's medical and ophthalmic histories, current medications, vitamin and mineral supplements and demographic information

- best corrected logMAR visual acuity (using the Early Treatment of Diabetic Retinopathy Study chart)
- evaluation of contrast sensitivity using the Pelli–Robson assessment procedure
- other macular psychophysical tests
- an ophthalmic examination of both eyes
- stereo pair digital colour fundus photographs with documentation
- patient eligibility on the basis of ARM severity confirmed by the fundus photograph reading centre at Belfast
- clinical data collected on appropriate data collection forms
- following completion of the screening procedures, patients will be randomised to receive the first course of supplemental antioxidant treatment or placebo treatment
- the following questionnaires will be completed: food frequency, general lifestyle and vision-related quality of life
- schedule patients for their next visit.

Visit 2: month 6 (± 7 days)

This visit will include the following:

- best corrected logMAR visual acuity (using the Early Treatment of Diabetic Retinopathy Study chart) measured
- evaluation of contrast sensitivity using Pelli–Robson assessment
- photopic interferometry
- an ophthalmic examination of both eyes
- stereo digital colour fundus photographs with documentation
- record of any changes in the patient's concomitant medications
- schedule patients for their next visit
- issue the second course of supplemental antioxidant treatment or placebo treatment.

Visit 3: month 12: exit (± 7 days)

This visit will include:

- best corrected logMAR visual acuity (using the Early Treatment of Diabetic Retinopathy Study chart) measured

- evaluation of contrast sensitivity using Pelli–Robson assessment
- photopic interferometry
- an ophthalmic examination of both eyes
- digital colour photographs with documentation
- record any changes in the patient's concomitant medications
- complete the exit form for the patient.

DISCONTINUATION OF PATIENTS

Discontinuations are defined as those patients who end the treatment phase of the study before completing all regularly scheduled study visits. Patients may discontinue from the study at any time for any reason.

Please note that an exit form must be completed for all discontinued patients, clearly stating the reason for their early exit from the study.

If a patient is to be discontinued from the study between scheduled visits, the following activities must occur:

- completion of an exit visit
- completion of an exit visit form.

Patients discontinued from the study will not be replaced and their patient and/or clinical unit number(s) will not be reused.

UNSCHEDULED EXAMINATIONS

Unscheduled visits may be conducted at the discretion of the investigator, recording the information on unscheduled-visit forms. If a patient discontinues at an unscheduled visit, an exit form must be completed.

DOSING GUIDELINES

Patients will be randomised to receive either supplemental antioxidants or placebo.

STANDARDISED METHODS

Distance visual acuity

Best corrected visual acuity measurements are performed in strict accordance with agreed procedure.

Pelli–Robson contrast sensitivity

All contrast sensitivity measurements will be performed in accordance with the agreed procedure.

Photopic interferometry

Visometry is undertaken using monochromatic light at a wavelength of 555 nm. To remove any effects of transverse chromatic aberration, interferometric acuity is measured (two alternative forced-choice orientation discriminations) using the green monochromatic light and an ascending method of limit resolution task where the subject must indicate the orientation of the gratings.

Resonance Raman spectroscopy

Recent studies have demonstrated that Raman spectroscopy, which is a non-invasive method for measuring the macular pigment signal in vivo, is highly reproducible and simple to use in older people.[2] Heterochromatic flicker, which is an alternative method, is time-consuming and difficult to use in older people. The Raman signal correlates well with macular carotenoid concentrations in in vitro studies. Measurements of in vivo macular carotenoid levels will therefore be performed using the Raman spectrometer.

STATISTICAL ANALYSIS

Primary analysis

The primary analysis will be a repeated-measures logistic regression analysis stratified by ARM category with outcomes measured every 6 months for 1 year.

The form will be a stratified block randomised design. Strata will be location (Belfast/Waterford), gender and patient category (category 1 = unilateral; category 2 = bilateral). It is anticipated that participants will be split equally across locations, that approximately 60% of participants will be female and 67% will be category 2 and potentially may have both eyes entered into the study. The size of the block will not be disclosed but will be set at a level to ensure reasonable balance within the smallest stratum.

Handling of data from category 2 participants

Several papers have cited the problem of statistical independence when dealing with outcomes on eyes.[3] Briefly, this arises because outcomes relating to two eyes within one individual are likely to be more closely related than outcomes on eyes from different individuals. Earlier references have tended to cite dichotomous outcomes and so the solution becomes a particular application of interclass correlation. In this study the main outcome will be treated as continuously distributed.

One possible solution is simply to use data from one eye only from subjects in whom both eyes fit the entry criteria. This method thereby imposes a strict regime of one eye per participant. The disadvantage of this approach is that it does not utilise all readily available data and is therefore cost-inefficient. Collecting all data and treating them as independent outcomes can also be flawed, for the reasons stated above. A compromise solution is suggested that follows parallel arguments to that for interclass correlation.

Category 1 patients will only have one study eye (the fellow eye having already been lost to exudative AMD). Let the variance associated with contrast sensitivity in this group be σ_1^2. Category 2 patients may have both eyes eligible for the study and thus have two components of variance that can be estimated. That between participants will be denoted σ_{2B}^2 and that between eyes within the same participant will be σ_{2W}^2. In practice the study will yield some large sample estimators: s_1^2, s_{2B}^2 and s_{2W}^2. A reasonable prior expectation might be for homogeneity of variance across all participants where $\sigma_1^2 = \sigma_{2B}^2 + \sigma_{2W}^2$.

However, the approach suggested will actually permit heterogeneity of variance between groups. It is usual, in situations of heterogeneity of variance, to weight cases by the reciprocal of the variation associated with each case. We propose, therefore, that all data be collected and the variance estimates described above calculated. Data will then be aggregated to one result per participant – the sole result will stand for category 1 participants and the mean of the two results will be applied to category 2 participants. The variance associated with category 1 participants will be s_1^2,

while that associated with the mean of category 2 participants will be $s_{2B}^2 + s_{2W}^2/2$. So in the main analysis, category 1 participants will be given a weight of 1, while category 2 participants will be given a weight:

$$w_2 = s_1^2 / (s_{2B}^2 + s_{2W}^2/2)$$

We note that, if most of the variation lies between participants, then w_2 will tend to be close to 1. Here the second eye from bilateral participants provides very little additional information. However, if most of the variation lies within participants then w_2 will tend to be close to 2. Here the second eye from bilateral participants provides much additional information and we are actually moving towards a situation where the two eyes have been entered as independent observations.

QUESTIONNAIRES

Questionnaires used include: (1) the food frequency questionnaire; (2) the general well-being questionnaire; and (3) vision-related quality-of-life questionnaire.

INVESTIGATOR RESPONSIBILITIES

Informed consent

All patients in this study are completely informed, according to informed consent guidelines, about the pertinent details and purpose of the study. A written informed consent form is signed and dated by each patient before enrolment into the study. The investigator keeps the original signed and dated consent forms in each patient's chart, and provides the patient with a copy. This study is conducted in accordance with principles set forth in the Declaration of Helsinki.

Data collection

The clinical investigator maintains detailed records on all study patients. Data for this study are recorded on the case report forms provided for each patient completely, promptly, accurately and legibly. The investigator makes one copy of all the case report forms and sends the original to the main study site. The investigator maintains a copy of all completed case report forms in his/her study files.

Study records

Investigator file content

The principal investigator maintains the following documentation in his/her study file:

- copy of the approved clinical protocol (and any amendments)
- approval letter from the local ethics committee (for study protocol and study consent form)
- approval letter(s) for any amendment(s)
- periodic/annual report to the local regional ethics committee
- final report to the local regional ethics committee
- original signed and dated informed consent forms for each patient
- copy of signed receipt of clinical supplies
- copy of clinical supplies dispensing records

- copy of all signed, completed case report forms
- copies of monitoring log
- study personnel log (list of all personnel involved in the study)
- patient enrolment log, showing the patient name and study patient number
- notification of any clinical supply expiry date extensions.

Inspection of investigator records

The investigator permits any trial-related monitoring visits, audits, local regional ethics committee review and inspections by regulatory agencies by providing direct access to data and documents. These inspections are for the purpose of verifying adherence to the protocol, the completeness and exactness of the data being entered in the case report form and compliance with regulations.

Test article storage

Test articles are stored in a secure area at the investigational site.

References

1. The Age-Related Eye Disease Study Group. A randomized, placebo-controlled, clinical trial of high-dose supplementation with vitamins C and E, beta carotene, and zinc for age-related macular degeneration and vision loss. AREDS report no. 8. Arch Ophthalmol 2001; 119:1417–1436.

2. Neelam K, O'Gorman N, Nolan J et al. Measurement of macular pigment: Raman spectroscopy versus heterochromatic flicker photometry. Invest Ophthalmol Vis Sci 2005; 46:1023–1032.
3. Ederer F. Shall we count numbers of eyes or numbers of subjects? Arch Ophthalmol 1973; 89:1–2.

SECTION 6

Contraindications, adverse reactions and ocular nutritional supplements

Chapter **6.1**

Contraindications, adverse reactions and ocular nutritional supplements

Hannah Bartlett and Frank Eperjesi

INTRODUCTION

People are increasingly taking an active interest in their well-being, and seeking alternative medical therapies.[1,2] Traditional health care providers have been perceived as having a negative attitude towards these therapies.[3] This may explain why many people do not consider their medical practitioner a major source of nutritional information[4-6] and do not always report unconventional therapy use to their physicians.[7]

Use of ocular nutritional supplementation has been investigated with regard to prevention of onset or progression of glaucoma, cataract and age-related macular disease. There is particular interest in the use of nutrition as a prevention and treatment strategy for age-related macular degeneration (AMD) as it is the leading cause of visual disability in the developed world,[8] and because treatment options are currently lacking.[9]

Eye care practitioners require information about the benefits, and potential hazards, of ocular nutritional supplements in order to be able to discuss their use with patients. It should be emphasised that the risk of side-effects from nutrients is much lower than from over-the-counter or prescription drugs. As an example, the National Health and Nutrition Examination Survey II estimated that 35% of the US population use vitamin A supplements,[10] and the rate of toxic reactions has been reported as 1 case per 1.1 million per year exposed.

Here, we aim to highlight possible contraindications and the potential for adverse reactions for those nutrients reported to be beneficial to ocular health. An overview of these nutrients can be found in Table 6.1, and drug interactions of nutrients considered beneficial for ocular health are summarised in Table 6.2.

CONTRAINDICATIONS

Provitamin A

In a review of the literature, β-carotene was promoted as a preferred source of vitamin A due to

Table 6.1 Summary of source, function, recommended daily allowance and safe upper limits for nutrients and herbs associated with ocular health

Nutrient	Sources	Main functions	Recommended daily allowance for adults	Safe upper limit	Tolerable upper intake level (US Food and Nutrition Board)
Vitamin A	As vitamin A: fish-liver oils, beef liver, egg yolk, butter and cream As carotenoids (provitamin A): dark-green leafy vegetables, yellow fruits and red palm oil	Maintenance of vision, skin, lining of intestine, lungs and urinary tract. Helps protect against infection. The basis of drugs called retinoids that are used to treat severe acne and some cancers	700–900 µg 1300 µg for pregnant and breast-feeding women	500–10 000* IU/day[11]	3000 g (retinol)
Vitamin E	Vegetable oil, wheatgerm, leafy vegetables, egg yolk, margarine and legumes	Acts as an antioxidant	15 mg	800 IU or 540 mg of D-α-tocopherol equivalents[90]	1000 mg
Vitamin B$_2$	Milk, cheese, liver, meat, fish, eggs and enriched cereals	Required for metabolism of carbohydrates and amino acids and for healthy mucous membranes	1.1 mg women 1.3 mg men	–	–

Table 6.1   *cont'd*

Vitamin B₆	Dried yeast, liver, organ meats, wholegrain cereals, fish and legumes	Required for metabolism of amino acids and fatty acids, for nerve function, for the formation of red blood cells and for healthy skin	1.5 mg women 1.7 mg men	10 mg/day,[90] although usually safe up to 200 mg/day[93]	25 mg
Vitamin B₁₂	Liver, meat, eggs, milk and milk products	Required for the metabolism of carbohydrates and fatty acids	2.4 µg	2 mg/day cyanocobalamin[90]	–
Vitamin C	Citrus fruits, tomatoes, potatoes, cabbage, and green peppers	Required for the formation and growth of bone and connective tissue, for healing of wounds and burns, and for normal function of blood vessels Acts as an antioxidant and helps the body to absorb iron	75 mg women 90 mg men 35 mg extra for smokers	2 mg[94]	2000 mg
Magnesium	Leafy green vegetables, nuts, cereals, grains and seafood	Required for the formation of bone and teeth, for normal nerve and muscle function, and for the activation of enzymes	300 mg/day men 270 mg/day women	Guidance level of 400 mg/day[90]	250 mg
Selenium	Meats, seafood, and cereals (depending on the selenium content of the soil where the grain was grown)	Acts as an antioxidant with vitamin E, protecting cells from oxidative damage. Also required for thyroid gland function	55 µg	500 µg[93]	300 µg

table continues

Table 6.1 *cont'd*

Zinc	Organ meats such as liver, eggs and seafood	Used to form many enzymes and insulin. Required for healthy skin, healing of wounds and growth	15 mg	25 mg supplemental zinc[90]	40 mg
Ginkgo biloba	*Ginkgo biloba* tree	Reduction in platelet aggregation and the production of free radicals. Role in neurotransmitter metabolism	Trials have used between 120 and 240 mg/day	–	–
Omega-3 essential fatty acids	Fish oils, including cod liver oil. Flaxseeds, linseeds, pumpkin seeds, soya bean, walnut oil, green leafy vegetables, grains, and oils made from linseed, rapeseed, and soya beans	Maintenance of cell membranes and production of prostaglandins	0.2–0.5 × amount of omega-6 essential fatty acid	–	–
Omega-6 essential fatty acids	Vegetables, fruits, nuts, grains, seeds and oils made from safflower, sunflower, corn, soya, evening primrose, pumpkin and wheatgerm. Also dairy products and beef	Maintenance of cell membranes and production of prostaglandins	3–6% of total calories, or 6–12 g	–	–

Table 6.2   Drug interactions of ocular nutritional supplements

Supplement	Drug	Explanation
Vitamin A	Anticonvulsant agents	Valproic acid may interfere with the body's ability to handle vitamin A[36]
Vitamin B$_6$	Folic acid	B$_6$ may reduce the absorption or activity of folic acid
Vitamin C	Paracetamol (pain relief)	High doses of vitamin C may interfere with normal breakdown of this drug. May result in liver-damaging accumulation of paracetamol[47]
Vitamin C	Anticoagulants	Impaired blood coagulation time[41] and interference with anticoagulant therapy[42] have been reported when large doses ($\geq$1 g) are routinely ingested for months or years
Vitamin E	Warfarin	800 IU daily vitamin E caused abnormal bleeding when added to the effects of warfarin[95]
Vitamin E	Non-steroidal anti-inflammatory drugs	Vitamin E appears to add to aspirin's blood-thinning effects[57,58]
Ginkgo biloba	Anticonvulsants	A natural nerve toxin has been found in the seeds of ginkgo biloba.[96] This toxin could prevent anticonvulsants from working as expected
Ginkgo biloba	Warfarin	Ginkgo biloba appears to reduce the ability of platelets to stick together.[97] It may add to the blood-thinning effects of warfarin[66]
Ginkgo biloba	Non-steroidal anti-inflammatory drugs	The combination of ginkgo biloba and aspirin may increase the chance of abnormal bleeding[65]
Magnesium	Amiloride (diuretic)	Amiloride may reduce urinary excretion of magnesium in animals.[98] People taking more than 300 mg magnesium and amiloride should consult their doctor
Magnesium	Fluoroquinoline antibiotics Tetracyclines Nitrofurantoin (antibiotic)	Magnesium can bind to these antibiotics, greatly decreasing the absorption of the drug[99]
Magnesium	Misoprostol (prostaglandin E$_1$ analogue that protects the mucosal lining of the stomach and intestines)	A common side-effect of misoprostol is diarrhoea, which is aggravated by magnesium[100]
Magnesium	Oral corticosteroids	Loss of magnesium from the body may be increased by magnesium.[99] Magnesium may interfere with absorption of dexamethasone[101]
Zinc	Fluoroquinolone antibiotics Tetracyclines	Zinc can bind to these antibiotics, greatly decreasing the absorption of the drug.[99] It is recommended to take the drugs 2 hours after consuming mineral-containing supplements[102]

the fact that it has virtually no adverse effects.[11] However, doses of 20 mg/day β-carotene, alone or in combination with α-tocopherol (vitamin E),[12] and 30 mg/day in combination with retinyl palmitate (vitamin A)[13] have been associated with an increased risk of lung cancer in smokers and those previously exposed to high levels of asbestos. The Physician's Health Study found no effect of 50 mg β-carotene every other day in a trial population comprising 11% smokers.[14] Hypotheses for the proposed increased risk of lung cancer in smokers include pro-oxidant behaviour by β-carotene initiated by the high oxygen tension within the lungs, and the production of damaging oxidation products by the components of cigarette smoke.

β-Carotene may be contraindicated in AMD patients as plasma lutein concentration is reduced following multiple[15] and single[16] doses. Other studies have, however, found no effect of β-carotene on serum levels of lutein.[17] In the Age-related Eye Disease Study (AREDS), serum levels of lutein and zeaxanthin decreased over 5 years, although changes in the treatment arm were not significantly different from the placebo arm.[18]

Preformed vitamin A

There are reports of lower bone mineral density with vitamin A supplementation,[19] as well as increased risk of osteoporotic fracture.[20] Studies suggest that bone reabsorption is stimulated by vitamin A,[21,22] and also that vitamin A toxicity decreases bone formation.[23,24] Vitamin A supplementation was inversely related to the rate of change of ulnar bone mineral content in postmenopausal women taking part in a 4-year clinical trial.[25] Intake of 1500 μg retinol equivalents (RE)/day compared with 500 μg RE/day was associated with a total body reduction in bone mineral density of 6% ($P = 0.009$) and twice the chance of hip fracture (odds ratio, 2.1, 95% confidence interval (CI), 1.1–4.0), although this study may be limited by information bias.[20] White women consuming ≥3000 μg RE/day had an increased relative risk for hip fractures (relative risk, 1.48; 95% CI, 1.05–2.07) compared to those taking <1250 μg RE/day,[26] and retinol intake has been associated with decreased bone mineral

density and increased bone loss at total daily intakes above 840 μg.[27]

However, daily supplementation with 7576 μg retinol palmitate for 6 weeks did not affect the serum markers of skeletal turnover in healthy men,[28] and no significant association between fasting serum retinyl esters and bone mineral density was found in a population of 5790 women aged 20 years or over.[29]

Teratogenic effects have been reported with high doses of retinoic acid consumed within the first 6 weeks of pregnancy.[30] It has been suggested that vitamin A doses should not exceed 10 000 IU/day during pregnancy;[31] this dosage has been shown to maintain blood vitamin A levels in the mother without increasing them in the newborn.[32]

Vitamin A supplements have been shown to increase the tendency towards abnormal bleeding in rats,[33–35] which may indicate that it interacts with vitamin K. Vitamin K is required for production of coagulation proteins, and so deficiency reduces blood coagulation. This effect has yet to be determined in humans.

Valproic acid (anticonvulsant) may interfere with the body's ability to handle vitamin A.[36]

Isotretinoin is a modified vitamin A molecule used to treat severe acne vulgaris, and it has above-average toxicity potential. People taking isotretinoin should avoid additional vitamin A supplements as little is known about how the two interact. Combined administration of isotretinoin and vitamin E may reduce the initial toxicity of high-dose isotretinoin without reducing its efficacy.[37] High-dose vitamin A and isotretinoin should be avoided by women who might become pregnant, patients with liver disease and those who drink heavily.

Vitamin C

Large doses of vitamin C are generally well tolerated. Vitamin C was investigated with regard to a possible interaction with oral anticoagulants following reports of an unexpected decrease in prothrombin time in people taking warfarin.[38,39] No change in coagulation status occurred in humans supplemented with 1g/day for 14 days.[40] Impaired blood coagulation time[41] and interference with anticoagulant therapy[42] have been reported when doses of ≥1 g are ingested routinely for months or years. Interestingly, studies suggest that the antiplatelet drug, aspirin, promotes loss of vitamin C via the urine.[43,44]

Reduced bactericidal activity of leukocytes,[45] reduced insulin production[46] may occur with routine doses ≥1 g over months or years. High doses of vitamin C have also been reported to interfere with the breakdown of acetaminophen.[47]

Vitamin E

A randomised controlled trial showed that 400 IU/day vitamin E may have an adverse effect on the progress of common forms of retinitis pigmentosa.[48] Participants taking this dosage of 400 IU/day vitamin E had a faster rate of decline in electroretinogram amplitude than those taking 3 IU/day. The decline rates were 11.8% and 10.0% for the dosage levels respectively. Investigators hypothesised that the 400 IU/day dosage of vitamin E may inhibit the absorption or transport of vitamin A, as the participants receiving this dosage of vitamin E had significantly decreased serum retinol levels compared with those not receiving vitamin E.

Vitamin E may exacerbate the effects of vitamin K deficiency and has been associated with an increased risk of haemorrhagic stroke, and a reduced risk of ischaemic stroke and ischaemic heart disease.[12] Other studies have found no relationship between vitamin E and haemorrhagic stroke,[49–55] and smokers with diabetes may represent a subset of the population that may benefit from 50 IU vitamin E per day without experiencing an increased risk of bleeding.[52]

Oral anticoagulants, such as warfarin, antagonise the effects of vitamin K and are indicated in deep-vein thrombosis and pulmonary embolism patients. The action of oral anticoagulants may be increased by concurrent administration of vitamin E. Concurrent vitamin E and warfarin use has been associated with abnormal bleeding,[56] and vitamin E appears to add to aspirin's blood-thinning effect.[57,58] However, vitamin E does not cause coagulation abnormalities in those who do not already have them.[59] It has been suggested that anticoagulant-treated patients should avoid megadoses of vitamin E.

Zinc

Patients with type 1 diabetes should consult their general medical practitioner before starting zinc supplementation as it has been reported to increase glycosylation.[60] Glycosylation refers to the addition of glucose to proteins, which is thought to be responsible for some of the clinical manifestations of type 1 diabetes.[61,62] Zinc supplementation has, however, been shown to reduce blood sugar levels in those with type 1 diabetes,[63] although it may not improve blood sugar levels in type 2 diabetes.[64]

Ginkgo biloba

Ginkgo biloba may thin the blood, and should be avoided before surgery, and also by those taking certain anticoagulant and antiplatelet drugs.[65,66]

ADVERSE REACTIONS

Provitamin A

Individuals consuming ≥30 mg β-carotene/day may experience hypercarotenaemia (high plasma β-carotene), which has also been observed in infants fed commercial foods containing large amounts of ground carrots.[67] The only adverse effect of hypercarotenaemia is a reversible yellowing of the skin (hypercarotenodermia). Babies born with hypercarotenaemia from high maternal intakes were otherwise normal, and so β-carotene is not considered significantly toxic to the human fetus.[68]

Preformed vitamin A

Globally, the incidence of vitamin A toxicity, or hypervitaminosis A, is a minor problem (200 cases per year) compared with the incidence of vitamin A deficiency (VAD) (1 million cases per year).[69] In 118 countries where foods lacking in carotene are staple, VAD is a serious public health problem,[70] combated by a successful World Health Organization supplementation programme.[71] In young children, 100 000 IU of vitamin A at 6–11 months and 200 000 IU given every 3–6 months for children aged between 12 and 60 months gives few side-effects and is effective for reducing mortality.[72] Nausea, vomiting, headache, diarrhoea and fever have, however, been reported in some children in the Philippines with doses of 100 000 and 200 000 IU.[73]

Symptoms of adult toxicity have, however, been reported with single or short-term doses of about 50 000 IU,[74] and include nausea, vomiting, increased cerebrospinal fluid pressure, headaches, blurred vision and lack of muscular coordination. Chronic toxicity, resulting from long-term consumption of high-dose vitamin A, includes vomiting, weight loss, bone abnormalities, headache, fever, an enlarged liver and raised intracranial pressure.[75] Women may experience menstrual disturbances. Response times for vitamin A toxicity range from 6 to 108 months for a dose of 100 000 IU/day, and days or weeks for doses of 1 000 000 IU/day.[69]

Vitamin A has been used therapeutically in retinitis pigmentosa.[48] A study showed that long-term supplementation with 15 000 IU/day vitamin A in healthy adults aged 18–54 years elicited no adverse effects, and no evidence of hepatic toxicity.[76]

Vitamin A has been shown to reduce vitamin E activity (an important antioxidant) by as much as 30%,[77] although plasma levels of vitamin E were not affected in a human study of 25 000 IU/day vitamin A given for 16 weeks.[78] In animal models, vitamin E has been shown to protect membranes against vitamin A hypervitaminosis-induced damage.[79] Animal studies have shown that vitamins A and D decrease the toxic effects of each other,[80] and also that zinc may be specifically involved in mobilising vitamin A from the liver to the circulation within a short period.[81]

The symptoms of hypervitaminosis A are usually relieved within a week of discontinuation, but long-term or irreversible effects can include cirrhosis[82] and bone changes.[69]

Vitamin C

Doses of vitamin C up to 2000 mg/day are well-tolerated, although stomach cramps, nausea and diarrhoea may occur with higher doses.[83] A review of the literature concluded that high doses of vitamin C are safe and free of side-effects.[59]

Zinc

Zinc interacts with copper by stimulating metallothionein levels of the intestinal wall. Metallothionein binds to dietary copper, preventing absorption, which leads to copper deficiency. This can result in copper-deficiency anaemia, since copper is required for the production of erythrocytes.[84–86]

Daily supplementation with more than 300 mg zinc per day has been associated with impairment of immune function.[87] There are reports of a potential role of zinc in Alzheimer-associated neuropathogenesis,[88] although more recent evidence from 4 patients showed an improvement in mental function with zinc supplementation.[89]

Acute zinc toxicity has been reported with doses of 200 mg or more.[90] In one study 20 female and 21 male volunteers were given 150 mg/day zinc for 6 weeks.[91] Symptoms including headaches, nausea, abdominal cramps, loss of appetite and vomiting were reported in 85% of the female and 18% of the male volunteers. These were particularly apparent when small meals or no food was taken with the supplements. The investigators suggested that the high percentage of females experiencing side-effects could be attributed to their lower body weight.

Ginkgo biloba

One case report associated long-term use of ginkgo biloba extract with bilateral subdural haematomas and increased bleeding time in a healthy 33-year-old female.[92]

SUMMARY

Practitioners should be particularly aware of potential relationships between vitamin A and reduced bone mineral density, β-carotene and an increased risk of lung cancer in smokers, and the anticoagulant and antiplatelet effects of vitamin E and ginkgo biloba respectively.[58] Vitamin A supplements should be avoided by women who may become pregnant, in those with liver disease and those who drink heavily.

When discussing ocular nutritional supplements with patients, practitioners should be aware of the contraindications and the potential for adverse reactions. Those contraindicated from certain supplements, or identified as at risk of adverse reaction, should be advised to discuss supplementation with their medical practitioner.

References

1. Eisenberg D, Davis R, Ettner S et al. Trends in alternative medicine use in the United States, 1990–1997: results of a follow-up national survey. JAMA 1998; 280:1569–1574.
2. Gilbert L. HealthFocus trend report. DesMoines, IA: HealthFocus; 1999.
3. Goodwin J, Tangum M. Battling quackery: attitudes about micronutrient supplements in American academic institutions. Arch Intern Med 1998; 158:2187–2191.
4. Barr S. Nutritional knowledge and selected nutritional practices of female recreational athletes. J Nutrition 1986; 18:167–174.
5. Levy A, Schucker R. Patterns of nutrient intake among dietary supplement users: attitudinal and behavioural correlates. J Am Diet Assoc 1987; 87:754–760.
6. Schutz H, Read M, Bendel R et al. Food supplement usage in seven western states. Am J Clin Nutr 1982; 36:897–901.
7. Eisenberg D, Kessler R, Foster C et al. Unconventional medicine in the United States: prevalence, costs, and patient use. N Engl J Med 1993; 328:246–252.
8. Klein R, Klein B, Jensen S, Meuer S. The five-year incidence and progression of age-related maculopathy: the Beaver Dam Eye Study. Ophthalmology 1997; 104:7–21.
9. Zarbin M. Current concepts in the pathogenesis of age-related macular degeneration. Arch Ophthalmol 2004; 122:598–614.
10. Koplan J, Annest J, Layde P, Rubin G. Nutrient intake and supplementation in the United States (NHANES II). Am J Public Health 1986; 76:287–289.
11. Meyers D, Maloley P, Weeks D. Safety of antioxidant vitamins. Arch Intern Med 1996; 156:925–935.
12. The ATBC Cancer Prevention Study Group. The effect of vitamin E and beta-carotene on the incidence of lung cancer and other cancers in male smokers. N Engl J Med 1994; 330:1029–1035.
13. Leo MA, Lieber CS. Risk factors for lung cancer and for intervention effects in CARET, the Beta-Carotene and Retinol Efficacy Trial. J Natl Cancer Inst 1997; 89:1722–1723.
14. Christen WG, Gaziano JM, Hennekens CH. Design of physicians' health study II – a randomized trial of beta-carotene, vitamins E and C, and multivitamins, in prevention of cancer, cardiovascular disease, and eye disease, and review of results of completed trials. Ann Epidemiol 2000; 10:125–134.
15. Micozzi M, Brown E, Edwards B et al. Plasma carotenoid response to chronic intake of selected foods and beta-carotene supplements in men. Am J Clin Nutr 1992; 55:1120–1125.
16. Kostic D, White W, Olson J. Intestinal absorption, serum clearance, and interactions between lutein and beta-carotene when administered to human adults in separate or combined oral doses. Am J Clin Nutr 1995; 62:604–610.
17. Fotouhi N, Meydani M, Santos M et al. Carotenoid and tocopherol concentrations in plasma, peripheral blood mononuclear cells, and red blood cells after long-term beta-carotene supplementation in men. Am J Clin Nutr 1996; 63:553–558.
18. The AREDS Research Group. A randomized, placebo-controlled, clinical trial of high-dose supplementation with vitamins C and E, beta carotene, and zinc for age-related macular degeneration and vision loss – AREDS report no. 8. Arch Ophthalmol 2001; 119: 1417–1436.
19. Sowers M, Wallace R, Lemke J. Correlates of mid-radius bone density among postmenopausal women: a community study. Am J Clin Nutr 1985; 41:1045–1053.
20. Melhus H, Michaelsson K, Kindmark A et al. Excessive dietary intake of vitamin A is associated with reduced bone mineral density and increased risk for hip fracture. Ann Intern Med 1998; 129:770–778.
21. Frame B, Jackson C, Reynolds W, Umphrey J. Hypercalcemia and skeletal effects in chronic hypervitaminosis A. Ann Intern Med 1974; 80:44–48.
22. Jowsey J, Riggs B. Bone changes in a patient with hypervitaminosis A. J Clin Endocrinol Metab 1968; 28:1833–1835.
23. Hough S, Avioli L, Muir H et al. Effects of hypervitaminosis on the bone and mineral metabolism of the rat. Endocrinology 1988; 122:2933–2939.
24. Frankel T, Seshadri M, McDowell D, Cornish C. Hypervitaminosis A and calcium regulating hormones in the rat. J Nutrition 1986; 116:578–587.
25. Freudenheim J, Johnson N, Smith E. Relationship between usual nutrient intake and bone-mineral content of women 35–65 years of age: longitudinal and cross-sectional analysis. Am J Clin Nutr 1986; 44:863–876.
26. Feskanich D, Singh V, Willet W, Colditz G. Vitamin A intake and hip fractures among postmenopausal women. JAMA 2002; 287:47–54.
27. Promislow J, Goodman-Gruen D, Slymen D, Barrett-Connor E. Retinol intake and bone mineral density in the elderly: the Rancho Bernardo Study. J Bone Mineral Res 2002; 17:1349–1358.

28. Kawahara T, Krueger D, Engelke J et al. Short-term vitamin A does not affect bone turnover in men. J Nutrition 2002; 132:1169–1172.

29. Ballew C, Galuska D, Gillespie C. High serum retinyl esters are not associated with reduced bone mineral density in the Third National Health and Nutrition Examination Survey, 1988–1994. J Bone Mineral Res 2001; 16:2306–2312.

30. Lammer E, Chen D, Hoar R. Retinoic acid embryopathy. N Engl J Med 1985; 313:837–841.

31. Bauernfeind J. Carotenoid vitamin A precursors and analogs in food and feeds. J Agric Food Chem 1972; 20:456–473.

32. Pereira S, Begum A. Vitamin A deficiency in Indian children. World Rev Nutr Diet 1976; 24:192–216.

33. Schrogie J. Coagulopathy and fat soluble drugs (letter). JAMA 1975; 232:19.

34. Walker S, Eylenberg E, Moore T. The action of vitamin A in hypervitaminosis A. Biochem J 1947; 41:575–580.

35. Doisey E. Nutritional hypoprothrombinemia and metabolism of vitamin K. Fed Proc 1961; 20:989–994.

36. Nau H, Tzimas GMM, Plum C, Spohr H. Antiepileptic drugs alter endogenous retinoid concentrations: a possible mechanism of teratogenesis of anticonvulsant therapy. Life Sci 1995; 57:53–60.

37. Dimery I, Hong W, Lee J et al. Phase 1 trial of alpha-tocopherol effects on 13-cis-retinoic acid toxicity. Ann Oncol 1997; 8:85–89.

38. Rosenthal G. Interactions of ascorbic acid and warfarin (letter). JAMA 1971; 215:1671.

39. Smith E, Skalski R, Johnson G, Rossi G. Interaction of ascorbic acid and warfarin (letter). JAMA 1972; 221:1166.

40. Hume R, Johnstone J, Weyers E. Interaction of ascorbic acid and warfarin (letter). JAMA 1972; 219:1479.

41. Barness L. Safety considerations with high ascorbic acid dosage. Ann NY Acad Sci 1975; 258:523–528.

42. Sigell L, Flessa H. Drug interactions with anticoagulants. JAMA 1970; 214:2035–2038.

43. Das N, Nebioglu S. Vitamin C aspirin interactions in laboratory animals. J Clin Pharm Ther 1992; 17:343–346.

44. Molloy T, Wilson C. Protein-binding of ascorbic acid 2. Interaction with acetylsalicylic acid. Int J Vitamin Nutr Res 1980; 50:387–392.

45. Shilotri P, Bhat K. Effect of mega doses of vitamin C on bactericidal activity of leucocytes. Am J Clin Nutr 1977; 30:1077–1081.

46. Levey S, Sutur B. Effect of ascorbic acid in diabetogenic activity of alloxan. Proc Soc Exp Biol Med 1946; 63:341–343.

47. Houston J, Levy G. Drug biotransformation interactions in man. VI: Acetaminophen and ascorbic acid. J Pharmacol Sci 1976; 65:1218–1221.

48. Berson E, Rosner B, Sandberg MA et al. A randomized trial of vitamin A and vitamin E supplementation for retinitis pigmentosa. Arch Ophthalmol 1993; 111: 761–772.

49. Gillian R, Mondell B, Warbassem J. Quantitative evaluation of vitamin E in treatment of angina pectoris. Am Heart J 1977; 93:444–449.

50. Ascherio A, Rimm E, Hernan M et al. Relation of consumption of vitamin E, vitamin C and carotenoids to risk of stroke among men in the United States. Ann Intern Med 1999; 130:963–970.

51. GISSI-Prevenzione Investigators. Dietary supplementation with n-3 polyunsaturated fatty acids and vitamin E after myocardial infarction: results of the GISSI-prevenzione trial. Lancet 1999; 354:447–455.

52. Leppala J, Virtammo J, Fogelholm R et al. Vitamin E and beta-carotene supplementation in high risk for stroke. Arch Neurol 2000; 57:1503–1509.

53. Yusuf S, Dagenais G, Pogue J et al. Vitamin E supplementation and cardiovascular events in high-risk patients. The Heart Outcomes Prevention Evaluation Study investigators. N Engl J Med 2000; 342:154–160.

54. Primary Prevention Project. Low-dose aspirin and vitamin E in people at cardiovascular risk: a randomised trial in general practice. Lancet 2001; 357:89–95.

55. Heart Protection Study Collaborative Group. MRC/BHF Heart Protection Study of antioxidant vitamin supplementation in 20 536 high-risk individuals: a randomised placebo-controlled trial. Lancet 2002; 360:23–32.

56. Corrigan J, Marcus F. Coagulopathy associated with vitamin E ingestion. JAMA 1974; 230:1300–1301.

57. Leppala J, Virtamo J, Fogelholm R. Controlled trial of alpha-tocopherol and beta-carotene supplements on stroke incidence and mortality in male smokers. Arterio Thromb Vasc Biol 2000; 20:230–235.

58. Liede K, Haukka J, Saxen L, Heinonen O. Increased tendency towards gingival bleeding caused by joint effect of alpha-tocopherol supplementation and acetylsalicylic acid. Ann Med 1998; 30:542–546.

59. Diplock A. Safety of antioxidant vitamins and beta-carotene. Am J Clin Nutr 1995; 62:1510S–1516S.

60. Cunningham JJ, Fu AZ, Mearkle PL, Brown RG. Hyperzincuria in individuals with insulin-dependent diabetes mellitus – concurrent zinc status and the effect of high-dose zinc supplementation. Metab Clin Exp 1994; 43:1558–1562.

61. Otsuji S, Kamada T. Biophysical changes in the erythrocyte membrane in diabetes mellitus. Rinsho Byori 1982; 30:888–897.

62. Huntley A. Diabetes mellitus: review. Dermatol Online J 1995; 1:2.

63. Rao K, Seshiah V, Kumar T. Effect of zinc sulfate therapy on control and lipids in type I diabetes. J Assoc Phys Ind 1987; 35:52.

64. Niewoehner CB, Allen JI, Boosalis M et al. Role of zinc supplementation in type II diabetes-mellitus. Am J Med 1986; 81:63–68.

65. Rosenblatt M, Mindel J. Spontaneous hyphema associated with ingestion of ginkgo biloba extract (letter). N Engl J Med 1997; 336:1108.

66. Matthews MJ. Association of ginkgo biloba with intracerebral haemorrhage. Neurology 1998; 50:1933–1934.

67. Lascari A. Carotenemia: a review. Clin Pediatr 1981; 20:25–29.

68. Mathews-Roth M. Lack of genotoxicity with beta-carotene. Toxicol Lett 1988; 3:185–191.

69. Bauernfeind J. The safe use of vitamin A: a report of the International Vitamin A Consultative Group. Washington, DC: Nutrition Foundation; 1980.

70. World Health Organization. Micronutrient deficiencies. Combating vitamin A deficiency. Available online at: www.who.int/nut/vad.htm; 2003.

71. Vijayaraghavan G, Naidu A, Rao N, Sritkantia S. A simple method to evaluate the massive dose vitamin A prophylaxis programme in preschool children. Am J Clin Nutr 1975; 28:1189–1193.

72. Beaton G, Martorell R, L'Abbe K et al. Effectiveness of vitamin A supplementation in the control of young child morbidity and mortality in developing countries. Nutrition policy discussion paper 13. Geneva: World Health Organization; 1993.

73. Florentino R, Tanchoco C, Ramos A et al. Tolerance of preschoolers to two dosage strengths of vitamin A preparation. Am J Clin Nutr 1990; 52:694–700.

74. Bendich A, Langseth L. Safety of vitamin A. Am J Clin Nutr 1989; 49:358–371.

75. Bush M, Dahms B. Fatal hypervitaminosis A in a neonate. Arch Pathol Lab Med 1984; 108:838–842.

76. Sibulesky L, Hayes KC, Pronczuk A et al. Safety of <7500RE (<25000 IU) vitamin A daily in adults with retinitis pigmentosa. Am J Clin Nutr 1999; 69:656–663.

77. Anonymous. Alpha-tocopherol influences tissue levels of vitamin A and its esters. Nutr Rev 1985; 43:55–56.

78. Willett W, Stampfer M, Underwood B et al. Vitamins A, E, and carotene: effects of supplementation on their plasma levels. Am J Clin Nutr 1983; 38:559–566.

79. Soliman M. Vitamin-A-Uberdosierung. I Mogliche teratogene Wirkungen. Int Z Vitam Ernahrungsforsch [Beih] 1972; 42:389–393.

80. Metz A, Walser M, Olson W. The interaction of dietary vitamin A and vitamin D related to skeletal development in the turkey poult. J Nutr 1985; 115:929–935.

81. Ette S, Basu T, Dickerson J. Short-term effect of zinc sulphate on plasma and hepatic concentrations of vitamins A and E in normal weanling rats. Nutr Metab 1979; 23:11–16.

82. Hruban Z, Russell R, Boyer J et al. Ultra-structural changes in livers of two patients with hypervitaminosis A. Am J Pathol 1974; 76:451–468.

83. Olson JA, Hodges R. Recommended dietary intakes (RDI) of vitamin C in humans. Am J Clin Nutr 1987; 45:693–703.

84. Dunlap W, James G, Hume D. Anaemia and neutropenia caused by copper deficiency. Ann Intern Med 1974; 80:470–476.

85. Flanagan P, Haist J, Valberg L. Zinc absorption, intraluminal zinc and intestinal metallothionein levels in zinc-deficient and zinc-replete rodents. J Nutr 1983; 113:962–972.

86. Fischer P, Giroux A, L'Abbe M, Effects of zinc on mucosal copper binding and on the kinetics of copper absorption. J Nutr 1983; 113:462–469.

87. Broun E, Greist A, Tricot G, Hoffman R. Excessive zinc ingestion – a reversible cause of sideroblastic anemia and bone marrow depression. J Am Med Soc 1990; 264: 1441–1443.

88. Bush A, Pettingell W, Multhaup G et al. Rapid induction of Alzheimer Ab amyloid formation by zinc. Science 1994; 265:1464–1467.

89. Potocnik F, van Rensburg S, Park C et al. Zinc and platelet membrane viscosity in Alzheimer's disease – the effect of zinc on platelet membranes and cognition. South Afr Med J 1997; 87:1116–1119.

90. Expert Group on Vitamins and Minerals. Safe upper limits for vitamins and minerals. Food Standards Agency 2003. Available online at www.foodstandards. gov.uk/multimedia/pdfs/vitamins2003/pdf (accessed 2003).

91. Samman S, Roberts D. The effect of zinc supplements on plasma zinc and copper levels and the reported symptoms in healthy volunteers. Med J Aust 1987; 146:246–249.

92. Rowin J, Lewis S. Spontaneous bilateral subdural hematomas associated with chronic ginkgo biloba ingestion. Neurology 1996; 46:1775–1776.

93. Gaby A. Literature review and commentary. Townsend Lett Doctors 1990; June:338–339.

94. Bloch A. Pushing the envelope of nutrition support: complementary therapies. Nutrition 2000; 16:236–239.

95. Cirrigan J, Marcus F. Coagulopathy associated with vitamin E ingestion. JAMA 1974; 230:1300–1301.

96. Arenz A, Klein M, Fiehe K. Occurrence of neurotoxic 4'-O-methylpyridoxin in ginkgo biloba leaves, ginkgo medications and Japanese ginkgo food. Planta Med 1996; 62:548–551.

97. Chung K, Dent G, McCusker M et al. Effect of a ginkolide mixture (BN 52063) in antagonising skin and platelet responses to platelet activating factor in man. Lancet 1987; i:248–251.

98. Devane J, Ryan M. The effects of amiloride and triamterene on urinary magnesium excretion in conscious saline-loaded rats. Br J Pharmacol 1981; 72:285–289.

99. Holt G. Food and drug interactions. Chicago: Precept Press; 1998.

100. Threlkeld D. Systemic anti-infectives, fluoroquinolones. In: Threlkeld D, ed. Facts and comparisons drug information. St Louis: Facts and Comparisons; 1994:2888–2891.

101. Sifton D. Physicians' desk reference. Montvale, NJ: Medical Economics; 2000.

102. Naggar V, Khalil S, Gouda M. Effect of concomitant administration of magnesium trisilicate on GI absorption of dexamethasone in humans. J Pharmacol Sci 1978; 67:1029–1030.

SECTION 7

Conclusions

Chapter **7.1**

Conclusions

Stephen Beatty and Frank Eperjesi

INTRODUCTION

In writing this book, it was our aim to present, in a readily accessible way, the current scientific evidence germane to the role of nutrition in vision. Following an introduction to the field of nutrition, we have discussed each nutrient and micronutrient with respect to the eye and with respect to vision, in a physiological context. Then, the ophthalmic manifestations of nutritional deficiencies were reviewed. Physiological and pathological ocular senescence have been considered, with particular emphasis on the role that nutrition plays in this ageing process. Finally, current evidence in support of dietary modification and/or supplementation in the prevention and/or management of ocular disease was reviewed, as well as potential adverse reactions to such dietary changes. The purpose of this concluding chapter is to contextualise the foregone discussions in a way that furnishes the front-line eye care professional with the ability to give patients sound, evidence-based nutritional advice.

CHANGES IN LIFESTYLE

There is no doubt that a healthy lifestyle, consisting of regular exercise, is associated with reduced morbidity and mortality attributable to cardiovascular disease. There are many mechanisms whereby a healthy lifestyle impacts positively on longevity, including a beneficial effect on blood pressure, adiposity and lipoprotein profile. As the eye is not an isolated organ, but rather a component of a multiorgan system, and since there is a considerable body of evidence implicating cardiovascular risk factors in eye diseases such as age-related macular degeneration (AMD), glaucoma, retinal vascular occlusion, diabetic maculopathy/retinopathy and cataract, it is reasonable to recommend a healthy lifestyle to people wishing to reduce their risk of such conditions. In other words, there is a biologically plausible rationale to suggest that diminution in risk for cardiovascular disease will be accompanied by reduced risk for eye diseases that share antecedents with cardiovascular disease. However, medical supervision of any fitness regime is advisable, especially in those at high risk of a cardiovascular event.

CHANGES IN DIET

Dietary modification in an attempt to reduce risk of ocular disease is best discussed in terms of restriction and fortification.

Dietary restriction

Dietary restriction of nutrients associated with cardiovascular disease, such as cholesterol and salt, may be advisable in selected patients under medical/dietetic supervision. For example, a high salt intake is associated with systemic hypertension, which in turn represents risk for many ophthalmic conditions, including hypertensive retinopathy, retinal vascular occlusion, glaucoma and anterior ischaemic optic neuropathy. Furthermore, systemic hypertension is known to aggravate diabetic retinopathy and maculopathy, and has been (in some studies at least) linked to cataract and AMD.

Dietary restriction of cholesterol may also be advisable in selected cases, and under medical/dietetic supervision. Hypercholesterolaemia is associated with increased risk of retinal vascular occlusion and anterior ischaemic optic neuropathy, as well as risk for a cerebrovascular accident with consequential loss of visual field. Furthermore, hypercholesterolaemia is known to aggravate diabetic retinopathy and maculopathy, and to be associated with carotid vascular disease with potential for emboli to the retinal vasculature. In other words, hypercholesterolaemia rep-

resents a risk for loss of vision by at least one of several mechanisms, and should be avoided. Means of reducing serum cholesterol include dietary restriction and the use of pharmacological agents, and should be supervised by a doctor and/or a dietician. Interestingly, there is some clinical evidence to suggest that those patients taking statin medication as part of their cholesterol reduction regime may be at less risk of developing AMD. This is thought to be due to a combination of increased blood flow (through reduced atherosclerosis) and the anti-inflammatory properties of these drugs.

Obesity is now recognised as a major cause of morbidity, and is associated with diabetes mellitus, cardiovascular disease and age-related maculopathy (ARM). Dietary restriction of selected foodstuffs, under medical/dietetic supervision, is required in many cases of obesity. Interestingly, adiposity is inversely related to macular pigment optical density (adipose tissue can act as a sink for lutein and zeaxanthin), possibly explaining the predisposition of obese subjects to ARM. Furthermore, some researchers have proposed that the tendency for women to have more adipose tissue than men (and therefore less macular pigment) may be one of the factors responsible for the increased prevalence of AMD in women.

In diabetics, restriction of sugar-containing foods is required. Clearly, such dietary restriction, if adhered to, will reduce the risk of sight-threatening diabetic eye disease, which is associated with poor diabetic control.

Dietary fortification

Dietary fortification with specific nutrients, in an attempt to prevent or modify eye disease(s), is more problematic because of the lack of an evidence base in support of such an approach. Certainly, a balanced diet rich in fresh fruit and vegetables is advisable for all persons, if only to maintain the physiological health and function of all body organs, including the eye. We have already discussed the need for adequate dietary intake of vitamins A and C if pathologic ophthalmic manifestations of deficiency are to be avoided, and the (albeit controversial) evidence in support of vitamin A supplements in patients with retinitis pigmentosa.

With respect to dry eye, there is a growing body of evidence in support of the view that a balanced diet is important in tear, conjunctival and corneal health. There is a biologically plausible rationale that would support dietary fortification with at least one of the following nutrients in an attempt to improve tear film characteristics: vitamin A, vitamin B_6, vitamin C and omega-3 fatty acids. However, a firm evidence base arising from a large scale randomised controlled trial in support of such dietary fortification is still lacking.

Similarly, there is no firm evidence that dietary fortification with specific nutrients, early or late in life, would reduce the incidence or severity of cataract or glaucoma.

AMD, which is the late stage of ARM, is the commonest cause of blind registration in the developed world. The Age-Related Eye Disease Study (AREDS) has provided firm evidence that appropriate dietary supplementation (vitamins C and E, zinc and β-carotene) in patients with ARM/AMD is associated with reduced risk of visual loss from this condition. However, it is worth emphasising that the doses used in AREDS could not realistically be achieved by dietary modification alone. Also, AREDS did not investigate the potential for these supplements in preventing the onset of ARM/AMD in subjects with healthy maculae. In other words, AREDS has provided us with a dilemma. Certainly, its results indicate a protective role for retinal antioxidants in terms of ARM/AMD progression, consistent with the biological rationale that stimulated that study. An extension of the same rationale would suggest that earlier intervention with retinal antioxidants would result in greater preservation of retinal health, given that ARM/AMD is believed to result from cumulative and chronic insult. However, there is no evidence base to support recommendations for supplements/dietary modification as a means of preventing/delaying the onset of ARM/AMD. Also, the doses used in AREDS are not achievable by dietary fortification in the absence of supplementation, and exceed European Union food safety guidelines. And finally, many investigators believe that the compounds used in AREDS were inappropriate, because β-

carotene is not found in retina, and lutein and zeaxanthin (believed to be the most biologically relevant retinal antioxidants for ARM/AMD) were not included in the supplement.

It would seem, therefore, that persons at risk of ARM/AMD should be encouraged to eat a healthy diet rich in fruit and vegetables, and that persons with AREDS stages 3 and 4 of ARM/AMD should be supplemented 'appropriately'. With respect to 'appropriate' supplementation, consideration should be given to local food safety guidelines and the smoking status of the patient. Ultimately, patients should be furnished with the relevant information, so that they can make an informed decision.

Dietary supplements

Using supplemental vitamins, minerals, trace elements and other nutrients, in an attempt to modify the course of ocular disease, is a controversial subject. Certainly, the AREDS supplement can be validly recommended for persons with AREDS stage 3 and 4 ARM/AMD, but only where such high doses comply with government guidelines. The Lutein Antioxidant Supplementation Trial (LAST) showed that visual function (visual acuity, contrast sensitivity and glare recovery) improved with lutein alone and lutein together with other nutrients for people with AMD. However, the researchers also noted that the results should be considered as preliminary given the small number of subjects, the short time period of observation and the lack of statistical significance among the three groups. Nevertheless, this was an important study, which showed that atrophic AMD is a nutrition-responsive disorder and that improvements in visual function can be obtained over a short period of time.

The question arises, however, whether supplemental nutrients are required, or whether these needs can be met by a healthy diet alone. The fact that AREDS doses could not be matched by diet alone is noteworthy.

Indeed, the vast majority of ocular diseases for which supplemental nutrients are currently under consideration are age-related, and are therefore escalating in prevalence because of increasing longevity. Also, there is a general consensus that these conditions (cataract, glaucoma and ARM/AMD) are the result of cumulative and chronic insult to the tissues involved. It is possible, therefore, that a balanced diet rich in fruit and vegetables provides adequate nutrient support for a healthy life until middle age, but that supplemental nutrients are required to prevent/delay the onset of age-related disorders that result from life-long insult. It is worth remembering that government guidelines such as dietary reference values (which replaced recommended daily allowances in the UK in 1991) are benchmark intakes of energy and nutrients – they can be used for guidance but should not be seen as exact recommendations. They show the amount of energy or an individual nutrient that a group of people of a certain age range (and sometimes sex) need for good health, but only apply to healthy people.

Older people or those who are ill are very likely to require higher levels of intake than those indicated by dietary reference values.

Eye care professionals will be best served by recommending a healthy lifestyle and diet to their patients. In cases where advice regarding nutrient supplements for specific ocular disease(s) is being sought, the health care professional should be guided by the current evidence base, in the context of local safety guidelines and with full appreciation of the nutrients' contraindications and potential adverse effects and seek advice from a diet specialist when appropriate. Where doubt exists, a full and frank discussion regarding the biological rationale, and the potential risks and benefits of nutritional supplementation, should furnish the patient with the wherewithal to make an informed decision.

Index